LIVING WELL
WITH CHRONIC ILLNESS

A Call for Public Health Action

Committee on Living Well with Chronic Disease: Public Health Action to
Reduce Disability and Improve Functioning and Quality of Life

Board on Population Health and Public Health Practice

INSTITUTE OF MEDICINE
OF THE NATIONAL ACADEMIES

THE NATIONAL ACADEMIES PRESS
Washington, D.C.
www.nap.edu

THE NATIONAL ACADEMIES PRESS • 500 Fifth Street, NW • Washington, DC 20001

NOTICE: The project that is the subject of this report was approved by the Governing Board of the National Research Council, whose members are drawn from the councils of the National Academy of Sciences, the National Academy of Engineering, and the Institute of Medicine. The members of the committee responsible for the report were chosen for their special competences and with regard for appropriate balance.

This study was supported by Contract No. DP000607 between the National Academy of Sciences and the Arthritis Foundation, and Contract No. 200-2005-13434, TO# 30 between the National Academy of Sciences and the Centers for Disease Control and Prevention. Any opinions, findings, conclusions, or recommendations expressed in this publication are those of the author(s) and do not necessarily reflect the view of the organizations or agencies that provided support for this project.

Library of Congress Cataloging-in-Publication Data

Living well with chronic illness : a call for public health action / Committee on Living Well with Chronic Disease: Public Health Action to Reduce Disability and Improve Functioning and Quality of Life, Board on Population Health and Public Health Practice, Institute of Medicine of the National Academies.
    p. ; cm.
  Includes bibliographical references.
  ISBN 978-0-309-22127-6 (pbk.) — ISBN 978-0-309-22128-3 (pdf)
    I. Institute of Medicine (U.S.). Committee on Living Well with Chronic Disease: Public Health Action to Reduce Disability and Improve Functioning and Quality of Life.
    [DNLM: 1.   Chronic Disease—prevention & control. 2.   Health Policy. 3.   Population Surveillance. 4.   Quality of Life. WT 30]

  362.1—dc23

                                2012012233

Additional copies of this report are available from the National Academies Press, 500 Fifth Street, NW, Keck 360, Washington, DC 20055; (800) 624-6242 or (202) 334-3313; http://www.nap.edu.

For more information about the Institute of Medicine, visit the IOM home page at: **www.iom.edu**.

The serpent has been a symbol of long life, healing, and knowledge among almost all cultures and religions since the beginning of recorded history. The serpent adopted as a logotype by the Institute of Medicine is a relief carving from ancient Greece, now held by the Staatliche Museen in Berlin.

Suggested citation: IOM (Institute of Medicine). 2012. *Living well with chronic illness: A call for public health action.* Washington, DC: The National Academies Press.

"Knowing is not enough; we must apply.
Willing is not enough; we must do."
—Goethe

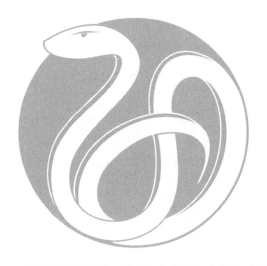

INSTITUTE OF MEDICINE
OF THE NATIONAL ACADEMIES

Advising the Nation. Improving Health.

THE NATIONAL ACADEMIES
Advisers to the Nation on Science, Engineering, and Medicine

The **National Academy of Sciences** is a private, nonprofit, self-perpetuating society of distinguished scholars engaged in scientific and engineering research, dedicated to the furtherance of science and technology and to their use for the general welfare. Upon the authority of the charter granted to it by the Congress in 1863, the Academy has a mandate that requires it to advise the federal government on scientific and technical matters. Dr. Ralph J. Cicerone is president of the National Academy of Sciences.

The **National Academy of Engineering** was established in 1964, under the charter of the National Academy of Sciences, as a parallel organization of outstanding engineers. It is autonomous in its administration and in the selection of its members, sharing with the National Academy of Sciences the responsibility for advising the federal government. The National Academy of Engineering also sponsors engineering programs aimed at meeting national needs, encourages education and research, and recognizes the superior achievements of engineers. Dr. Charles M. Vest is president of the National Academy of Engineering.

The **Institute of Medicine** was established in 1970 by the National Academy of Sciences to secure the services of eminent members of appropriate professions in the examination of policy matters pertaining to the health of the public. The Institute acts under the responsibility given to the National Academy of Sciences by its congressional charter to be an adviser to the federal government and, upon its own initiative, to identify issues of medical care, research, and education. Dr. Harvey V. Fineberg is president of the Institute of Medicine.

The **National Research Council** was organized by the National Academy of Sciences in 1916 to associate the broad community of science and technology with the Academy's purposes of furthering knowledge and advising the federal government. Functioning in accordance with general policies determined by the Academy, the Council has become the principal operating agency of both the National Academy of Sciences and the National Academy of Engineering in providing services to the government, the public, and the scientific and engineering communities. The Council is administered jointly by both Academies and the Institute of Medicine. Dr. Ralph J. Cicerone and Dr. Charles M. Vest are chair and vice chair, respectively, of the National Research Council.

www.national-academies.org

Study Staff

E. LORRAINE BELL, Senior Study Director
PAMELA LIGHTER, Research Assistant
CHELSEA FRAKES, Senior Program Assistant
ANDREW LEMERISE, Research Associate
HOPE HARE, Administrative Assistant
AMY PRZYBOCKI, Financial Associate
ROSE MARIE MARTINEZ, Senior Director, Board on Population
    Health and Public Health Practice

Reviewers

This report has been reviewed in draft form by persons chosen for their diverse perspectives and technical expertise, in accordance with procedures approved by the National Research Council's Report Review Committee. The purpose of this independent review is to provide candid and critical comments that will assist the institution in making its published report as sound as possible and to ensure that the report meets institutional standards for objectivity, evidence, and responsiveness to the study charge. The review comments and draft manuscript remain confidential to protect the integrity of the deliberative process. We wish to thank the following individuals for their review of this report:

Susan Babey, University of California, Los Angeles, Center for Health Policy Research
R. Don Blim, Retired Physician Executive
Noreen M. Clark, University of Michigan Center for Managing Chronic Disease
Christine C. Ferguson, George Washington University School of Public Health and Health Services
George R. Flores, The California Endowment
Linda P. Fried, Columbia University Joseph L. Mailman School of Public Health
Patricia A. Ganz, University of California, Los Angeles, Jonsson Comprehensive Cancer Center
Lisa I. Iezzoni, Harvard Medical School

Although the reviewers listed above have provided many constructive comments and suggestions, they were not asked to endorse the conclusions or recommendations nor did they see the final draft of the report before its release. The review of this report was overseen by **Antonia M. Villarruel,** University of Michigan, and **Eric B. Larson,** Group Health Research Institute. Appointed by the National Research Council, they were responsible for making certain that an independent examination of this report was carried out in accordance with institutional procedures and that all review comments were carefully considered. Responsibility for the final content of this report rests entirely with the authoring committee and the institution.

Foreword

Chronic illness in America imposes an enormous and growing burden on individuals, families, communities, and the nation as a whole. An aging population is one key driver, and rising rates of obesity are making matters worse. Insufficient physical activity and persistent smoking in about 20 percent of the adult population contribute to the problem. For those who are living with chronic disease, access to suitable disease management programs is uneven, disparities among racial and ethnic groups persist, and shortcomings in the quality of care are all too common.

Public health programs have made important inroads in the prevention of several types of cancer, heart disease, and other chronic conditions. However, much remains to be done in primary prevention, initial treatment, and long-term follow-up to deter the onset of disease, reduce the incidence of complications, and diminish the severity of illness. This report examines the role of public health services in accomplishing these goals.

Public health systems have a variety of tools that can be brought to bear on chronic illness. Some are direct public health functions, such as surveillance and regulation; others involve outreach to patients and families through education; some entail closer coordination with those who deliver personal health services; and still others involve enlisting the cooperation of diverse leaders in the public and private sectors. Despite substantial gaps in knowledge and insufficient resources, public health has the capacity to help reduce, manage, and control chronic diseases. This report shows how.

Coping with chronic illness is not America's challenge alone. In September 2011, for the first time, the United Nations took up the topic of chronic diseases as a principal theme at a plenary gathering. The rising burden of chronic disease affects countries at every position on the economic spectrum. Each has much to learn from others, recognizing that differences in culture, conditions, and circumstances will demand distinctive solutions. We hope that the report that follows can help the United States bring new leadership to mitigating the burden of chronic illness at home and for the global community.

Harvey V. Fineberg, M.D., Ph.D.
President, Institute of Medicine

Contents

ABSTRACT   xv

SUMMARY   1

INTRODUCTION   21

1   LIVING WELL WITH CHRONIC ILLNESS   27
    The Timely Relevance of a Push Toward Living Well with
        Chronic Illness, 28
    The Population Health Perspective, 29
    Chronic Diseases and Their Impact on Health and Function, 30
    Doing Something About It, 33
    Conclusion, 44
    References, 45

2   CHRONIC ILLNESSES AND THE PEOPLE WHO LIVE
    WITH THEM   51
    Introduction, 51
    The Spectrum of Chronic Illnesses: Differences in Time
        Course/Chronicity, Health Burden, and Consequences, 52
    The Spectrum of Chronic Illnesses: Common Consequences, 57
    Exemplar Chronic Illnesses, 68
    Who Are the People with Chronic Illnesses?, 90
    Recommendations 1–5, 97

Chronic Illness and the Nation's Health and Economic
  Well-Being, 100
Recommendation 6, 104
References, 105

3 POLICY   119
Introduction, 119
Contextualizing Health Policy Interventions: Frieden's Pyramid, 124
The Affordable Care Act, 132
Health in All Policies and Health Impact Assessments, 137
Conclusion, 140
Recommendations 7–8, 141
References, 148

4 COMMUNITY-BASED INTERVENTION   151
Introduction, 151
Preventive Interventions, 151
Monitoring, Evaluation, and Research, 170
Conclusion, 174
Recommendations 9–12, 175
References, 176

5 SURVEILLANCE AND ASSESSMENT   187
Introduction, 187
Conceptual Framework for Chronic Disease Surveillance, 189
Use of Surveillance to Inform Public Policy Decisions, 194
Current Data Sources and Surveillance Methods, 195
Public Health Surveillance System Integration, 207
Future Data Sources, Methods, and Research Directions, 213
Conclusion, 220
Recommendations 16–17, 222
References, 222

6 INTERFACE OF THE PUBLIC HEALTH SYSTEM, THE
   HEALTH CARE SYSTEM, AND THE NON–HEALTH
   CARE SECTOR   229
Introduction, 229
Public Health System Structures and Approaches, 230
Health Care System Approaches, 238
The Community-Based and Non–Health Care Sector, 244
Conclusion, 250
Recommendations 13–15, 252
References, 253

7   **THE CALL FOR ACTION**   **257**
    References, 260

APPENDIXES

A   Improving Recognition and Quality of Depression Care in
    Patients with Common Chronic Medical Illnesses,
    Wayne J. Katon   261
B   New Models of Comprehensive Health Care for People with
    Chronic Conditions, *Chad Boult and Erin K. Murphy*   285
C   Agendas of Public Meetings Held by the Committee   319
D   Committee Biographies   323

Abstract

The report *Living Well with Chronic Illness: A Call for Public Health Action* is a guide for immediate and precise action to reduce the burden of all forms of chronic illness through the development and implementation of cross-cutting and coordinated strategies to help Americans live well.

The committee developed original and incorporated established conceptual models to provide a framework for the report. The report describes the economic consequences of chronic illnesses for individuals, their families, the health care system, and the nation; provides a concerted approach to understanding the dimensions of prevention as they relate to chronic disease control in the community; highlights the populations that experience chronic illnesses disproportionately; considers a wide spectrum of chronic diseases and their clinical stages, their patterns and anticipated course, and the common or cross-cutting burden and consequences of living with chronic illness; details how to improve surveillance systems to better assess and address chronic illnesses; describes the role of public health and community-based interventions for chronic disease management and control; considers the importance of federal policy in enhancing chronic disease control; and highlights the critical role of aligning public health, health care system, and non–health care community services as a system change to better control chronic illnesses.

The committee concludes that all chronic illnesses have the potential to reduce population health by limiting individual capacity to live well. Maintaining or enhancing quality of life for individuals living with chronic illnesses has not been given the attention it needs by health care funders, health systems, policy makers, and public health programs and agencies.

There are domains of chronic disease management from a public health perspective for which there is not enough research or program evaluation. Much more needs to be done.

The committee does not recommend a specific set of diseases on which to focus for public health action. Instead, we describe nine exemplar diseases, health conditions, and impairments that have notable implications for the nation's health and economy; impact quality of life and functional status; cut across many chronic illnesses; complicate and/or increase risks for multiple chronic conditions (MCCs); and impact the community, families, and caregivers of those with chronic illnesses. Each represents an important challenge to public health. Therefore, the committee recommends that a variety of illnesses be selected for public health action based on a planning process that emphasizes the inclusion of chronic illnesses with cross-cutting clinical, functional, and social implications that impact the individuals who live with them. The committee provides specific criteria for illness selection.

The committee concludes that there are many intervention issues and opportunities related to the prevention and management of MCCs. The committee recommends that surveillance techniques more likely to capture MCCs effectively be explored, and that public health interventions aimed at preventing or altering the course of new illness occurrences in individuals with MCCs, or who are at risk for them, be tested and evaluated. Also, the committee recommends that the states be supported to develop comprehensive population-based strategic plans that focus on the management of chronic illnesses among their residents, including community-based efforts to address the health and social needs of individuals living with chronic illnesses and experiencing disparities in health outcomes.

The committee recommends greater use of new and emerging economic methods in making policy decisions that will promote living well with chronic illnesses. In addition, the committee recommends that evidenced-based interventions that help individuals with chronic illness live well be widely disseminated, particularly in communities with disparities in health outcomes. Barriers for translating research into practice need to be identified and resolved. Furthermore, the committee recommends that federal, state, and privately funded programmatic and research initiatives in health include an evaluation of their effect on health-related quality of life and functional status, particularly in persons with chronic illness. The committee also recommends a Health in All Policies approach, with Health Impact Assessments as a promising practice to be piloted and evaluated for a set of major federal legislation, regulations, and policies for its impact on health, health-related quality of life and functional status for individuals with chronic illness, and relevant efficiencies.

Surveillance systems need to be improved to assess health-related quality of life and functional status and inform the planning, development, implementation, and evaluation of public health policies, programs, and interventions relevant to individuals living with chronic illness. Therefore, the committee recommends that a standing national work group be established to oversee and coordinate multidimensional chronic illnesses surveillance activity.

To improve living well with chronic illness, the committee recommends the testing and evaluation of existing, emerging, and/or new models of chronic disease care that align the resources of community-based organizations, the health care delivery system, employers and businesses, the media, and the academic community. Additional important recommendations are presented in this report regarding research and evaluation, interventions, policies, and surveillance to promote public health action around chronic illness.

1

Summary

Chronic diseases have emerged in recent decades as the major cluster of health concerns for the American people. A chronic disease or illness, in general terms, is a condition that is slow in progression, long in duration, and void of spontaneous resolution, and it often limits the function, productivity, and quality of life of someone who lives with it.[1] According to the Centers for Disease Control and Prevention (CDC), in the United States, chronic diseases currently account for 70 percent of all deaths (Kung et al., 2008; Wu and Green, 2000). Close to 48 million Americans report a disability related to a chronic illness (CDC, 2009).

In the past few centuries, extraordinary advances in developed countries in medicine and public health, as well as economic growth leading to more widely accessible social welfare programs, have changed the chronic disease landscape dramatically. Hygienic and sanitary advances have prevented many previously common infectious diseases. Immunizations and clinical and community interventions have substantially controlled many past causes of chronic illness, such as tuberculosis and polio. Pharmacotherapy has enabled many persons with chronic mental illness to live in their communities. Chronic cardiovascular diseases have become less disabling in many important ways. Therapeutic approaches have improved the function

---

[1]For the purpose of this report, the committee has chosen to use the term "chronic disease(s)" when referring to the population at large; communities; groups of illnesses or conditions; or when the term properly describes a program, service, and/or an agency; or is derived from cited research. The term "chronic illness(es)" is used when referring to or closely associated with individuals or families living with one or more medical conditions.

and overall health for some persons with chronic illness through advances in corrective surgery, new approaches in analgesia, better rehabilitation and physical and occupational therapy, improved nutrition management, and adaptation of home and community environments for functionally impaired persons.

However, these advances have been compromised by parallel increases in physical inactivity, unhealthful eating, obesity, tobacco use, and other chronic disease risk factors. Today, more than one in four Americans has multiple (two or more) chronic conditions (MCCs), and the prevalence and burden of chronic illness among the elderly and racial and ethnic minorities are notably disproportionate. Chronic disease has now emerged as a major public health problem, and it threatens not only population health but also social and economic welfare.

Cardiovascular disease, many cancers, stroke, and chronic lung disease are the most common causes of death in America. But there are also other chronic diseases, such as arthritis, asthma, depression, and epilepsy, which have less substantial contributions to mortality but can severely diminish the health-related quality of life of the individuals who live with them, and effective disease prevention programs are not well developed.

Chronic illnesses not only impact the social and economic lives of millions of Americans and their families but also are a major contributor to health care costs. The medical care costs of people with chronic illnesses represent 75 percent of the $2 trillion the United States spends annually on health care (Kaiser Family Foundation, 2010). By 2030, the global economic burden of noncommunicable chronic diseases is estimated to be $47 trillion (Bloom et al., 2011).

In 2010, CDC and the Arthritis Foundation sought assistance from the Institute of Medicine (IOM) to identify the population-based public health actions that can help reduce disability and improve functioning and quality of life among individuals who are at high risk of developing a chronic illness and those with one or more chronic illnesses.

The Statement of Task (Box S-1) suggested the following diseases for the committee to consider: heart disease and stroke, diabetes, arthritis, depression, respiratory problems (asthma, chronic obstructive pulmonary disease [COPD]), chronic neurological conditions, and cancer. These diseases or categories of disease were not intended as a prescriptive set of diseases to include in the report. In fact, the committee was advised by the sponsors of this study not to focus on the common high-mortality diseases, but rather consider diseases that have the potential to cause or that actually cause functional limitations and/or disabilities. This guidance thus allowed the committee to consider all chronic diseases in the context of living well. With respect to primary prevention, the committee was advised to consider prevention only among individuals with high-risk factors (e.g., prediabetes).

BOX S-1
Statement of Task

The Statement of Task for this consensus study provides that the IOM establish a committee to examine the nonfatal burden of chronic disease and the implications for population-based public health action.

Questions to be considered by the committee for persons with single as well as multiple chronic diseases include

1. What consequences of chronic diseases are most important (criteria to be decided and justified by the committee) to the nation's health and economic well-being?
2. Which chronic diseases should be the focus of public health efforts to reduce disability and improve functioning and quality of life?
3. Which populations need to be the focus of interventions to reduce the consequences of chronic disease including the burden of disability, loss of productivity and functioning, health care costs, and reduced quality of life?
4. Which population-based interventions can help achieve outcomes that maintain or improve quality of life, functioning, and disability?
   - What is the evidence on effectiveness of interventions on these outcomes?
   - To what extent do the interventions that address these outcomes also affect clinical outcomes?
   - To what extent can policy, environmental, and systems change achieve these outcomes?
5. How can public health surveillance be used to inform public policy decisions to minimize adverse life impacts?
6. What policy priorities could advance efforts to improve life impacts of chronic disease?
7. What is the role of primary prevention (for those at highest risk), secondary, and tertiary prevention of chronic disease in reducing or minimizing life impacts (e.g., preventing diabetes in pre-diabetics, preventing incidence of disability in people with arthritis, preventing recurrence of cancer, managing complications of cardiovascular disease)?

Chronic diseases related to congenital disorders, infectious diseases, substance abuse, and childhood conditions are not the focus of the study.

CONCEPTUAL FRAMEWORKS

Chronic disease is a public health as well as a clinical problem. Therefore, a population health perspective for developing strategies, interventions, and policies to combat it is critical. A population perspective considers how individuals' genes, biology, and behaviors interact with the social, cultural, and physical environment around them to influence health outcomes for the entire population. It is this perspective that informed the development and use of four frameworks in this study.

First, building on prior frameworks, is an integrated framework on determinants of health, health outcomes, and policy; the interactions in this framework help identify which strategies are likely to offer the greatest promise to improve health for individuals living with chronic illness. This integrated framework addresses a principal aim of interventions to reduce chronic illness morbidity: helping each affected person and the population as a whole to "live well" regardless of the illness in question or an individual's present state of disablement. For this study, the concept of living well reflects the best achievable state of health that encompasses all dimensions of physical, mental, and social well-being.

Second, a living-well framework was developed to inform the consideration of policies and the allocation of resources about the interactions among individual, behavioral, social, and environmental characteristics that shape important problems related to chronic illness.

Third, a framework depicting a pyramid of layered intervention strategies to promote living well presents the nature and scope of public health policies and other interventions. The pyramid attempts to frame different intervention strategies not only in terms of their target level (i.e., population-wide versus individually based) but also in terms of the relative intensity of a strategy to meet the needs of the people who shoulder the greatest burden of nonfatal chronic illness.

Fourth, a framework is used to describe the great variation in the causes, onset, clinical patterns, and outcomes of specific chronic diseases.

CHRONIC ILLNESSES AND THE PEOPLE WHO LIVE WITH THEM

Chronic illnesses can be characterized by stages of clinical severity, patterns of symptoms, and anticipated courses of progression. The stage of clinical severity (i.e., early, moderate, late) for any chronic illness has the largest impact on health and social function, including the symptoms, degree of impairment and/or disability, level of self-management, and burden to caregivers, family, and significant others. The burden of chronic illness is often compounded by MCCs, or comorbidities, that contribute to worse outcomes, multiple organ systems involvement, complex treatment approaches, and decreased adherence to treatment. In addition, the adverse effects of clinical treatment and secondary conditions contribute to the development of MCCs and disability.

The prevalence of MCCs increases substantially among adults over age 65. Although the relationship between aging and chronic illness is complex and variable, the difference between older and younger persons must be considered in population-based approaches to living well with chronic illness. Similarly, to address the disproportionate prevalence of chronic illness among some racial and ethnic groups, the social determinants of health as the context for a population-based approach to living well must be considered.

The question "Which chronic disease should be the focus of public health efforts to reduce disability and improve functioning and quality of life?" is difficult to answer because of the many illnesses from which to choose and many forms of suffering and disability. Fundamentally, the determination of priorities for public health intervention begins with the population burden of disease and preventability (Sainfort and Remington, 1995). Other considerations include the perceptions of urgency around the problem; the severity of the problem; the potential for economic loss; the impact on others; effectiveness, proprietorship, economics, acceptability, and the legality of solutions; and the availability of resources (Vilnius and Dandoy, 1990).

The very considerable costs that chronic diseases impose on society are due to many factors, including their high—and, in many cases, apparently increasing—prevalence; the aging of the population; advances in treatment that help sustain many individuals; their occurrence across the life course; and the highly disabling nature of many chronic illnesses, especially when inadequately treated.

POLICY

Numerous health and other public policies have an impact on the well-being of high-risk populations living with chronic illness. These social policies have proven critical to maintaining function and independence for chronically ill populations that are most disadvantaged in terms of income and/or disability. Many of these policies and laws—such as clean indoor air laws and support for smoking cessation interventions—prevent disease in the general population and help facilitate function as well as deter disease progression in those who are already chronically ill. Recently passed federal health reform, the Patient Protection and Affordable Care Act (ACA), represents the most significant changes to health care policy since the establishment of Medicare and Medicaid. Some provisions targeted to improving health care delivery and population health in the ACA are particularly relevant to the well-being of those with chronic illness.

Federal, state, and local government policies have important impacts on the population's health status, including those living with a chronic illness. To promote synergistic improvements in public policies that have the potential to impact health, the Health in All Policies (HIAP) approach, supported by Health Impact Assessments (HIAs), seeks to assess the health implications of both health and nonhealth public- and private-sector policies. HIAP is emerging as a credible public health policy approach toward health promotion and disease prevention to improve the lives and reduce the disability of people living with chronic illness.

COMMUNITY-BASED INTERVENTIONS

Evidence-based preventive interventions recommended for the general population are relevant to living well with chronic illnesses. Even when a particular health behavior is not directly related to a person's chronic illness (e.g., smoking and arthritis), adoption of a healthy lifestyle by individuals with chronic illness can serve to improve their overall health and make them less vulnerable to further health threats and disability. Lifestyle behaviors, such as physical activity, appropriate eating habits, smoking and tobacco use cessation, disease screening, vaccination, and chemoprevention (the use of chemical agents, drugs, or food supplements to prevent disease), are valuable health maintenance and promotion measures for individuals in the community. What is needed, however, is better evidence from existing public health programs regarding their impact on the long-term health outcomes of those with overt chronic illness.

Other potentially useful interventions with community dimensions include self-help management programs, disease management programs, complementary and alternative medicine, cognitive training programs, and access and mobility strategies for individuals with disabilities. These types of interventions are community-based and patient-driven and need further evaluation of their benefit to population health.

There are rigorously evaluated interventions that have not been widely disseminated. More attention needs to be paid to the barriers to translating research into practice, including research design; resources; and sociocultural, physical, economic, and environmental barriers. Also, it is difficult to assess the long-term impact of community and public health interventions, including identifying any adverse effects of such interventions. Nevertheless, the barriers to translating research into practice need to be addressed in order to provide more community-based intervention options for people living with chronic illness and disability.

SURVEILLANCE AND ASSESSMENT

Although the best way to meet the goal of living well is to effectively manage the illness, improve quality of life, and prevent the development of additional chronic illness, the difficulties of doing this persist. In order to determine if the program and community goals are being met, a comprehensive surveillance system is required that includes incentives for individuals and organizations to participate in surveillance activities. The characteristics of surveillance systems used to enhance living well with chronic illness are complex. They integrate a number of measures of the multiple determinants and dimensions of outcomes most relevant to patients, including measures of public health program structure and outcomes, the presence of policy initiatives, and the activities of the health care system. However, many barriers continue to prevent optimal integration and use of these data for program planning and evaluation. In addition to the need for fundamental research on measurement reliability, validity, and responsiveness to change, many questions remain regarding which measurements are needed and how frequently data should be collected for surveillance to be effective.

Although further research is needed, surveillance using a composite of relatively simple measures of life satisfaction and well-being and comprehensively assessing health-related quality of life, combined with health care system (e.g., access) and population-level measures (e.g., clinical, access, and funding policies), will be necessary to monitor the effectiveness of relevant health care and public health interventions to promote living well among patients with chronic illness. Longitudinal approaches to population health surveillance will also be necessary for determining the impact of interventions aimed at living well with chronic disease.

INTERFACE OF THE PUBLIC HEALTH SYSTEM, THE HEALTH CARE SYSTEM, AND THE NON–HEALTH CARE SECTOR

Most of the literature related to population-based approaches to health improvement is not specifically focused on chronic illness. In addition, although models to align population-based public health interventions with health care have been widely proposed, they are largely untested.

The type of payment system used in health care systems can have a significant effect on the effectiveness of chronic disease prevention and control services. Regardless of the type of payment system, however, few systems provide incentives for chronic disease prevention or improvements in the health outcomes of patients with chronic illness. Nevertheless, an aligned system with a strong interface among public health, health care, and the community and nonhealth care sectors could produce better prevention and treatment outcomes for populations living with chronic illness. In part, these systems are natural allies, as they often serve the same populations and see themselves as contributing to the public's health, and they often share the burden of poor chronic disease outcomes. They could serve as powerful partners, because only together can they achieve living well across populations and across chronic illnesses.

RECOMMENDATIONS AND RESPONSE TO THE CHARGE

The committee makes 17 recommendations without priority order or measured ranking, as all of them are thought to be important strategies and steps to undergird public health action to help individuals living with chronic illnesses. The recommendations are presented under the seven questions from the statement of task. The committee found that answering each question worked best with a different logical flow, so the recommendations are presented in order below, but the seven questions are not.

> Which chronic diseases should be the focus of public health efforts to reduce disability and improve functioning and quality of life?

In view of the many chronic diseases and the great heterogeneity of their clinical manifestations and outcomes in different individuals, communities, and populations, the committee does not recommend a specific set of diseases on which to focus for public health action. Instead, we chose nine exemplar diseases, health conditions, and impairments that have notable implications for the nation's health and economy; impact function and disability; often cut across chronic illnesses; complicate and/or increase risks for MCCs; and impact the community, families, and caregivers of those with chronic illness. Each represents an important challenge to public health.

CDC's announced theme of "winnable battles," which generally leads to selection of diseases for which risk factor interventions lead to some level of primary prevention, is logical and valuable. However, to be more inclusive of the wide variety of chronic conditions and people who live with them, and to emphasize the need to optimize "living well" in these individuals, the committee chose exemplars that reflect the tremendous variation in chronic diseases shown in the fourth framework (see Table 2-1). The exemplar approach gives CDC the medical, social, and public health latitude to address many conditions, with varied anatomic, physiological, functional, and complex outcomes. Although each of the nine diseases is important for specific reasons, the committee wished to avoid comparing their importance relative to other, also important, chronic diseases, in the belief that competition for the "worst diseases in society" is destructive and pointless.

The committee's multidimensional approach to selecting exemplars is intended to address these perceived limitations in the current approach to selecting diseases for public health attention:

1. Selecting diseases for control activity based on such criteria as prevalence, mortality, disability, and economic cost to the care sys-

tem is useful, but these criteria are often orthogonal to each other, and thus the selection algorithm is in several ways arbitrary.

2. Selecting specific diseases inadequately addresses the great variation in clinical manifestations and trajectories that makes public health approaches complex and challenging.
3. A large number of people have less common illnesses that impact individuals and communities in important ways but are not included in disease-by-disease approaches.
4. The recognized problem of MCCs cannot be adequately addressed in current disease control activities.

The nine exemplars did not come from a list but were chosen on the basis of the clinical and research experience of committee members to highlight some important features of chronic diseases that have received less emphasis in the past, including

1. Great diversity in clinical manifestations within and among chronic diseases, as well as the great variation in their manifestations as illnesses continue their natural histories.
2. The inclusion of illnesses that can be manifest across the life course, raising the possibility of public health interventions that may be effective at various life stages of disease. The life course approach also more effectively deals with the occurrence of recurrent or additional, different conditions (MCCs).
3. The highlighting of important psychological and social consequences that come with many chronic illnesses, including primary mental illnesses and those that are secondary to other conditions.
4. The highlighting of the chronic, multiple, degenerative age-related conditions, for which public health approaches are perhaps less well developed.

The committee endorses CDC's emphasis on "winnable battles" and thinks that the exemplar approach will help identify new types of battles and population-based interventions in the management and control of chronic diseases.

The nine exemplar diseases are arthritis, cancer survivorship, chronic pain, dementia, depression, type 2 diabetes, posttraumatic disabling conditions, schizophrenia, and vision and hearing loss. Because different chronic illnesses affect social participation and health-related quality of life in varied ways, the committee uses examples of different chronic illnesses to illustrate key concepts. This should not, however, be viewed as an assertion that some illnesses are more burdensome or more important than others.

In response to the question about which chronic diseases should be the focus of public health efforts to reduce disability and improve functioning and quality of life, and based on the discussion in Chapter 2, the committee makes two recommendations.

Recommendation 1

The committee recommends that CDC select a variety of illnesses for special consideration based on a planning process that first and foremost emphasizes the inclusion of chronic illnesses with cross-cutting clinical, functional, and social implications that impact the individuals who live with them. In addition, the committee suggests that other important criteria for illness selection include

- nonduplication with major illnesses for which public health programs have already been developed (e.g., cardiovascular disease, stroke);
- those with important implications for various models of chronic illness care, such as public health, health system, and self-care programs, especially when effective health service interventions are possible;
- variation in organ systems and long-term clinical manifestations and outcomes; and
- those for which the effective public health preventive interventions are either most feasible or at least the subject of promising research.

Also, there are many important intervention issues for living well with MCCs.

Recommendation 2

Although research has attempted to characterize MCCs, the complexity of single chronic illnesses over time has not allowed for MCC taxonomies that will be easily applicable to public health control of chronic diseases. Thus, the committee recommends that CDC:

1. Continue to review the scientific literature to monitor for potential MCC taxonomies that are useful for planning, executing, and evaluating disease control programs of MCC occurrences.
2. Explore surveillance techniques that are more likely to capture MCCs effectively. This should include counting not merely the co-occurrence of diseases and conditions but also the order of occurrence and the impact on quality of life and personal function.

3. Emphasize MCC prevention by selecting for execution and evaluation one or more exploratory public health interventions aimed at preventing or altering the course of new disease occurrences in patients with MCCs or who are at risk for them. This might include established approaches, such as tobacco control, or experimental approaches, such as metabolic or genetic screening.

4. Increase demonstration programs for chronic disease control that cut across specific diseases or MCCs and emphasize mitigating the secondary consequences of a variety of chronic conditions, such as falls, immobility, sleep disorders, and depression.

Which populations need to be the focus of interventions to reduce the consequences of chronic disease including the burden of disability, loss of productivity and functioning, health care costs, and reduced quality of life?

Numerous studies have documented differences in the prevalence of chronic diseases and outcomes among racial and ethnic groups across the life cycle in the United States. In general, African Americans have the highest rates of chronic diseases and the worst outcomes. Hispanic Americans, Asian Americans, and American Indians have some higher and some lower risks for chronic health problems when compared with white Americans. The most extreme disparities in health are based on socioeconomic status.

The implementation of evidence-based public health interventions is needed to help people with chronic illness in populations with the greatest disparities. However, there are considerable difficulties to assessing community and public health interventions. Population-based interventions aimed at increasing health-promoting lifestyles that fail to give attention to differential response capabilities by race, ethnicity, socioeconomic position, and geographical location may inadvertently exacerbate health disparities, even as overall population health improves (IOM, 2010). Therefore, so that interventions designed to help individuals with chronic illness live well can be brought to the maximal number of people, more attention needs to be paid to the barriers to translating research into practice.

Effective strategies to improve living well with chronic illness will consider the potential impact of health outcomes across population subgroups, as well as policies and social determinants that impact health and function.

Recommendation 3

The committee recommends that the secretary of U.S. Department of Health and Human Services (HHS) support the states in developing comprehensive population-based strategic plans with specific goals, objectives, actions, time frames, and resources that focus on the management of chronic illness among their residents, including community-based efforts to address the health and social needs of people living with chronic illness and experiencing disparities in health outcomes. Such strategic plans should also include steps to collaborate with community-based organizations, the health care delivery system, employers and businesses, the media, and the academic community to improve living well for all residents with chronic illness, including those experiencing disparities in health outcomes.

All major chronic illnesses have the potential to impose an adverse impact on personal, family, and community economic status and the cost of medical care. At a time when the nation's ability to address widespread economic hardship is challenged, it is extremely important for public health programs to reach out to all with such illnesses. In addition, research has shown that almost all chronic illnesses are associated with various disparities, such as socioeconomic, race/ethnicity, and geographic status. For the sake of political enfranchisement and social justice, it is important to invoke feasible and appropriate surveillance and evidence-based control programs that touch the greatest number of persons living with chronic illnesses.

Recommendation 4

The committee recommends that, in addition to addressing individual illnesses in the community, all relevant federal and state agencies charged with public health and community approaches to control chronic illness, to the extent feasible, extend surveillance, evaluation, and mitigation programs to the widest possible range of chronic illnesses. This approach recognizes the commonality of important health, functional, and social outcomes for the population of individuals who live with different chronic illnesses.

> What is the role of primary prevention (for those at highest risk), secondary, and tertiary prevention of chronic disease in reducing or minimizing life impacts?

Although there are authoritative sources of effective primary and secondary preventive interventions for persons in clinical practice (e.g., the U.S. Preventive Services Task Force reports) and in the community (e.g., the Community Guide), neither of these resources systematically or comprehensively addresses these important interventions for persons with overt chronic illnesses. The committee found major gaps in research-based recommendations for routine preventive activities for those with common and important chronic illnesses.

Recommendation 5

The committee recommends that the federal health and related agencies that create and promulgate guidelines for general and community and clinical preventive services evaluate the effectiveness of these services for persons with chronic illness and specifically catalog and disseminate these guidelines to the public health and health care organizations that implement them.

> What consequences of chronic diseases are most important to the nation's health and economic well-being?

The economic consequences of chronic illnesses for individuals, families, the health care system, and the nation are related to many factors, including the natural history and progression of the illness; secondary consequences of care; levels of treatment of adverse effects; the treatability of the primary illnesses; the economic, social, and medical care resources available to the patient; the chronic care models available; the direct cost of care; the presence of comorbidity; the impact on family function and economic productivity; and, to some extent, the impact of public health interventions on the illnesses. In Chapter 2, the committee describes a number of ways to improve the quality and utility of information on the economic burdens of chronic illness, and—importantly—on opportunities to prevent or reduce them.

Recommendation 6

The committee recommends that CDC support the greater use of new and emerging economic methods, as well as those currently in use, in making policy decisions that will promote living well with chronic illnesses, including

1. **those with greater use of cost-effectiveness techniques;**
2. **more exploitation of methods used in determining national health accounts, but for specific and important chronic illnesses with long-term outcomes;**
3. **enhanced consideration of opportunity costs for various program decisions; and**
4. **those with a greater focus on economic evaluation of interventions that involve MCCs and cut across a variety of community settings.**

> What policy priorities could advance efforts to improve life impacts
> of chronic disease?

As policy makers have focused on the implementation of various features of the ACA, the public health community may see this as an opportunity to refocus efforts on those interventions at the population level essential to the prevention of chronic illness, thus reducing their role in interventions aimed at the management of chronic illness. As detailed in Chapters 3 and 6, the ACA provides a number of reforms and opportunities that have the potential to improve the lives of individuals with chronic illness. The ACA has new care concepts to improve the coordination and delivery of care to persons living with chronic illness, insurance coverage options and subsidies to purchase insurance, as well as chronic disease prevention policies. Provisions in the ACA can be used to help align public health and clinical care services in order to promote living well for those with chronic illness. The ACA also contains important provisions for the development of programs related to healthier nutrition choices, reduction of risky behaviors, and increasing healthy behaviors. Therefore, the ACA can be leveraged as an existing law with important implications for living well with chronic illness at both the clinical and the community level.

Recommendation 7

The committee recommends that CDC routinely examine and adjust relevant policies to ensure that its public health chronic disease management and control programs reflect the concepts and priorities embodied in the current health and insurance reform legislation that are aimed at improving the lives of individuals living with chronic illness.

There is a growing recognition that policies enacted by government agencies beyond the health sector have substantial effects on the health of the population (IOM, 2011). The concept of HIAP recognizes and underscores the importance of considering the links between health and a wide set of government policies. This approach requires policy makers and other stakeholders to adopt collaborative and structured approaches to consider the health effects of major public policies in all government sectors. A HIAP approach has been successfully adopted in the European Union and in several Canadian providences. HIAs are a primary population health promotion tool for the achievement of a HIAP approach. HIAs require an assessment of the health impacts of policies, plans, and projects in diverse economic sectors, using quantitative, qualitative, and participatory techniques (World Health Organization, [a]). To improve national health outcomes and reduce health risks, HHS recommends HIAs as an important planning resource for implementing *Healthy People 2020*.

Recommendation 8

The committee recommends that the secretary of HHS and CDC explore and test a HIAP approach with HIAs as a promising practice on a select set of major federal legislation, regulations, and policies and evaluate its impact on health-related quality of life, functional status, and relevant efficiencies over time.

Which population-based interventions can help achieve outcomes that maintain or improve quality of life, functioning, and disability?

- What is the evidence on effectiveness of interventions on these outcomes?
- To what extent do the interventions that address these outcomes also affect clinical outcomes?
- To what extent can policy, environmental, and systems change achieve these outcomes?

Most of the literature related to population-based approaches to health improvement is not specifically focused on chronic disease. Although there is ample evidence of the effectiveness of widely disseminated wellness or lifestyle programs at community sites, there is inadequate evaluation of their impact on the health-related quality of life and health outcomes of individuals living with chronic illness. Although some interventions, such as physical activity, have been well studied and shown to improve the lives of persons living with many types of chronic illness, all interventions could benefit from further research on effectiveness, adaptation, and maintenance. Once interventions for both prevention of additional illness and control of existing illness are developed and shown to be effective, the public health community should join with health care systems and community organizations in giving much more attention to disseminate and implement those interventions.

Recommendation 9

The committee recommends that CDC conduct rigorous evaluations of its funded chronic disease prevention programs to include the effects of those programs on health-related quality of life and functional status.

Recommendation 10

The committee recommends that all major CDC-funded research programs aimed at primary community-based chronic disease prevention
or interventions be evaluated for their effect on persons with existing
chronic illness to assess health- and social-related quality of life, management of existing illness, and efforts to prevent subsequent illnesses.

Recommendation 11

The committee recommends that public and private research funders
increase support for research on and evaluation of the adoption and
long-term maintenance of healthy lifestyles and effective preventive
services (e.g., promoting physical activity, healthy eating patterns, appropriate weight, effective health care) in persons with chronic illness.
Support should be provided for implementation research on how to disseminate effective long-term lifestyle interventions in community-based
settings that improve living well with chronic illness.

The context for inequities and disparities in living well with chronic
illness is described in Chapter 1 and highlighted again in Chapter 2. Addressing these inequities will require that strategies to improve living well
with chronic illness, as well as policies and social determinants that impact
health and function, consider their potential impact on health outcomes
across population subgroups.

Recommendation 12

The committee recommends that federally supported efforts to improve
living with chronic illness have as an explicit goal the reduction of
health disparities across affected populations.

- Barriers to obtaining complete assessments of community and public health interventions for populations experiencing health disparities should be identified and addressed.
- When interventions typically result in positive health outcomes
  for the general population of individuals living with chronic illness, they should be assessed and modified for adaptation and
  implementation in communities experiencing disparities in health
  outcomes.

The goal of health care is to improve the health outcome of individuals
based on a medical regime and treatment. In contrast, the goal of public

health is to improve the health status of the population through health promotion and disease prevention measures (Hardcastle et al., 2011). The ACA offers several opportunities to support improved coordination between public health and health care. Community-based non–health care sector organizations contribute significantly to the prevention and treatment of chronic disease. Serious efforts to reduce morbidity and to realize improved outcomes in chronic disease can benefit from cooperation among the public health, health care, and community non–health care sectors (Hardcastle et al., 2011). Such cooperation may also be a promising approach to cost efficiencies. There are also new and emerging models of care and public health initiatives, as described in Appendix B, designed to improve the functional status and quality of life for persons living with chronic illness that need to be tested, expanded, and evaluated.

Recommendation 13

The committee recommends that HHS agencies and state and local government public health agencies (GPHAs) evaluate existing (e.g., chronic care model, expanded chronic care model), emerging, and/or new models of chronic disease care that promote cooperation among community-based organizations, the health care delivery system, employers and businesses, the media, and the academic community to improve living well with chronic illness.

- CDC and state and local GPHAs should serve convening and facilitating functions for developing and implementing emerging models.
- HHS agencies (e.g., the Health Resources and Services Administration, the Centers for Medicare and Medicaid Services, the Administration on Aging, CDC) and GPHAs should fund demonstration projects and evaluate these emerging models.
- Federal, private, and other payors should create new financing streams and incentives that support maintaining and disseminating emerging models that effectively address persons living well with chronic illness.

Recommendation 14

The committee recommends that CDC develop and promote, in partnership with organizations representing health care, public health, and patient advocacy, a set of evidenced-based policy goals and objectives specifically aimed at actions that decrease the burden of suffering and improve the quality of life of persons living with chronic illness.

Worksite wellness programs have grown tremendously in the past decade, not only with government agencies but also with a diverse set of large self-insured employers and insurers. There are very limited data on such programs from small employers or businesses. The focus of worksite wellness programs is often improvement in lifestyle behaviors. Evaluation of the effectiveness of these programs in several systematic reviews and meta-analyses suggests a robust and significant effect on improvement of targeted lifestyle behaviors (e.g., diet, weight loss, physical activity). As discussed in Chapter 3, there is very scant evidence of worksite programs targeted at people living with chronic illness.

Recommendation 15

The committee recommends that federal and state policy makers develop and implement pilot incentives programs for all employers, particularly low-wage employers, small businesses, and community-based organizations, to provide health promotion programs with known effectiveness for those living with chronic illness.

> How can public health surveillance be used to inform public policy decisions to minimize adverse life impacts?

In the change process driving interventions to help patients with chronic illness live well and to improve the nation's health and economic well-being by reducing disability and improving quality of life and functioning, surveillance is the first step. This shift in focus from merely extending life to living well has the potential to facilitate decision making at the individual, health care system, and population levels, improving outcomes not only for patients and families but also for society. Integrating multiple measures of health status and detailed measures of determinants of health is required for an optimal surveillance system to assess how well individuals are living with chronic illness.

Recommendation 16

The committee recommends that the secretary of HHS encourage and support pilot tests by health care systems to collect patient-level information, share deidentified data across systems, and make them available at the local, state, and national levels in order to monitor and improve chronic illness outcomes. These data should include patient self-reported outcomes of health-related quality of life and functional status in persons with chronic illness.

Recommendation 17

The committee recommends that the secretary of HHS establish and support a standing national work group to oversee and coordinate multidimensional chronic diseases surveillance activity, including obtaining patient-level data on health-related quality of life and functional status from electronic medical records and data on the implementation and dissemination of effective chronic disease interventions at the health care system and the community levels, including longitudinal health outcomes.

CONCLUSION

The burden of chronic disease in America today is indeed vast and continues to grow. The sheer magnitude of this burden for society; the striking inequalities in living well among minorities, the elderly, and the disadvantaged; and the simple fact that numerous chronic illnesses are leading causes of death and disability are all emblematic of the considerable limitations of existing policies, programs, and systems of care and support for people living with chronic illness today.

Government public health agencies have the ability to take action to help people live better with chronic illness. They have the expertise to assess a public health problem, develop an appropriate program or policy, and ensure that programs and policies are effectively delivered and implemented. The committee thinks that its recommendations are rooted in a population-based approach, underscore the importance of public health action in the management and control of chronic disease, and offer strategies to support public health efforts.

As the nation strives to consider and implement new strategies for understanding and addressing the burden of chronic illness, it is imperative that those strategies give ample consideration to all chronic illnesses and all dimensions of suffering. Indeed, all chronic illnesses have the potential to reduce population health not only by causing premature death but also by limiting people's capacity to live well during all the years of their lives. For society, living well is impacted both by the numbers of persons living with chronic illnesses and by the effects of those illnesses on the quality of life of patients, their peers, and their caregivers. In this context, the overall burden of chronic illness could be drastically reduced through coordinated efforts toward both primary prevention and other interventions and policies designed to improve health for persons already living with chronic illness.

REFERENCES

Bloom, D.E., E.T. Cafiero, E. Jané-Llopis, S. Abrahams-Gessel, L.R. Bloom, S. Fathima, A.B. Feigl, T. Gaziano, M. Mowafi, A. Pandya, K. Prettner, L. Rosenberg, B. Seligman, A. Stein, and C. Weinstein. 2011. *The Global Economic Burden of Non-Communicable Diseases.* Geneva: World Economic Forum.

CDC (Centers for Disease Control and Prevention). 2009. Prevalence and most common causes of disability among adults—United States, 2005. *Morbidity and Mortality Weekly Report* 58(16):421-426. http://www.cdc.gov/mmwr/preview/mmwrhtml/mm5816a2.htm (accessed October 4, 2011).

Hardcastle, L.E., K.L. Record, P.D. Jacobson, and L.O. Gostin. 2011. *Improving the population's health: The Affordable Care Act and the importance of integration.* http://papers.ssrn.com/sol3/papers.cfm?abstract_id=1932724 (accessed October 4, 2011).

IOM (Institute of Medicine). 2010. *A Population-Based Policy and Systems Change Approach to Prevent and Control Hypertension.* Washington, DC: The National Academies Press.

IOM. 2011. *For the Public's Health: Revitalizing Law and Public Policy to Meet the New Challenge.* Washington, DC: The National Academies Press.

Kaiser Family Foundation. 2010. *U.S. Health Care Costs.* http://www.kaiseredu.org/Issue-Modules/US-Health-Care-Costs/Background-Brief.aspx (accessed October 12, 2011).

Kung, H.C., D.L. Hoyert, J.Q. Xu, and S.L. Murphy. 2008. Deaths: Final data for 2005. *National Vital Statistics Reports* 56(10). http://www.cdc.gov/nchs/data/nvsr/nvsr56/nvsr56_10.pdf (accessed October 4, 2011).

Sainfort, F., and P.L. Remington. 1995. *The Disease Impact Assessment System (DIAS).* Public Health Reports 110(5):639–644.

Vilnius, D., and S. Dandoy. 1990. A priority rating system for public health programs. *Public Health Reports* 105(5):463–470.

World Health Organization (a). *Health Impact Assessment (HIA).* http://www.who.int/hia/en/.

Wu, S.Y., and A. Green. 2000. *Projection of Chronic Illness Prevalence and Cost Inflation.* Santa Monica, CA: RAND Health.

Introduction

Chronic diseases have emerged in recent decades as the major cluster of health concerns of the American people. A chronic condition or illness, in general terms, is a condition that is slow in progression, long in duration, and void of spontaneous resolution, and it often limits the function, productivity, and quality of life of those who live with them.

Globally, chronic diseases will account for 69 percent of all global deaths by 2030, and 80 percent of these deaths will occur in low-income and middle-income countries. According to the Centers for Disease Control and Prevention (CDC), in the United States, chronic diseases currently account for 70 percent of all deaths (Kung et al., 2008). In fact, close to 48 million Americans report a disability related to a chronic illness (Brault et al., 2009). Arthritis is the most common cause of disability, affecting about 8.6 million people, followed by back or spine problems, which affect about 7.6 million people. In addition, heart problems impede the functioning of about 3 million people (Brault et al., 2009).

Looking toward the future, the first baby boomers reach age 65 in 2011, and, of these, 37 million, or 6 out of 10, will be managing more than one chronic disease by 2030. For certain chronic diseases, the burden will be substantial; it is estimated that 14 million baby boomers will live with diabetes, and almost half will live with arthritis (expected to hit just over 26 million in 2020) (HHS, 2010).

Some chronic illnesses do not contribute significantly to mortality but can severely impact the quality of life of the individuals who live with them. Asthma, for example, affects more than 16 million American adults. Individuals who identify asthma as their main disabling condition report more physically unhealthy days, mentally unhealthy days, and days with activity limitations in the previous month than people who do not have asthma. Data from the California Health Interview Survey, for example, indicate that about 30 percent of adults with asthma experienced daily or weekly asthma symptoms. In 2005, asthma accounted for 2 million days of missed work among Californians.

Epilepsy, another example, is a chronic neurological condition identified by recurring seizures. Epilepsy can be caused by different conditions that affect a person's brain, such as stroke, head trauma, and infection, and those with the condition are at higher risk for injuries (both unintentional and self-inflicted) and other chronic illnesses. Epilepsy affects about 2 million people in the United States, which makes it one of the most common neurological conditions. Epilepsy accounts for $15.5 billion in medical costs and loss or reduction in earnings and productivity. Despite medical attention and treatment, more than one-third of individuals with epilepsy continue to have seizures, a situation that significantly affects the quality of life for those living with this chronic illness. In addition, many people who suffer from seizure disorders also live with the burden and risk of a phenomenon known as sudden unexpected death from epilepsy (CDC, 2011).

Chronic illnesses not only impact the lives of millions of people in America but also are a major contributor to health care costs. The medical care costs of people with chronic illness represent 75 percent of the $2 trillion spent annually in the United States on health care (Kaiser Family Foundation, 2010). The substantial costs in terms of the number of lives lost, quality of life diminished, and medical expenditures mean that public health interventions are needed to reduce the burden of chronic disease, especially among those at highest risk (e.g., those with prediabetes, hypertension, high cholesterol) and in preventing further consequences among those with chronic illnesses (secondary prevention).

In 2010, the CDC and the Arthritis Foundation sought assistance from the Institute of Medicine (IOM) to identify population-based public health actions that can help reduce disability and improve functioning and quality of life among individuals who are at high risk of developing a chronic illness and those with one or more chronic illnesses.

STATEMENT OF TASK

The statement of task for this consensus study provides that the IOM will establish a committee to examine the nonfatal burden of chronic disease and the implications for population-based public health action. A set of questions was to be considered for persons with single as well as multiple chronic diseases:

1. What consequences of chronic diseases are most important (criteria to be decided and justified by the committee) to the nation's health and economic well-being?
2. Which chronic diseases should be the focus of public health efforts to reduce disability and improve functioning and quality of life?
3 Which populations need to be the focus of interventions to reduce the consequences of chronic disease including the burden of disability, loss of productivity and functioning, health care costs, and reduced quality of life?
4. Which population-based interventions can help achieve outcomes that maintain or improve quality of life, functioning, and disability?
   • What is the evidence on effectiveness of interventions on these outcomes?
   • To what extent do the interventions that address these outcomes also affect clinical outcomes?
   • To what extent can policy, environmental, and systems change achieve these outcomes?
5. How can public health surveillance be used to inform into public policy decisions to minimize adverse life impacts?
6. What policy priorities could advance efforts to improve life impacts of chronic disease?
7. What is the role of primary prevention (for those at highest risk), secondary, and tertiary prevention of chronic disease in reducing or minimizing life impacts (e.g., preventing diabetes in pre-diabetics, preventing incidence of disability in people with arthritis, preventing recurrence of cancer, managing complications of cardiovascular disease)?

In conducting this work, the committee was asked to consider the following diseases: heart disease and stroke, diabetes, arthritis, depression, respiratory problems (asthma, chronic obstructive pulmonary disease [COPD]), chronic neurological conditions, and cancer. These diseases or categories of disease were included in the statement of task as examples of diseases for the committee to consider, not as a prescriptive set of diseases to include in the report. In fact, the committee was advised by the sponsors of this report not to focus on the common high-mortality diseases, but rather to consider diseases that have the potential to cause or actually do cause functional limitations and/or disabilities. This guidance thus allowed the committee to consider a wide range of chronic diseases, including all chronic diseases, in the context of living well. With respect to primary prevention, the committee was asked to consider prevention only among individuals with high-risk factors (e.g., prediabetes). Chronic illnesses related

---

Additional Guidance from the Sponsors

Acknowledging the depth and breadth of the statement of task and the time and resources needed, the sponsors advised the committee to focus the deliberations and recommendations in the report to:

- Identify the consequences of chronic diseases that are most important to the nation's health and economic well-being.
- Identify which chronic diseases and populations should be the focus of public health efforts to reduce disability and improve quality of life.
- Identify which population-based interventions can help achieve outcomes that maintain or improve quality of life, functioning, and disability.
- Identify ways to highlight the morbidity of arthritis and influence systematic change to improve the lives of those living with arthritis.
- Recommend population-based public health actions and strategies for implementation.

---

to congenital disorders, infectious diseases, substance abuse, and childhood conditions are not the focus of this study.

COMMITTEE APPROACH

Over a 12-month period, a 17-member committee held 5 in-person meetings, convened a series of small-group, chapter-focused conference calls, and conducted extensive literature reviews and Internet searches regarding an array of topic areas related to chronic illness. These topics ranged from disease-specific articles to social determinants of health discussions; from surveillance methods to various chronic care models; from health care economics to public health policies; from suffering to health-related quality of life; from patient-centered approaches to writings on caregiver burden; from health care system efforts to public health approaches; from evidenced-based interventions to promising community-based models; and from CDC studies to a series of IOM reports related to the topic—and much more.

Some committee members attended meetings related to public health and chronic disease prevention, and others participated in relevant meetings on chronic disease as part of the information-gathering process. The committee conducted two public workshops in which we listened to a variety of perspectives on living well with chronic illness to use in our deliberations and development of this report. In addition, the committee commissioned two experts to develop papers on specific topics to supplement the report.

The paper topics include depression and chronic illness and community care models for chronic disease. These papers are found in Appendixes A and B.

ORGANIZATION OF THE REPORT

The introductory chapter provides the background and premise for this report, the charge to the committee, the scope of the study, and the method for this report.

Chapter 1, "Living Well with Chronic Illness," describes the conceptual frameworks and population-based approach used for development of this report. It also provides a contextual construct for discussion and information in the chapters to follow.

Chapter 2, "Chronic Illnesses and the People Who Live with Them," explores the differences, similarities, and clinical stages among many chronic illnesses; discusses the burden of chronic illness on both those who live with them and their communities; highlights nine exemplar conditions that are clinically important, impact function and disability, impact the community, families, and caregivers, and represent an important challenge to public health; and discusses the economic consequences of chronic illness on the nation's health.

Chapter 3, "Policy," describes the challenges and opportunities for developing and testing promising policies and approaches, and using current legislation that supports community-level programs and actions to help people who are living with chronic illness live better.

Chapter 4, "Community-Based Intervention," provides an overview of the state of the art of community-based interventions aimed at helping people live well with chronic illness.

Chapter 5, "Surveillance and Assessment," describes the conceptual framework for chronic disease surveillance and explains how appropriate surveillance methods can enhance living well with chronic illness by providing information and data for public health policies and interventions. This chapter also examines and identifies gaps in the current data sources and methods for surveillance of certain chronic illnesses and discusses future data sources, methods, and research directions for surveillance to enhance living well with chronic illness.

Chapter 6, "Interface of the Public Health System, the Health Care System, and the Non–Health Care Sector," examines how the public health and health care systems and non–health care organizations could align to improve outcomes in prevention and management of chronic diseases.

Chapter 7, "The Call for Action," describes the committee's findings and conclusions.

Appendix A is a paper by Wayne J. Katon called "Improving Recognition and Quality of Depression Care in Patients with Common Chronic Medical Illnesses."

Appendix B is a paper by Chad Boult and Erin K. Murphy called "New Models of Comprehensive Health Care for People with Chronic Conditions."

Appendix C contains the agendas for the public workshops held by the committee, and Appendix D contains biographical sketches of committee members.

REFERENCES

Brault, M.W., J. Hootman, C.G. Helmick, K.A. Theis, and B.S. Armour. 2009. Prevalence and most common causes of disability among adults—United States, 2005. *Morbidity and Mortality Weekly Report* 58(16):421–426. http://www.cdc.gov/mmwr/preview/mmwrhtml/mm5816a2.htm (accessed October 4, 2011).

CDC (Centers for Disease Control and Prevention). 2011. *Targeting Epilepsy. Improving the Lives of People with One of the Nation's Most Common Neurological Conditions. At a Glance.* http://www.cdc.gov/chronicdisease/resources/publications/aag/pdf/2011/Epilepsy_AAG_2011_508.p df (accessed October 12, 2011).

HHS (U.S. Department of Health and Human Services). 2010. *News Release. Secretary Sebelius Awards Funding for Chronic Disease Self-Management Programs for Older Americans.* http://www.hhs.gov/news/press/2010pres/03/20100330a.html (accessed November 16, 2011).

Kaiser Family Foundation. 2010. *U.S Health Care Costs.* http://www.kaiseredu.org/Issue-Modules/US-Health-Care-Costs/Background-Brief.aspx (accessed October 12, 2011).

Kung, H.C., D.L. Hoyert, J. Xu, and S.L. Murphy. 2008. Deaths: Final data for 2005. *National Vital Statistics Reports* 56(10). http://www.cdc.gov/nchs/data/nvsr/nvsr56/nvsr56_10.pdf (accessed October 4, 2011).

1

Living Well with Chronic Illness

Americans value health and the capacity to live with a sense of physical, mental, and social well-being. For many, having health also implies access to social and personal resources that enable them to live well on a day-to-day basis (WHO, 1986). Generally, people tend to place less value on simply living longer if added years of life come without the security of health and well-being. Indeed, there is a limit to people's willingness to accept physical and psychosocial discomfort or to compromise functional independence, the capacity to enjoy relationships with others, or financial security in exchange for longer life expectancy (Miller and Levy, 2000; Tengs et al., 1995).

Chronic diseases are long-term health conditions that threaten well-being and function in an episodic, continuous, or progressive way over many years of life (NCCDPHP, [a]; WHO, [a]). Not only have chronic diseases emerged as leading causes of death; they also represent enormous and growing causes of impairment and disability (WHO, 2004). Tremendous advances in public health and health care over the past century have extended average life expectancies, but these advances have been compromised by parallel increases in physical inactivity, unhealthful eating, obesity, tobacco use, and other chronic disease risk factors (McGinnis and Foege, 1993; Mokhad et al., 2004; WHO, 2009). As a result of this combination, more individuals are living longer but with one or more chronic illnesses (HHS, 2010). In fact, living for many years with a chronic disease is now common, and this presents a growing threat not only to population health but also to the nation's economic and social welfare. Although much work is under way to address the burden of chronic disease, resources are limited and the problem is growing. In this context, there is a clear danger that these efforts will prove unsuccessful unless they can be prioritized, aligned, and coordinated in a way that achieves the greatest benefit at a cost that is acceptable to society. Addressing the toll of all chronic diseases, from a population health perspective, is the subject of this report.

THE TIMELY RELEVANCE OF A PUSH TOWARD LIVING WELL WITH CHRONIC ILLNESS

Chronic illnesses have always been a great burden not only to those living with them but also to their societies and cultures, taking a tremendous toll on welfare, economic productivity, social structures, and achievements. Individuals with chronic illnesses have historically sought varied healers and healing institutions in their communities to alleviate suffering, but over past centuries there were few management aids for severe and progressive conditions, and survivorship was often modest at best. This problem was exacerbated by frequent lack of access to supportive or palliative care, and death often came quickly. However, even in these unfortunate historical circumstances, the state, along with many nongovernmental organizations, played important roles in the response to chronic diseases, providing almshouses and hospitals for impoverished, disabled, and otherwise sick individuals who may not have had the fiscal or social resources to remain in the community or who had been ostracized from community life because of their conditions.

In the past century, extraordinary advances in developed countries in medicine and public health, as well as economic growth leading to more widely accessible social welfare programs, have changed the chronic disease landscape dramatically. Hygienic and sanitary advances have prevented many previously common diseases. Immunizations and clinical and community interventions have substantially controlled many past causes of chronic illness, such as tuberculosis and syphilis. Good progress in reducing tobacco use has occurred, even if incomplete. Pharmacotherapy has enabled most persons with chronic mental illnesses to be deinstitutionalized, even in the absence of prevention or cure. Although there is more work to do, chronic cardiovascular diseases have been diminished in many important ways. Importantly, additional therapeutic approaches have improved the function and overall health for some persons with chronic illnesses through advances in corrective surgery, new approaches in analgesia, better rehabilitation and physical and occupational therapy, improved nutrition management, and adaptation of home and community environments for functionally impaired persons.

Despite these advances, many community-wide problems with chronic diseases remain major public health concerns. Individuals with congenital disabling conditions now survive longer into adulthood. Numerous important chronic diseases still have no known or controllable causes and continue unabated, such as mental illnesses, chronic skin conditions, inflammatory bowel diseases, collagen vascular diseases, and degenerative neurological illnesses. Chronic illnesses resulting from injuries or burns or from infectious agents (e.g., hepatitis B and C, HIV, *H. pylori*) also continue to take an important long-term toll on those affected. The control of many chronic illnesses among young and middle-aged adults, even with some important successes, has delayed the onset of these illnesses to older ages. Amid medical progress, enhanced population survival has also permitted the emergence of more degenerative illnesses at older ages, such as arthritis, dementia, and end-stage kidney disease. Moreover, the availability and application of more intensive medical therapies has increased treatment costs and the probability of adverse events. Some examples include deep vein thrombosis following joint replacement surgery for hip or knee arthritis; increases in type 2 diabetes during treatment with some common mental health medications; more cardiovascular events with intensive glucose lowering in some patients with diabetes; antibiotic resistant infections of kidney dialysis catheters; and increased risk of falls or fractures among frail elders treated with sedative-hypotic medications intended for improving sleep or reducing agitation.

In addition, some population risk factors for chronic diseases are going in the wrong direction. Obesity levels have increased dramatically, along with physical inactivity and unhealthful eating, accounting for a considerable proportion of prevalent chronic diseases, such as diabetes and cardiovascular diseases (McGinnis and Foege, 1993; Mokdad et al., 2004). As a result, the average life expectancy for Americans living in most U.S. counties has decreased over the past decade relative to gains being made in other leading nations around the world (Kulkarni et al., 2011). Thus, in the modern era, the toll of chronic diseases on physical, mental, and social health, health care, and the economy continues to a problem of critical magnitude in America today (Center for Healthcare Research and Transformation, 2010; DeVol and Bedroussian, 2007; Michaud et al., 2006; NCCDPHP, 2009).

THE POPULATION HEALTH PERSPECTIVE

Taking a population health perspective means considering the magnitude and distribution of health outcomes from the viewpoint of societal groups or populations (Kindig, 2007). From such a perspective, genes, biology, behavior, and environment are all seen to interact in their impact on health and function. Older adults are biologically prone to being in poorer health than adolescents because of the physical and cognitive effects of aging. Individuals can also inherit a higher probability of developing many illnesses, such as sickle cell anemia, breast cancer, heart disease, and diabetes. People interact with one another and their environments through behaviors that can also impact health. For example, a person who is physically inactive is more likely to develop obesity, depressive illness, heart disease, type 2 diabetes, and many cancers (HHS, 1996). Conversely, an individual who quits smoking can reduce his or her risk of developing heart disease, chronic obstructive lung diseases, and many cancers. Social influences and the physical environments in which people are born, live, learn, play, work, and age influence health in important ways. Educational and job opportunities; poverty; social norms and attitudes; discrimination; social support; exposure to mass media and technologies, such as the internet or cell phones; transportation options; and access to healthy foods, safe physical activities, or health care services are all important examples of environmental conditions that play important roles in determining health and function.

CHRONIC DISEASES AND THEIR IMPACT ON HEALTH AND FUNCTION

In 2005, 133 million Americans—almost half of all adults—had at least one chronic illness, causing 7 in 10 deaths in the United States each year (CDC, [a]). More than one in four Americans have concurrent multiple chronic conditions (two or more) (MCCs) (Anderson, 2010), including, for example, arthritis, asthma, chronic respiratory conditions, diabetes, heart disease, HIV infection, and hypertension. Regardless of the severity, pattern of effects, or duration of the disease, many diseases typically last at least a year, require ongoing medical attention, and limit activities of daily living (HHS, 2010).

"Morbidity" is a term commonly used to describe the burden of suffering, in terms of impairment or disability, caused by an illness or health condition. Morbidity can be measured at the individual level or summed to reflect the aggregate health of a population. Chronic diseases cause considerable population morbidity, which is reflected in often striking statistics regarding the frequency of various complications and subsequent high levels of health care utilization, health care costs, and missed days of work due to illness or disability. The degree of population morbidity caused by a chronic illness is often challenging to define, however, since some conditions are less common but lead to devastating consequences, whereas others affect millions of individuals in more subtle yet meaningful ways. Chronic illnesses also cause morbidity by impacting the quality of life of not only those who have the condition but also their families, friends, and caregivers. For society, chronic diseases take a large toll by imposing psychosocial stress, lowering economic prosperity, and increasing costs in both the health care and the public health sector (DeVol and Bedroussian, 2007; Thorpe, 2006).

In terms of a toll on quality of life, chronic disease morbidity can be assessed along multiple dimensions, such as pain, fatigue, physical impairment, lack of sleep, emotional distress, and decreased social health, or as a summative effect across all of these dimensions (NIH, 2011). Not surprisingly, different chronic diseases also impact dimensions of health in varied ways. For example, both schizophrenia and rheumatoid arthritis have a dramatic impact on the quality of life of individuals and their caregivers, but the scope of those impacts is very different. Persons with schizophrenia must deal with the stigma and often relapsing and remitting symptoms of a lifelong mental illness, causing many to never reach such milestones as getting married, having children, forming strong relationships with family, or being gainfully employed. In contrast, persons with rheumatoid arthritis suffer a variable course of physical concerns, changes in role function, and loss of specific abilities that often increase over time. It is important to appreciate the many facets of chronic disease morbidity and to recognize that all chronic diseases, whether common or rare, are of considerable importance to those who are affected.

It is also important to recognize that the degree of impairment or disability imposed by a particular chronic illness is subject to change over time, as the illness's course and the affected individual's coping responses evolve. Some chronic diseases, such as arthritis or type 2 diabetes, begin to impact quality of life even prior to their diagnosis, by causing psychological stress or physical symptoms. Other diseases that are typically considered chronic, such as high blood pressure or prediabetes, may continue for years without symptoms or measurable signs of illness per se. Having these illnesses, however, can still cause various forms of impairment. For example, quality of life can be reduced by the added stress of coping with the diagnosis itself, as individuals must perform new and sometimes complex self-care behaviors or to engage more intensively in health services designed to treat or prevent complications of the condition. Moreover, despite even the best of intentions, therapies for chronic illnesses can have unintended consequences, such as increasing stress or physiological symptoms or even by causing direct harm. Many of these consequences are easily overlooked. The full spectrum of health and morbidity for persons with chronic illnesses has been depicted previously in several frameworks (Nagi, 1965). By combining these past frameworks in a way that highlights a perspective of population health along the full spectrum of health and morbidity, the committee constructed an integrated framework to serve as a reference for discussing which strategies are likely to offer the greatest promise to improve health for individuals living with chronic illness, depicted in Figure 1-1.

A key feature of this integrated framework is that a principal aim of

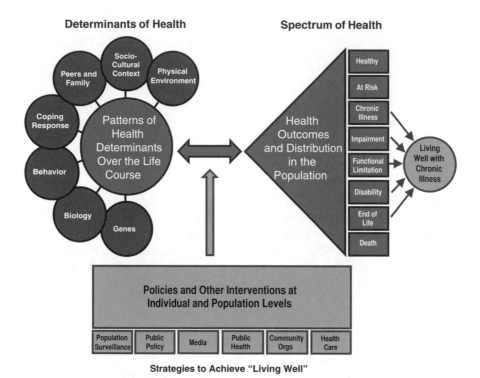

FIGURE 1-1 Integrated framework for living well with chronic illness.
SOURCE: Committee on Living Well with Chronic Disease: Public Health Action to Reduce Disability and Improve Functioning and Quality of Life.

addressing chronic illness morbidity is to help each affected person and the population as a whole to live well, regardless of the illness in question or an individual's own current state of disablement. The committee adopted the concept of living well, as proposed previously by other chronic disease experts (Lorig et al., 2006), to reflect the best achievable state of health that encompasses all dimensions of physical, mental, and social well-being. For each individual with chronic illness, to live well takes on a unique and equally important personal meaning, which is defined by a self-perceived level of comfort, function, and contentment with life. Living well is shaped by the physical, social, and cultural surroundings and by the effects of chronic illness not only on the affected individual but also on family members, friends, and caregivers. In this way, progress toward living well can be achieved through the combination of all efforts enacted across individual and societal levels to reduce disability and improve functioning and quality of life, regardless of each unique individual's current state of health or specific chronic illness diagnosis.

This concept of living well, integrated within a broader population health framework, is intended to promote a more holistic perspective beyond the traditional focus on other important goals, such as primary prevention or the prolongation of life expectancy alone. Moreover, it is intended also to heighten awareness that interventions and policies that promote function, reduce pain, remove obstacles for the disabled, or alleviate suffering at the end of life play an essential role in providing a more complete response for addressing chronic diseases in the United States today.

DOING SOMETHING ABOUT IT

In this report the committee elected to use the "living well framework" to inform the consideration of policies and the allocation of resources to solve important issues related to chronic diseases in a manner that is tied to a more complete understanding of the interactions among individual, behavioral, social, and environmental characteristics. Specific strategies designed to help individuals live well must also be considered in the context of a broader array of activities targeting primary, secondary, and tertiary prevention for all persons, regardless of whether they already have a chronic illness (Figure 1-2).

Many strategies that are promoted for primary prevention, such as vaccination, tobacco cessation, physical activity promotion, healthful eating, and injury prevention, can also help persons who have already developed a chronic illness or disability to live more healthfully. In addition, strategies that prevent or delay complications, build coping skills, improve function, or alleviate pain and suffering may serve a dual purpose of reducing the magnitude of illness burden over an individual's remaining years of life as well as reducing and/or delaying the development of additional complications or comorbidities in a way that serves to compress the period of morbidity until later in life (Hubert et al., 2002). Indeed, it is likely that the greatest societal benefit will emerge not from singular approaches, but from a deeper understanding of how different approaches might be coordinated to achieve the greatest progress toward living well for all persons with chronic illness.

Regardless of their scale or focus, most policies or programs to improve health require some form of investment that is both human and monetary. Moreover, even strategies that yield overall societal benefits may have adverse effects for some individuals or groups, including unforeseen and/or unintended consequences. All strategies should be fashioned with careful consideration of anticipated impacts, resource inputs, implementation steps, and plans for surveillance of both intended and unintended conse-

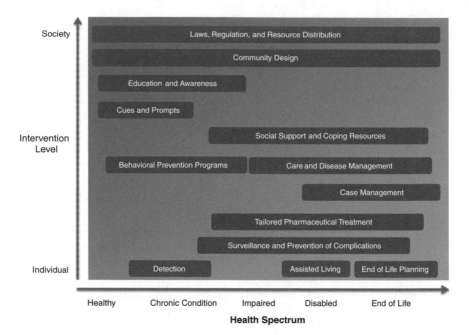

Society — Laws, Regulation, and Resource Distribution
Community Design
Education and Awareness
Cues and Prompts
Social Support and Coping Resources
Intervention Level — Behavioral Prevention Programs / Care and Disease Management
Case Management
Tailored Pharmaceutical Treatment
Surveillance and Prevention of Complications
Individual — Detection / Assisted Living / End of Life Planning

Healthy   Chronic Condition   Impaired   Disabled   End of Life

Health Spectrum

FIGURE 1-2 Interaction of multilevel interventions and policies to achieve living well across the spectrum of health and chronic disease.

SOURCE: Adapted from Copyright © Fielding, J.E., and S.M. Teutsch. 2011. An opportunity map for societal investment in health. *Journal of the American Medical Association* 305(20):2111. All rights reserved.

quences. In this report, we attempt to highlight important considerations of a thoughtful population health approach for living well with chronic illness. Before introducing those concepts, however, it is important first to consider the evolution of American strategies designed to understand illness burden and how existing resources and strategies available to promote population health might help to guide the nature and scope of future living-well interventions.

A Brief History

The capacity of society to respond to health threats, chronic or otherwise, is influenced by the way in which it documents and interprets the magnitude and distribution of health outcomes. From its earliest colonial beginnings, Americans have paid particular attention to such life events as births, marriages, and burials as a part of religious or cultural traditions. At the outset, disease ranked with starvation as a primary threat to the existence of many of the colonies. Infectious outbreaks, such as malaria, dysentery, typhoid, smallpox, and yellow fever, decimated many early colonial settlements (CDC and NCHS, [a]). Outbreaks of disease were met as emergencies with varied responses.

In the years just prior to the turn of the 19th century, large cities, such as Baltimore and Philadelphia, established boards of health as the forerunners of modern local health departments. Those boards attempted to introduce more systematic, population-based efforts to identify and track causes of serious health threats and to guide the public health response to epidemics. During the mid-19th century, states began enacting laws to expand and improve approaches to track causes of death. In 1879, the U.S. Congress created the National Board of Health, tasked to centralize information, engage in sanitary research, and collect vital statistics. Over time, the methods for documenting and interpreting the numbers and more precise causes of deaths in America continued to evolve, and this ultimately led to the establishment of the National Office of Vital Statistics of the Public Health Service in 1946 and the National Center for Health Statistics (NCHS) in 1963. Since that time, NCHS has produced reports of vital statistics and has worked with other agencies to advance methods to capture and analyze population health in America.

For the past half-century, efforts by organizations, such as the CDC (including NCHS), the World Health Organization (WHO), the National Institutes of Health (NIH), the Agency for Healthcare Research and Quality (AHRQ), and others, have used data from an evolving list of population health indicators to inform a variety of strategies by governmental public health entities, community-based nongovernmental organizations, and the health care system to address illness and promote health and function.

Recently, the increasing burden of chronic diseases globally has expanded the attention of these efforts to focus well beyond simply prolonging life, with an increasing emphasis on wellness and function. Implicit in this shift is a growing recognition that American society places less value on a longer life if additional years also bring additional pain and suffering or leave individuals without a capacity for independent decision making, the ability to perform activities of daily living independently, or enjoy relationships or financial security.

Today HHS, through CDC, AHRQ, NIH, and other centers, routinely tracks data and publishes reports on such outcomes as health behaviors; biological indicators of health; health care access, quality, utilization, disparities, and costs; prevalence of diseases; and vital statistics (BRFSS, [a]; CDC and NCHS, [a]; HCUPnet, [a]; MEPS, [a]). Beginning in the mid-1990s, the U.S. Council of State and Territorial Epidemiologists (CSTE) began working with epidemiologists and chronic disease program directors at the state and federal levels to select, prioritize, and define 73 chronic disease indicators. These data are intended to summarize available information from surveys, registries, and other surveillance systems about the incidence, prevalence, events, and efforts to detect and treat select chronic diseases and their behavioral risk factors (CDC, [a]). The first set of indicators was published in 1999, with state-specific data published the following year. In 2001, the content of both reports became available online. In 2002, the CSTE adopted a revised and expanded set of indicators. Although this reflects progress in shining light on the magnitude of morbidity imposed by chronic illnesses, the current efforts do not encompass all chronic diseases and do not capture many of the meaningful negative effects on quality of life caused by different forms of functional impairment and disability.

Since 2004, NIH has funded the development of the Patient Reported Outcomes Measurement Information System (PROMIS) to create, test, and recommend a more uniform set of tools for the measurement and surveillance of patient-reported health status indicators reflecting physical, mental, and social well-being (PROMIS, [a]). Although evidence-based and publicly accessible, PROMIS and similar tools have not yet been adopted more broadly for surveillance of quality of life or well-being for the U.S. population.

In parallel with PROMIS, other initiatives have tried to consider how population health indicators could be measured practically and used to inform local policies to address chronic disease (Parrish, 2010; Wold, 2008). Some examples of this work include the IOM's State of the USA Health Indicators report (2008) and the University of Wisconsin's Mobilizing Action Toward Community Health (MATCH) Project (Kindig et al., 2010). Although these initiatives are attempting to advance the capacity to understand the impact of chronic diseases and their risk factors on population health, practical considerations have led them to recommend only very brief metrics that are already being collected and are in the public domain. An example of one such metric is CDC's HRQOL-4, which has been collected at the state level since 1993. Although readily available today, this metric lacks specific information about activity limitation, functional status, and experiential state. Over the coming decade, one key goal for the Healthy People 2020 initiative is to evaluate the use of PROMIS and other available metrics for monitoring health-related quality of life and well-being in the United States (Healthy People 2020, [a]). Indeed, as discussed throughout this report, without the implementation of a more robust system for population-level surveillance of indicators that reflect the full depth and distribution of chronic disease morbidity on different dimensions of quality of life and well-being, it will prove challenging to prioritize, evaluate, and refine strategies that aim to help all Americans to live well with chronic illness.

Summary Measures of the Burden of Chronic Illness

In addition to considering the societal burden of chronic disease in terms of specific dimensions of health status, well-being, social participation, or survivorship, methods are also available to quantify morbidity using summary measures that combine information on both mortality and nonfatal health outcomes into a single numerical index (Murray et al., 2002). Such measures are broadly intended to quantify not only mortality but also the impact of impairment or disability on population health when individuals are living with a particular illness. Typically, these summary measures express "either the expected number of future years of healthy life after a given age or the number of years that chronic disease and disability subtract from a healthy life" (Parrish, 2010).

One example of a population-health summary measure, developed by the WHO, expresses health states in terms of disability-adjusted life-years (DALYs), in which one less DALY is equal to the loss of one healthy life-year. The impact of a particular chronic health state on disability is often estimated from information collected from individuals in the population and then summed to reflect the burden of a particular disease on a group or population. In this context, the DALY burden or human toll associated with a given illness for a population becomes a function of the numbers of persons affected; the age at onset, the pattern of its natural history (i.e., duration, chronicity, and episodic nature); and its effects over time on disability, functioning, and premature mortality. Based on the DALY metric, Michaud and colleagues reported in 2006 that noncommunicable diseases cost the United States 33.1 million DALYs per year, based on data collected by WHO. Common chronic illnesses, including ischemic heart disease, cerebrovascular disease, major depression, chronic obstructive pulmonary disease, asthma, HIV, diabetes mellitus, osteoarthritis, and chronic neurological disorders together accounted for about 35 percent of this total, which corresponds to about 16 days of healthy life lost for every person in the U.S. population that year (Michaud et al., 2006).

Another common way to express the summative impact of chronic diseases for a population is through a cost of illness approach, which attempts to monetize the direct and indirect financial costs incurred by society for a particular chronic disease. The cost of illness method typically views direct costs as those associated with health care per se (e.g., clinic visits, hospitalizations, medications, medical devices, and therapy/rehabilitation services as well as public health initiatives focused on primary or secondary prevention). Conversely, indirect costs are those that are incurred through effects on premature mortality, reduced labor output (including consideration of public and private income assistance programs, which serve to replace labor income for the disabled), and other consequences that lie beyond the health care system.

At the national level, direct health care spending in the United States can be assessed using the National Health Expenditure Accounts (NHEAs) (CMS, [a]). Currently, the NHEAs report health expenditures overall, by type of service delivered (e.g., hospital care, physician services), and by source of funding (e.g., private, Medicaid, Medicare), but not by categories of illness (Rosen and Cutler, 2009). The only exception is mental health and substance abuse treatment, which are reported separately by the Substance Abuse and Mental Health Services Administration (SAMHSA, 2007). However, some estimates of the costs associated with major chronic diseases do exist from other sources.

For example, in a 2007 report, the Milken Institute examined treatment costs for seven common chronic diseases in the United States in 2003: cancers, diabetes, heart disease, hypertension, stroke, mental disorders, and pulmonary conditions. This report estimated direct treatment expenditures to be $277 billion across those seven conditions, corresponding to 16 percent of total 2003 national health expenditures of $1.7 trillion (DeVol and Bedroussian, 2007; Smith et al., 2005). The authors further estimated that these seven conditions alone imposed indirect costs of $1.047 trillion on the U.S. economy in 2003 via reduced labor productivity (DeVol and Bedroussian, 2007). As concern has emerged about the fiscal burden of chronic diseases on the health care sector, the findings of this report underscore that this burden is indeed considerable. However, it is also striking that these estimates suggest the fiscal impact of chronic diseases on other sectors of the economy to be equal to or perhaps several-fold greater than their impact on direct medical spending alone.

Although such summary estimates are both striking and potentially more interpretable for decision makers and the public, there are notable limitations to the use of such measures for chronic disease morbidity. That said, the identification and wide-scale adoption of a common set of meaningful indicators that reflect the nonfatal burden of chronic diseases could prove instrumental in advancing efforts to enact, evaluate, and refine policies and other interventions to maximize progress toward living well. In this context, the discussion regarding how best to address the burden of chronic diseases might rise above a prioritized list based on different diagnoses, which tends to pit different diseases against one another for limited societal resources. The result of coordinated action that is focused instead on the common dimensions of living well might serve to align policies, programs, and the groups that advocate for them to achieve a more complete solution that advances quality of life and well-being for all of society. Subsequent chapters of this report discuss in more detail how metrics of living well can be used to guide policies toward a more complete solution to address the burden of nonfatal chronic diseases in America today.

Inequalities in Living Well with Chronic Illness

Health inequalities are formed by cultural, historical, economical, and political structures in the United States (Lewis et al., 2011). Health and economic outcomes for individuals living with chronic illnesses vary by race and ethnicity. Understanding the distributions of health indicators at a population level assists in recognizing key health determinants and population groups. Reducing inequalities in health not only helps the individual but also improves the overall health of the population.

In 2010, racial and ethnic minorities made up 35.1 percent of the U.S. population. Hispanics contributed to the largest portion of minorities with 16 percent; second, African Americans at 12.2 percent; and, third, Asians at 4.5 percent (Kaiser Family Foundation, 2010). These rates are expected to grow. It is anticipated that by 2050 these groups will make up almost half of the U.S. population (U.S. Census Bureau, 2004).

Compared with whites, African Americans are twice as likely to be diagnosed with diabetes (HHS, [a]). In 2009, arthritis and coronary heart disease affected African Americans slightly more than whites (CDC, 2010b). African Americans have a significantly higher prevalence of hypertension and stroke than all other race and ethnic groups. Compared with whites (the second-largest group living with both hypertension and stroke), 32.2 percent of African Americans have hypertension versus 23 percent of whites, and 3.8 percent experience stroke, compared with 2.5 percent of whites (CDC, 2010b).

American Indians/Alaskan Natives have lower rates of coronary heart disease but extremely high rates of diabetes in certain subgroups (CDC, 2010b; HHS, [b]). They also have higher chronic joint symptoms compared with whites (CDC, 2010b). Self-rated health status also differs by ethnic group. In 2003, approximately 7.4 percent of Asian Americans and 8.5 percent of white Americans consider themselves to be in fair or poor health, compared with 14.7 percent of African American, 16.3 percent of American Indians/Alaskan Natives, and 13.9 percent of Hispanic Americans (Cowling, 2006).

Serious psychological distress is reported at 30 percent more in African Americans than whites (HHS, [c]). Asian American women have the highest rate of suicide of all American women over 65 years old. Hispanic girls, grades 9–12, have 60 percent more suicide attempts than their white counterparts (HHS, [d]).

Research demonstrates drastic differences by socioeconomic status (SES) and, to a lesser extent, by race/ethnicity in health behaviors that represent dominant risk factors for the development and progression of chronic diseases. In the United States, tobacco use is the most preventable cause of disease and disability (CDC, 2011). Over 8 million Americans have a disease or disability caused by smoking (Hyland et al., 2003). Smoking is related to a wide range of chronic diseases, including chronic obstructive pulmonary disease, coronary heart disease, stroke, peripheral vascular disease, and peptic ulcer disease (Fagerström, 2002). There is an increased prevalence of tobacco use among lower income individuals. Almost 30 percent of adults living below the poverty line smoke, compared with 18.3 percent of adults who are at or above the poverty line. In addition, tobacco use increases in populations with less education. Just over 25.1 percent of adults who do not have a high school diploma smoke, whereas 9.9 percent of college graduates smoke, compared with only 6.3 percent of adults with a graduate degree (CDC, 2011). American Indians/Alaskan Natives have the highest prevalence of smoking at 31.4 percent (CDC, 2011).

The distributions of obesity show a very different pattern, varying both by race/ethnicity, SES, and gender. Socioeconomic status, defined by educational levels and income, is linked to obesity (McLaren, 2007). In 2001, 31.1 percent of blacks and 23.7 percent of Hispanics were obese, compared with 19.6 percent of white Americans and 15.7 percent of others, including Asians. A similar range is shown by education, for which 15.7 percent of college graduates are obese compared with 27.4 percent of those who did not graduate from high school (IOM, 2006). Obesity is more prevalent in women with lower income. And 42 percent of women living at 130 percent of the poverty level or below are obese, compared with 29 percent living at or above the poverty level (CDC, 2010a).

Underlying population differences in social and environmental conditions affect racial and ethnic inequalities in distributions of chronic disease risk factors and morbidity, not genetic factors alone (IOM, 2006). Although health care plays a crucial role in the treatment of disease, disparities in health care are estimated to account for only a small fraction of premature mortality among racial and ethnic minorities. On average, disadvantaged ethnic minorities complete fewer years of formal education, have lower income, and are less likely to have health insurance. This leads to less access to beneficial health services and an overall lower quality of care received (IOM, 2003). Disadvantaged individuals have greater exposure to crowding and noise (Kawachi and Berkman, 2003), constrained conditions for exercise, and less access to well-stocked grocery stores (McGinnis et al., 2002). In contrast, social environments with more social capital and social cohesion are more available in advantaged communities (Cohen et al., 2003; Kawachi and Berkman, 2000). In this context, it is imperative that strategies to improve living well with chronic illness consider the potential impact on *distributions* of health outcomes across population subgroups, as well as the way in which policies across other sectors, such as education, transportation, farming, and other areas, can indirectly impact health and contribute to disparities in health.

Frameworks to Guide Action Across Sectors

It can be daunting to consider how best to ensure a policy development process that promotes population health while considering the unequal distributions of chronic disease burden as well as the potential ripple effects when policies from different sectors collide. In this context, the committee thought it helpful to introduce another concept, which depicts a pyramid of layered intervention strategies to achieve living well (Figure 1-3). This pyramid attempts to frame different potential intervention strategies not only in terms of their target level (i.e., population-wide versus individually based) but also in terms of their relative intensity to meet the needs of those who shoulder the greatest burden of nonfatal chronic illnesses. This framework is used in subsequent chapters to communicate the nature and

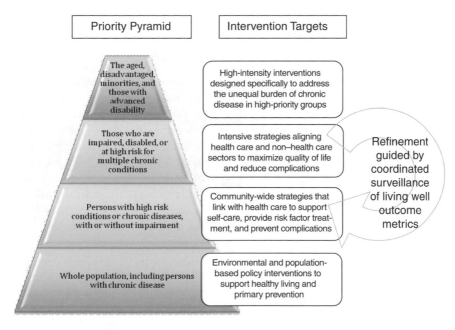

FIGURE 1-3 Prioritization scheme for policies and other interventions to address the burden of nonfatal chronic diseases across the population.
SOURCE: Committee on Living Well with Chronic Disease: Public Health Action to Reduce Disability and Improve Functioning and Quality of Life.

scope of different policy and other intervention recommendations made by the committee.

At the base of the priority pyramid are broad societal strategies to promote health and prevent disease for the entire population. At the very broadest level is the Health in All Policies (HIAP) perspective. This perspective acknowledges that health is fundamental to every sector of the economy and that every policy, large and small, whether focused primarily on transportation, education, agriculture, energy, trade, or another area, should take into consideration its impact on health (Aspen Institute, [a]; Blumenthal, 2009). Clearly, achieving such a goal is no trivial pursuit and is likely to require top-down coordination of policy sectors at the national, state, and local levels (The Strategic Growth Council, [a]) as well as a shared sense of participation and accountability among individuals, groups, institutions, businesses, communities, and governments to preserve, protect, and advance population health at every level. WHO and numerous other entities worldwide have promoted the development of frameworks and strategies to advance the HIAP perspective (WHO, [a]). From an operational perspective, the implementation of such a high-level and coordinated focus on health is likely to take considerable time to mature and will clearly require fundamental changes in policy development processes across both governmental and private sectors.

With slightly more focus, the acceleration of public and health system policies specifically intended for promoting health through the support of healthier lifestyle behaviors and access to evidence-based preventive services is also urgently needed. Although dedicated health policies are also typically directed at a population level, it is important to recognize that they can have meaningful (and often greater) benefits for individuals already affected by a chronic illness or high-risk condition (e.g., high cholesterol, prediabetes). Moreover, the presence of policies that enhance support and accessibility can amplify the impact of other environmental, social, and health care resources to help chronically ill persons live more healthful and higher quality lives. In this context, policy interventions serve as the very foundation of the priority pyramid and are discussed in greater depth in Chapter 3.

Moving up the priority pyramid, it is important to recognize that individuals who have already been diagnosed with a chronic illness can also benefit from access to additional care management and support resources in both health care and non–health care sectors. Such resources may include more intensive risk factor surveillance, medication therapies, medical procedures, educational and behavioral programs, and other support systems. The intensity of these resources needs increases among individuals who have MCCs and those who have progressed to develop impairment or disability. Exposure to multiple care providers and use of care management resources in multiple settings, though often needed, may introduce new problems if poorly aligned or fragmented. Poor coordination of services for the chronically ill can lead to care that, although intensive, is both ineffective and wasteful. Moreover, such care can also increase the possibility of harm caused by conflicting therapies or poor communication among affected individuals and providers (IOM, 1999).

Because many treatment and self-care resources for persons with nonfatal chronic illnesses can be complementary, they are likely to offer the greatest benefit for an individual and for the population if they are coordinated across sectors in ways that reach more individuals, reinforce behaviors throughout communities, provide the most efficient use of limited resources, and avoid harms. For several years, professionals in both the health care and the public health sector have worked to develop and evaluate frameworks for the coordination of resources to prevent and manage chronic diseases. The Chronic Care Model (CCM), for example, is a conceptual framework designed to identify structural elements in the health system that are believed to impact chronic disease outcomes through their ability to create productive interactions among informed, activated patients and prepared, productive care providers. Increasingly, the CCM is being used as a foundation for efforts to define the model elements of a patient-centered medical home (NCQA, [a]) and to guide broader concepts related to transformation of health systems into "accountable care" organizations. In this context, the CCM is an important consideration in the discussion of how best to implement strategies that will transform the structure and process of health care delivery.

Although used initially as a tool to improve chronic health care services, the CCM does attempt to overlay health care delivery on a broader landscape of community resources and policies. Since its initial introduction in the 1990s, several groups have attempted to refine the CCM to place even stronger emphasis on community influence and prevention (Barr et al., 2003). One such adaption, the Expanded Chronic Care Model (Barr et al., 2003), depicted in Figure 1-4, advances the perspective that care model elements bridge across health care and non–health care sectors and that an overarching goal of those bridging support structures and programs is to improve population health outcomes not only by impacting the health and behaviors of individual patients and their health care providers but also by activating communities and preparing community partners.

Although integration frameworks, such as the Expanded Chronic Care Model, may prove helpful in coordinating care resources for persons with nonfatal chronic illnesses, much more work is needed not only to understand the best approaches for developing clinical-community linkages (Ackermann, 2010; Etz et al., 2008) but also to guide higher level strategies that ensure an efficient interface across policy sectors and among public and

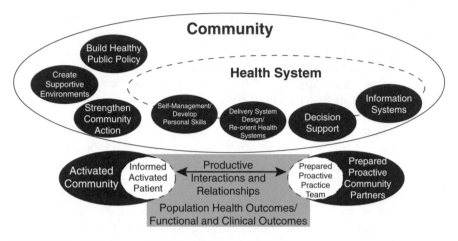

FIGURE 1-4 The Expanded Chronic Care Model.
SOURCE: Barr, V., S. Robinson, B. Marin-Link, L. Underhill, A. Dotts, D. Ravensdale, and S. Salivaras. 2003. The expanded chronic care model: An integration of concepts and strategies from population health promotion and the chronic care model. *Healthcare Quarterly* 7(1):73–82.

private partners to advance population health and living well with chronic illness on a much larger scale. It is the position of the committee that such progress will require not only new structures and processes for collaborative policy development but also the careful alignment of incentives to promote accountability toward population health and greater coordination of efforts to achieve that goal. A more robust description of interventions in communities and strategies for coordinating interventions across non–health care and health care settings appears in Chapters 4 and 6.

CONCLUSION

The burden of chronic disease in America today is indeed vast and continues to grow. The sheer magnitude of this burden for society; the striking inequalities in living well among minorities, the elderly, and the disadvantaged; and the simple fact that numerous chronic diseases are leading causes of death and disability are all emblematic of the considerable limitations of existing policies, programs, and systems of care and support for Americans living with chronic illness today.

New strategies for understanding and addressing this burden must give ample consideration to all chronic illnesses and all dimensions of suffering. Indeed, all chronic diseases have the potential to reduce population health not only by causing premature death but also by limiting people's capacity to live well during the remaining years of their lives. For society, living well is impacted not only by the numbers of persons who suffer from chronic illnesses but also by the effects of those illnesses on their quality of life and that of their peers, caregivers, children, and dependents. In this context, the overall burden of chronic diseases could be drastically reduced through co-ordinated efforts toward both primary prevention and other interventions and policies that are designed to improve health for persons already living with chronic illness. Although both of these overarching goals are essential to the health of America, the remainder of this report focuses on the goal of living well with chronic illness.

In the chapters that follow, the committee consistently adopts a popu-lation health perspective to guide discussions of how individuals' genes, biology, and behaviors interact with the social, cultural, and physical envi-ronment around them to influence health outcomes for the entire popula-tion. Subsequent chapters consider and recommend practical steps toward advancing efforts to coordinate action across sectors to help society live well with all forms of chronic illness and to address gaping inequalities in their distribution and their complications among vulnerable population subgroups. Because different chronic illnesses impact social participation and quality of life in varied ways, the committee also uses examples of dif-ferent chronic diseases to illustrate key concepts. This, however, should not be viewed as an assertion that some diseases are more burdensome or more important than others. In the end, it is our hope that this report will guide immediate and precise action to reduce the burden of all forms of chronic disease through the development of cross-cutting and coordinated strategies that can help all Americans to live well.

REFERENCES

Ackermann, R.T. 2010. Description of an integrated framework for building linkages among primary care clinics and community organizations for the prevention of type 2 diabetes: Emerging themes from the CC-Link study. *Chronic Illness* 6(2):89–100.

Anderson, G. 2010. *Chronic Care: Making the Case for Ongoing Care*. Princeton, NJ: Robert Wood Johnson Foundation. http://www.rwjf.org/files/research/50968chronic.care.chart book.pdf (accessed December 2, 2010).

Aspen Institute (a). *Health in All Policies*. http://www.aspeninstitute.org/policy-work/health-biomedical-science-society/health-stewardship-project/principles/health-all (accessed Oc-tober 19, 2011).

Barr, V.J., S. Robinson, B. Marin-Link, L. Underhill, A. Dotts, D. Ravensdale, and S. Salivaras. 2003. The expanded Chronic Care Model: An integration of concepts and strategies from population health promotion and the Chronic Care Model. *Hospital Quarterly* 7(1):73–82.

Blumenthal, S. 2009. Health in all policies. *Huffington Post*, July 31. http://www.huffington post.com/susan-blumenthal/health-in-all-policies_b_249003.html (accessed October 4, 2011).

BRFSS (Behavioral Risk Factor Surveillance System) (a). http://www.cdc.gov/brfss/ (accessed October 14, 2011).

CDC (Centers for Disease Control and Prevention) (a). *Chronic Disease Prevention and Health Promotion.* http://www.cdc.gov/chronicdisease/overview/index.htm (accessed October 4, 2011).

CDC. 2010a. *Obesity and Socioeconomic Status in Adults: United States, 2005–2008.* Atlanta, GA: Centers for Disease Control and Prevention. http://www.cdc.gov/nchs/data/databriefs/db50.htm#ref3 (accessed December 19, 2011).

CDC. 2010b. *Summary Health Statistics for U.S. adults: National Health Interview Survey, 2009.* Washington, DC: Centers for Disease Control and Prevention.

CDC. 2011. Vital signs: Current cigarette smoking among adults aged ≥ 18 years—United States, 2005–2010. *Morbidity and Mortality Weekly Report* 60(35):1207–1212.

CDC and NCHS (National Center for Health Statistics) (a). *U.S. Vital Statistics System. Major Activities and Developments, 1950-95.* http://www.cdc.gov/nchs/data/misc/usvss.pdf (accessed October 4, 2011).

Center for Healthcare Research and Transformation. 2010. *Issue Brief January 2010. The Cost Burden of Disease. U.S. and Michigan.* http://www.chrt.org/assets/price-of-care/CHRT-Issue-Brief-January-2010.pdf (accessed October 4, 2011).

CMS (Centers for Medicare and Medicaid Services) (a). *National Health Expenditure Data. Overview.* https://www.cms.gov/nationalhealthexpenddata/ (accessed October 4, 2011).

Cohen, D.A., T.A. Farley, and K. Mason. 2003. Why is poverty unhealthy? Social and physical mediators. *Social Science and Medicine* 57:1631–1641.

Cowling, L.L. 2006. Chapter 17. Health and dietary issues affecting African Americans. In *California Food Guide: Fulfilling the Dietary Guidelines for Americans.* Sacramento, CA: California Department of Health Care Services and California Department of Public Health. http://www.dhcs.ca.gov/dataandstats/reports/Documents/CaliforniaFoodGuide/17HealthandDietaryIssuesAffectingAfricanAmericans.pdf (accessed October 18, 2011).

DeVol, R., and A. Bedroussian. 2007. *An Unhealthy America: The Economic Burden of Chronic Disease: Charting a New Course to Save Lives and Increase Productivity and Economic Growth.* Santa Monica, CA: Milken Institute.

Etz, R.S., D.J. Cohen, S.H. Woolf, J.S. Holtrop, K.E. Donahue, N.F. Isaacson, K.C Stange, R.L. Ferrer, and A.L. Olson. 2008. Bridging primary care practices and communities to promote healthy behaviors. *American Journal of Preventive Medicine* 35(Suppl 5):S390–S397.

Fagerström, K. 2002. The epidemiology of smoking: Health consequences and benefits of cessation. *Drugs* 62(Suppl 2):1–9.

HCUPnet (a). *Welcome to HCUPnet.* http://hcupnet.ahrq.gov/ (accessed October 14, 2011).

Healthy People 2020 (a). *Health-Related Quality of Life and Well-Being.* http://www.healthypeople.gov/2020/about/QoLWBabout.aspx (accessed October 4, 2011).

HHS (U.S. Department of Health and Human Services) (a). *African American Profile.* http://minorityhealth.hhs.gov/templates/browse.aspx?lvl=2&lvlid=51 (accessed December 19, 2011).

HHS (b). *Diabetes and American Indians/Alaska Natives.* http://minorityhealth.hhs.gov/templates/content.aspx?ID=3024 (accessed October 18, 2011).

HHS (c). *Mental Health and African Americans.* http://minorityhealth.hhs.gov/templates/content.aspx?ID=6474 (accessed January 5, 2012).

HHS (d). *Mental Health Data/Statistics.* http://minorityhealth.hhs.gov/templates/browse.aspx?lvl=3&lvlid=9 (accessed January 5, 2012).

HHS. 1996. *Surgeon General Report Physical Activity and Health.* Atlanta, GA: U.S. Department of Health and Human Services, Centers for Disease Control and Prevention, National Center for Chronic Disease Prevention and Health Promotion. http://profiles. nlm.nih.gov/NN/ListByDate.html (accessed October 13, 2011).

HHS. 2010. *Multiple Chronic Conditions: A Strategic Framework Optimum Health and Quality of Life for Individuals with Multiple Chronic Conditions.* http://www.hhs.gov/ ash/initiatives/mcc/mcc_framework.pdf (accessed October 4, 2011).

Hubert, H.B., D.A. Bloch, J.W. Oehlert, and J.F. Fries. 2002. Lifestyle habits and compression of morbidity. *Journals of Gerontology: Series A, Biological Sciences and Medical Sciences* 57(6):M347–M351.

Hyland, A., C. Vena, J. Bauer, Q. Li, G.A. Giovino, J. Yang, K.M. Cummings, P. Mowery, J. Fellows, T. Pechacek, and L. Pederson. 2003. Cigarette smoking-attributable morbidity— United States, 2000. *Morbidity and Mortality Weekly Report* 52(35):842–844.

IOM (Institute of Medicine). 1999. *To Err Is Human: Building a Safer Health System.* Washington, DC: National Academy Press.

IOM. 2003. *Unequal Treatment: Confronting Racial and Ethnic Disparities in Health Care.* Washington, DC: The National Academies Press.

IOM. 2006. *Examining the Health Disparities Research Plan of the National Institutes of Health: Unfinished Business.* Washington, DC: The National Academies Press.

IOM. 2008. *State of the USA Health Indicators: Letter Report.* Washington, DC: The National Academies Press.

Kaiser Family Foundation. 2010. *Distribution of U.S. Population by Race/Ethnicity, 2010 and 2050.* Menlo Park, CA: Kaiser Family Foundation. http://facts.kff.org/chart.aspx?ch=364 (accessed December 19, 2011).

Kawachi, I., and L.F. Berkman. 2000. Social cohesion, social capital, and health. In *Social Epidemiology,* edited by I. Kawachi and L.F. Berkman. New York: Oxford University Press. Pp. 174–190.

Kawachi, I., and L.F. Berkman. 2003. *Neighborhoods and Health.* New York: Oxford University Press.

Kindig, D. 2007. Understanding population health terminology. *Milbank Quarterly* 85(1): 139–161.

Kindig, D.A., B.C. Booske, and P.L. Remington. 2010. Mobilizing Action Toward Community Health (MATCH): Metrics, incentives, and partnerships for population health. *Preventing Chronic Disease* 7(4):A68. http://www.cdc.gov/pcd/issues/2010/jul/10_0019. htm (accessed November 16, 2011).

Kulkarni, S.C., A. Levin-Rector, M. Ezzati, and C.J. Murray. 2011. Falling behind: Life expectancy in U.S. counties from 2000 to 2007 in an international context. *Population Health Metrics* 9(16). http://www.pophealthmetrics.com/content/9/1/16 (accessed November 16, 2011).

Lewis, J.M., M. DiGiacomo, D.C. Currow, and P.M. Davidson. 2011. Dying in the margins: Understanding palliative care and socioeconomic deprivation in the developed world. *Journal of Pain and Symptom Management* 42(1):105–118.

Lorig, K., H.R. Holman, D. Sobel, D. Laurent, V. González, and M. Minor. 2006. *Living a Healthy Life with Chronic Conditions.* 3rd ed. Boulder, CO: Bull Publishing.

McGinnis, J.M., and W.H. Foege. 1993. Actual causes of death in the United States. *Journal of the American Medical Association* 270(18):2207–2212.

McGinnis, J.M., P. Williams-Russo, and J.R. Knickman. 2002. The case for more active policy attention to health promotion. *Health Affairs* (Millwood) 21(2):78–93.

McLaren, L. 2007. Socioeconomic status and obesity. *Epidemiological Reviews* 29(1):29–48.

MEPS (Medical Expenditure Panel Survey) (a). http://www.meps.ahrq.gov/mepsweb/ (accessed October 14, 2011).

Michaud, C.M., M.T. McKenna, S. Begg, N. Tomijima, M. Majmudar, M.T. Bulzacchelli, S. Ebrahim, M. Ezzati, J.A. Salomon, J.G. Kreiser, M. Hogan, and C.J. Murray. 2006. The burden of disease and injury in the United States 1996. *Population Health Metrics* 4(11). http://www.pophealthmetrics.com/content/4/1/11 (accessed November 16, 2011).

Miller, T.R., and D.T. Levy. 2000. Cost-outcome analysis in injury prevention and control: Eighty-four recent estimates for the United States. *Medical Care* 38(6):562–582.

Mokdad, A.H., J.S. Marks, D.F. Stroup, and J.L. Gerberding. 2004. Actual causes of death in the United States, 2000. *Journal of the American Medical Association* 291(10):1238–1245.

Murray, C.J., J.A. Salomon, C.D. Mathers, and A.D. Lopez. 2002. *Summary Measures of Population Health: Concepts, Ethics, Measurement and Applications.* Geneva, Switzerland: World Health Organization. http://whqlibdoc.who.int/publications/2002/9241545518.pdf (accessed October 14, 2011).

Nagi, S. 1965. Some conceptual issues in disability and rehabilitation. In *Sociology and Rehabilitation,* edited by M.B. Sussman. Washington, DC: American Sociological Association.

NCCDPHP (National Center for Chronic Disease Prevention and Health Promotion) (a). *Chronic Diseases and Health Promotion.* http://www.cdc.gov/chronicdisease/overview/index.htm (accessed October 13, 2011).

NCCDPHP. 2009. *Chronic Diseases. The Power to Prevent, The Call to Control. At a Glance 2009.* http://www.cdc.gov/chronicdisease/resources/publications/AAG/pdf/chronic.pdf (accessed October 4, 2011).

NCQA (National Committee for Quality Assurance) (a). *NCQA Patient-Centered Medical Home.* http://www.ncqa.org/Portals/0/PCMH%20brochure-web.pdf (accessed August 10, 2011).

NIH (National Institutes of Health). 2011. *PROMIS Instruments Available for Use.* http://www.nihpromis.org/Documents/Item_Bank_Tables_Feb_2011.pdf (accessed October 4, 2011).

Parrish, R.G. 2010. Measuring population health outcomes. *Preventing Chronic Disease* 7(4):A71. http://www.cdc.gov/pcd/issues/2010/jul/10_0005.htm (accessed November 16, 2011).

PROMIS (Patient Reported Outcomes Measurement Information System) (a). http://www.nihpromis.org/ (accessed October 14, 2011).

Rosen, A.B., and D.M. Cutler. 2009. Challenges in building disease-based national health accounts. *Medical Care* 47(7 Suppl 1):S7–S13.

SAMHSA (Substance Abuse and Mental Health Services Administration). 2007. *National Expenditures for Mental Health Services and Substance Abuse Treatment. 1993–2003.* http://www.samhsa.gov/spendingestimates/samhsafinal9303.pdf (accessed October 4, 2011).

Smith, C., C. Cowan, A. Sensenig, A. Catlin, and the Health Accounts Team. 2005. Health spending growth slows in 2003. *Health Affairs* 24(1):185–194.

The Strategic Growth Council (a). *Health in All Policies Task Force—About Us.* http://sgc.ca.gov/hiap/about.html (accessed October 4, 2011).

Tengs, T.O., M.E. Adams, J.S. Pliskin, D.G. Safran, J.E. Siegel, M.C. Weinstein, and J.D. Graham. 1995. Five-hundred life-saving interventions and their cost-effectiveness. *Risk Analysis* 15(3):369–390.

Thorpe, K.E. 2006. Factors accounting for the rise in health-care spending in the United States: The role of rising disease prevalence and treatment intensity. *Public Health* 120(11):1002–1007.

U.S. Census Bureau. 2004. *U.S. Interim Projections by Age, Sex, Race, and Hispanic Origin: 2000–2050.* http://www.census.gov/population/www/projections/usinterimproj/ (accessed January 5, 2012).

WHO (World Health Organization) (a). *HEALTH21: An Introduction to the Health for All Policy Framework for the WHO European Region. European Health for All Series No. 5.* Geneva, Switzerland: World Health Organization. http://www.euro.who.int/__data/assets/pdf_file/0003/88590/EHFA5-E.pdf (accessed October 4, 2011).

WHO. 1986. *Ottawa Charter for Health Promotion. First International Conference on Health Promotion. Ottawa, 21 November 1986—WHO/HPR/HEP/95.1.* http://www.who.int/hpr/NPH/docs/ottawa_charter_hp.pdf (accessed October 4, 2011).

WHO. 2004. *The Global Burden of Disease: 2004 Update.* Geneva, Switzerland: World Health Organization. http://www.who.int/healthinfo/global_burden_disease/2004_report_update/en/index.html (accessed October 4, 2011).

WHO. 2009. *Global Health Risks: Mortality and Burden of Disease Attributable to Selected Major Risks.* Geneva, Switzerland: World Health Organization. http://www.who.int/healthinfo/global_burden_disease/global_health_risks/en/index.html (accessed October 4, 2011).

Wold, C. 2008. *Health Indicators: A Review of Reports Currently in Use.* Pasadena, CA: Wold and Associates. http://www.cherylwold.com/images/Wold_Indicators_July08.pdf (accessed November 16, 2011).

2

Chronic Illnesses and the People Who Live with Them

INTRODUCTION

Some chronic diseases are well known as "causes" of mortality. Cardiovascular disease, many cancers, stroke, and chronic lung disease are the most common causes of death in the United States (Mokdad et al., 2004; Thacker et al., 2006). There are many other chronic illnesses, however, that may or may not directly cause death but may have multiple effects on quality of life. The quality of life impact of these chronic illnesses is not as widely appreciated in public health, clinical practice, or health policy planning. Chronic illnesses often cause bothersome health problems for those affected and/or those around them, problems that persist over time. These include problems with physical health (e.g., distressing symptoms, physical functional impairment), mental health (e.g., emotional distress, depression, anxiety), or social health (e.g., social functional impairment), all of which are associated with lower quality of life (Cella et al., 2010). In many people with chronic illnesses, a mild impairment in any single one of these aspects of health leads to impairments in other aspects and may progress further to disability.

There is, in fact, a spectrum of chronic diseases that are in some ways quite disparate, yet they share certain commonalities that merit their being listed together. They are disparate in that they affect different organ systems and are frequently characterized by different time courses and the severity of disease burden. They are similar in that their effects on health and individual functioning share common pathways and outcomes. This chapter explores the differences and similarities among many chronic diseases, considers several exemplar diseases, health conditions, and impairments in more detail, and examines the people living with these illnesses and the ways in which they are affected.[1]

THE SPECTRUM OF CHRONIC ILLNESSES: DIFFERENCES IN TIME COURSE/CHRONICITY, HEALTH BURDEN, AND CONSEQUENCES

In this section, we first consider the nature of chronic diseases, including their similarities and differences. We then discuss the effects of these illnesses on the ability to live well with them.

The National Center for Health Statistics has defined chronic diseases as those that persist for 3 months or longer or belong to a group of conditions that are considered chronic (e.g., diabetes), regardless of when they began. Although some (e.g., polymyalgia rheumatica, depression) may resolve, most are lifelong diseases. Chronic diseases can vary in multiple ways, including their stage at presentation and characteristic clinical symptoms and their natural history (time course). Some specific conditions have typical time courses for clinical progression. Other chronic diseases, such as treated breast or prostate cancers, may follow a quiescent pattern for many years. Similarly, the health burden in terms of symptoms and functional impairment, requirements for self-management, effects on significant others, and individual economic impact vary. This results in disparate patterns of human suffering across the spectrum of chronic illnesses. Table 2-1 displays selected patterns of chronic illnesses along important dimensions. For example, some illnesses (e.g., diabetes) have high self-management requirements, whereas others (e.g., Alzheimer's disease) may require substantial care from others. Age of onset may also influence complications and burden; for example, older onset rheumatoid arthritis is associated with more shoulder involvement and symptoms of polymyalgia rheumatica and less frequent hand deformities compared with younger onset disease (Turkcapar et al., 2006). The stability of the condition over time is also an important determinant of overall health burden.

Below we summarize the spectrum of chronic diseases as early, moderate, and late stage. As highlighted in Table 2-1, individuals with certain chronic illnesses, such as congestive heart failure, chronic obstructive pulmonary disease (COPD), Parkinson's disease, and diabetes mellitus, may

---

[1]Some chronic illnesses have a recognized precursor state (e.g., osteopenia, hyperlipidemia, ductal carcinoma in situ) that may or may not progress to a chronic condition that people sense and suffer from. Although these presymptomatic states, if diagnosed, may cause symptoms (e.g., worry) or socioeconomic consequences (e.g., inability to obtain insurance), this report focuses on persons who actually have and are living with a chronic illness, not just a precursor state. Thus, such states as asymptomatic hypothyroidism or stage 3 chronic kidney disease are not considered.

present at various stages during the course of their illness with different health and economic consequences.

Chronic illnesses can be characterized by the stage (i.e., clinical severity), pattern (i.e., continuous versus intermittent symptoms), and anticipated course (i.e., stable, fixed deficit versus progressive). Because the stage of the condition has the largest impact on health and social consequences, we have organized this section around condition stages.

Early-Stage Chronic Illnesses

We define early-stage chronic illnesses as ones that cause little or no functional impairment and impose a low burden on others. This often characterizes certain chronic illnesses early after their diagnosis or in their uncomplicated stages. For example, such illnesses as benign prostatic hypertrophy (BPH) or early Parkinson's disease have mild symptoms and burden. Some chronic early stage illnesses, such as uncomplicated diabetes or New York Heart Association stage I (i.e., individuals with heart disease with no physical limitations) or II heart failure (i.e., individuals with heart disease with slight physical activity limitations), although associated with low functional impairment and burden to others, are associated with a high self-management burden (e.g., the need to monitor sodium and fluid intake and daily weight in heart failure, the need for self-monitoring of blood glucose in diabetes). Other early-stage chronic illnesses, such as mild asthma or osteoarthritis, may cause physical symptoms and functional limitation only intermittently, with asymptomatic periods in between, requiring a low to moderate degree of self-management.

Moderate-Stage Chronic Illnesses

Moderate-stage illnesses can be characterized by moderate, as opposed to low, degree of functional impairment and disability and moderate to high self-management and caregiver burden. At this stage, symptoms often interfere with usual lifestyles. Examples include painful hip or knee osteoarthritis and stage 2 or 3 Parkinson's disease.

Several illnesses are associated with disabling episodic flares, although they may have low burden between flares. They are distinguished from early-stage illnesses following this pattern in that they cause moderate to severe, episodic disability (e.g., hospitalization for a flare of COPD), increased self-management and caregiver burden, and moderate to high economic impact. COPD, rheumatoid arthritis, depression, and migraine headache are conditions that often follow this pattern. Some people with complicated diabetes may have functional impairment due to peripheral neuropathy or a lower extremity amputation yet remain stable for some years, despite high

TABLE 2-1 Selected Patterns of Chronic Illnesses: Stage, Chronicity, Burden, and Example Illnesses

Stage	Chronicity/Time Course	Health Burden and Consequences (not including economic)				Example Illnesses
		Symptoms[a]	Functional impairment/disability	Self-management burden	Burden to others	
Early	Chronic with episodic flares	Minimal or none between flares	Low	Variable	Low	Asthma in adults, mild degenerative joint disease
	Chronic	Mild	Low	Low	Low	BPH, mild Parkinson's disease
	Chronic	Mild	Low	High	Low	Uncomplicated but symptomatic diabetes, NYHA I or II heart failure
Moderate	Chronic with episodic flares	Mild or minimal between flares, moderate or severe during flares	Moderate	Moderate	Moderate	COPD, RA, depression, migraine headache
	Chronic, quiescent	None to moderate	Low	Low	Low	Breast or prostate cancer in remission
	Chronic, stable	Moderate	Moderate	High	Moderate	Complicated diabetes, mild to moderate stroke, mild to moderate posttraumatic states, RA with some joint deformities

	Chronic, progressive	Moderate	Moderate	Moderate	High	Severe osteoarthritis, severe Parkinson's disease, progressive Alzheimer's disease, progressive macular degeneration, progressive hearing impairment
Late	Chronic, progressive	Moderate or severe	High	Variable	High	Severe dementia, severe diabetes with extensive vascular disease
	Chronic, slowly progressive	Moderate or severe	High	High	High	NYHA Class III or IV heart failure, COPD with chronic respiratory failure, end-stage renal disease on dialysis
	Terminal	Severe	High	High	High	Metastatic cancer, patients in hospice

NOTE: BPH = benign prostatic hyperplasia; COPD = chronic obstructive pulmonary disease; NYHA = New York Heart Association; RA = rheumatoid arthritis.

aSpecific symptoms vary by condition.

self-management burden, moderate caregiver burden, and moderate to high economic impact on the individual. Similarly, people with a posttraumatic disabling condition or previous mild to moderate stroke may have a chronic pattern that remains stable over some time despite having moderate functional impairment and disability and moderate to high self-management and caregiver burden and individual economic impact.

Another pattern shown by moderate-stage chronic illnesses is more progressive. Alzheimer's disease typically begins with memory loss and is later associated with functional impairment and behavioral and psychological complications, leading to moderate to high self-management and caregiver burden and individual economic impact. People with Parkinson's disease and some with macular degeneration or hearing impairment may also experience this time course and burden. Amyotrophic lateral sclerosis (ALS) often begins with milder symptoms and burden but may progress rapidly to severe disability and death.

Late-Stage Chronic Illnesses

We define late-stage chronic illnesses as those that are slowly or rapidly progressive or terminal and are characterized by high functional impairment and disability and self or caregiver management burden. People with late-stage chronic illnesses often have multiple chronic conditions (MCCs) and may suffer a rapidly progressive decline in multiple functions. For example, people with severe dementia or people with diabetes and severe vascular disease often have a progressive course with high burden on significant others. In its terminal stage, metastatic cancer is often accompanied by a rapidly progressive, downhill course. In contrast, some people with late-stage chronic illnesses progress more slowly. For example, some people with end-stage renal disease who are on dialysis or some people with severe COPD and require chronic oxygen may remain stable for years. Other chronic conditions (e.g., those with spinal cord injuries) may result in high functional impairment and remain stable for many years.

Variation in a Chronic Illness in Time Course, Health Burden, and Consequences

Although Table 2-1 indicates differences in commonly encountered patterns among chronic illnesses, it also highlights the marked variation within them. A single chronic illness may, in different people, demonstrate its own range of time course and burden. Some people with the same condition may progress from mild burden to severe limitation to disability or death at a constant, rapid rate, and others may progress slowly or not at all. For example, although the median survival for a person younger than age 75 with Alzheimer's disease is 7.5 years, a quarter do not survive 4.2 years and another quarter live beyond 10.9 years (Larson et al., 2004). Similarly, some people with diabetes progress inexorably to severe visual impairment, and others show little evidence of severe ocular complications or retinopathy regression even years after diagnosis (Klein et al., 1989). Only a few illnesses have a "typical" type of progression in that the vast majority of affected people show the same rate of worsening status. Most chronic illnesses are more variable, with different individuals with the same illness progressing at widely varying rates. The variation in progression rates is often independent of medical treatment. As a result of the variability of the natural history of individual illnesses, comorbidity, interactions between illness and environment, and adverse effects of treatments, the true burden of chronic illness in an individual is inconsistent and sometimes unpredictable. Thus, typical illness patterns of consequences are only rough guides. Any individual person may have a health burden that varies from the typical situation.

THE SPECTRUM OF CHRONIC ILLNESSES: COMMON CONSEQUENCES

In addition to demonstrating differences among chronic illnesses, Table 2-1 also displays their common consequences. It is useful to consider that all of these illnesses create a common human burden of suffering. Although these illnesses have multiple mechanisms leading to suffering with variable time courses and severity, they all affect the same aspects of health: physical, mental, and social (Cella et al., 2010). A variety of models have been used to describe the process leading from disease to consequences in these aspects, including the Disablement Model that includes pathology; impairment at the tissue, organ, or body level, functional limitations; and disability (Nagi, 1976). More recently, the World Health Organization's (WHO's) International Classification of Functioning, Disability and Health (known as ICF) has classified health and health-related domains from "body, individual and societal perspectives by means of two lists: a list of body functions and structure, and a list of domains of activity and participation. Since an individual's functioning and disability occurs in a context, the ICF also includes a list of environmental factors" (WHO, [a]). Regardless of the model used to explain the pathway from disease to consequences, chronic illnesses all lead, in their own ways, to human suffering (Cassell, 1983). In Table 2-1, we have rated the health burden and consequences of chronic illnesses along four dimensions: functional impairment/disability, self-management burden, and burden to others. The economic impact of chronic illness to the individual is described separately later in the chapter.

Below we discuss important dimensions of the health burden of chronic illnesses and mention a measurement approach developed by the Patient Reported Outcomes Measurement Information System (PROMIS). The PROMIS instruments also measure related constructs of social support, interpersonal attributes, and global health but do not include management burden directly or caregiver burden (Cella et al., 2010). In a pilot study of a large but unrepresentative sample of the general population, PROMIS selected five domains to assess health-related quality of life in people with chronic illnesses: physical function, fatigue, pain, emotional distress, and social function (Rothrock et al., 2010). They found that people with chronic illnesses reported poorer scores on these domains than did people without such illnesses and that people with two or more chronic illnesses had poorer scores than people with only one had.

Symptoms

These are medical or psychiatric symptoms that can be measured quantitatively and/or qualitatively. Examples include pain, fatigue, immobility, dyspnea on exertion, claudication (lameness), foot dysesthesia (numbness), depressive symptoms, seizures, and behavioral and psychological symptoms of dementia. The PROMIS approach measures physical symptoms, emotional distress, cognitive function, and positive psychological function (Cella et al., 2010).

Functional Impairment/Disability

Functional impairment can relate to restrictions in physical, mental, or social function. Disability is a more severe impairment that limits the performance of functional tasks and fulfillment of socially defined roles (handicap). For example, physical disability is the inability to complete specific physical functional tasks, called activities of daily living (ADLs) and instrumental activities of daily living (IADLs), that are important to daily life. The PROMIS measures assess both physical function and social function.

Chronic illnesses can cause functional impairment or disability through any of the three following health pathways:

1. Directly causing impairment or disability
2. Causing other medical complications that lead to impairment and disability
3. Causing mental health complications that lead to impairment and disability

Below we consider examples of each.

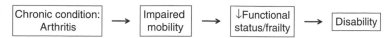

FIGURE 2-1 Osteoarthritis.

Chronic Illnesses Directly Causing Disability

Osteoarthritis causes impairment or disability directly through reduced mortality or pain in such joints as the knee or hip. Knee osteoarthritis results in 25 percent of affected individuals having difficulty performing activities of daily living due to pain and limited mobility (CDC, [c]). Knee and hip osteoarthritis are the third leading cause of years lived with disability in the United States (Figure 2-1) (Michaud et al., 2006).

Chronic Illnesses Leading to Other Medical Conditions

Diabetes can lead to impairment and disability indirectly, such as its effects on blood vessels. For example, visual impairment and end-stage renal disease are often microvascular complications, and coronary heart and cerebrovascular disease are frequently macrovascular complications (Figure 2-2).

Data from the National Health and Nutrition Examination Survey show that cardiovascular disease (i.e., coronary heart disease or chronic

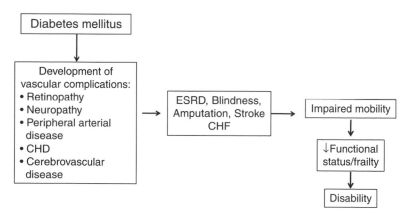

FIGURE 2-2 Diabetes mellitus and coronary heart disease as examples of complications leading to disability.
NOTE: CHD = chronic heart disease; CHF = chronic heart failure; ESRD = end stage renal disease.

heart disease [CHD], heart failure, and stroke) and obesity among older adults with diabetes were associated with greater disability in several areas, including lower extremity mobility, general physical activity, activities of daily living, and instrumental activities of daily living (Kalyani et al., 2010). Data from the Women's Health and Aging Study show that women with diabetes had a higher prevalence of mobility disability and severe walking limitation and that this was partially explained by peripheral arterial disease and peripheral nerve dysfunction (Volpato et al., 2002).

Chronic Illnesses Leading to Mental Health Conditions

Chronic medical illnesses, such as diabetes, may also lead to mental health illnesses, such as depression and dementia, which have an adverse effect on health behaviors, leading to increased risk of clinical complications (Figure 2-3).

Both diabetes and cardiovascular disease are associated with an increased risk of developing depression (Mezuk et al., 2008; Rugulies, 2002). Conversely, depressive disorders in persons with diabetes are also associated with poor adherence to therapy (Gonzalez et al., 2008), worse control of glycemia and cardiovascular risk factors (Lustman et al., 2000), and greater diabetes complications (De Groot et al., 2001). Thus, individuals who develop depression are at higher risk of disability secondary to their greater propensity to develop vascular complications. Similarly, population-based studies indicate that type 2 diabetes is a risk factor for age-related cognitive decline (Biessels et al., 2008) with a 1.5- to 2.0-fold increased

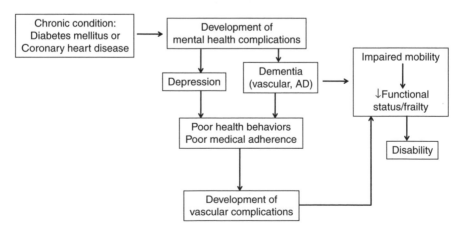

FIGURE 2-3 Association of chronic illnesses with mental health consequences.
NOTE: AD = Alzheimer's disease.

risk of all-cause dementia (Cukierman et al., 2005). Studies also show that cognitive impairment is associated with poor diabetes self-management behaviors (Sinclair et al., 2000; Thabit et al., 2009) hyperglycemia (Munshi et al., 2006), and higher prevalence of diabetes complications (Roberts et al., 2008), which are predicted to contribute to functional, in addition to cognitive, impairment in this population.

In 2011, the Centers for Disease Control and Prevention's (CDC's) National Center for Chronic Disease Prevention and Health Promotion released a public health action plan on mental health promotion and chronic disease prevention, which contains eight strategies to integrate mental health and public health programs that address chronic disease (CDC, 2011c). The eight strategy categories include surveillance, epidemiology research, prevention research, communication, education of health professionals, program integration, policy integration, and systems to promote integration. In recognizing the complexity of living well and effectively managing a chronic illness when a serious mental health condition is present, the committee has included a separate article highlighting depression care in patients with medical chronic illness (see Appendix A).

Chronic Illness Management Burden

In many cases, patients themselves must deliver their own care to effectively manage the chronic illnesses they live with, demanding consistent participation from patients and caregivers (Bayliss et al., 2003). In doing so, patients put forth substantial time, effort, and inconvenience that accompany day-to-day management of the illness. To properly manage their condition, patients typically run through the process of joining in physically and psychologically beneficial activities, working with health professionals to ensure adherence to treatment guidelines, monitoring health and making appropriate care decisions, and managing the effects of the illness on their physical, psychological, and social well-being (Bayliss et al., 2003). Any disruption to this process can have negative consequences on an individual's health and livelihood (Bayliss et al., 2003).

To effectively address the multiple determinants behind almost all chronic illnesses, self-management regimens dictate appropriate medical guidelines as well as psychological and social functioning (Newman et al., 2004). Chronic illnesses factor into patient lifestyle choices, such as diet, level of physical activity, and suitable living environments, forcing self-management regimens for those illnesses to cross over multiple domains and affect the quality of a patient's life (Newman et al., 2004). Patients with diabetes, for example, maintain day-to-day self-management routines typically including multiple components (e.g., self-monitoring of blood glucose, carbohydrate counting/awareness, home dialysis, home oxygen use, and daily weights and check-ins with disease management programs). With all these activities, diabetes patients understandably perceive management of their condition as burdensome, frustrating, and overwhelming, which can have further negative consequences on their health (Weijman et al., 2005).

As Weijman et al. (2005) found, adherence to self-management activities has strong ties to the perceived burden. Patients who do not see these activities as burdensome perform them more frequently with close regard to proposed guidelines and reported better health outcomes in relation to their diabetes (Weijman et al., 2005). In contrast, patients who saw these activities as burdensome reported poorer health outcomes in relation to their diabetes, higher rates of depression and fatigue, and overall poorer quality of life (Weijman et al., 2005). Despite consistent evidence in support of self-management (Warsi et al., 2004), barriers still exist and complicate the self-care strategy. Many patients, such as those living with heart failure, are elderly, highly symptomatic with frequent hospitalizations, and without strong financial and social support, making self-management regimens difficult to maintain (Gardetto, 2011). In addition, issues with physical and financial limitations, health literacy, logistical complications, and lack of social and financial support interrupt and prevent effective progression through the self-management process (Bayliss et al., 2003). Without greater investment in addressing these barriers, patients will continue to face the burden behind self-management regimens designed to promote living well with chronic illness.

Social Isolation and Chronic Illness

The social consequence of chronic illness is a significant burden and impacts the ability to live well, especially when a chronic illness presents a visible functional impairment or limitation. In *Social Isolation: The Most Distressing Consequence of Chronic Illness* (Royer, 1998), the author eloquently describes the essence of social isolation as experienced by many individuals living with disabling chronic illnesses. Individuals living "with long-term health problems are at high risk for lessened and impaired social interactions and social isolation." Lessened and impaired social contact and a sense of social isolation are among the more detrimental consequences of chronic illness (Royer, 1998):

> Impaired social interaction relates to the state in which participation in social exchanges occurs but is dysfunctional or ineffective because of discomfort in social situations, unsuccessful social behaviors, or dysfunctional communication patterns. Indeed, social relationships are frequently disrupted and usually disintegrate under the stress of chronic illness and its management because chronic illnesses often involve disfigurement, limitations in mobility, the need for additional rest, loss of control of some body

functions, and an inability to maintain steady employment. These factors tend to reduce a person's ability to develop and maintain a network of supportive relationships. As the illness takes up more and more of a person's time and energy, only the most loyal family members and friends persist in offering support. . . . [T]he worse the illness (and/or its phases), then the more probability exists that the ill persons will feel or become isolated. Social isolation probably also occurs because family and friends need to withdraw from the ill person to gain emotional distance and protect themselves from a painful situation, particularly if they are unable to help in alleviating the problems of the sufferer. Thus, social isolation can happen in two ways: either the ill person, given the symptoms, unexpected crises, lengthy hospitalizations and convalescence, additional financial burdens, difficult regimens and loss of energy, withdraws from most social contact, or the ill person is avoided or even abandoned by friends and relatives.

The committee thinks that social isolation is not only an important consequence of long-term debilitating chronic illnesses; it is also a burden that cuts across a host of chronic illnesses, thus highlighting the commonality among many of them and presenting an opportunity to develop, disseminate, and evaluate relevant community-based interventions to help people with chronic illness.

Caregivers of Individuals with Chronic Illness

The burden of chronic illness reaches beyond the person with the illness, affecting family members as well, particularly those involved in caregiving. The National Alliance for Caregiving (NAC) and AARP conducted a national survey of caregivers in the United States to assess the issues they faced in 1997, 2004, and 2009 (NAC and AARP, 2009). The 2009 survey indicated that approximately 28.5 percent—or an estimated 65.7 million people in the United States—served as a family caregiver to an ill or disabled child or adult in the past 12 months. Caregivers of adults spend an average of 18.9 hours per week providing care. And 66 percent of caregivers are women, and women caregivers report more time spent in caregiving than men caregivers.

The burden on informal caregivers is highly variable (see Table 2-1), but as the severity of illness-related impairment increases, caregiver burdens increase as well. Research has documented numerous physical and mental health effects of caregiving. The NAC and AARP report (2009) documents that 17 percent of caregivers consider their health to be fair or poor compared with 13 percent of the general population. Health is particularly affected among low-income caregivers, 34 percent of whom report fair or poor health (NAC and AARP, 2009). Female caregivers in the Nurses' Health Study were more likely to report a history of hypertension, diabetes, high cholesterol, and poorer health behaviors (more likely to smoke, eat more saturated fat, and have a higher body mass index). When controlling for these factors, the study found an 82 percent higher incidence of CHD in those who cared for a spouse than in noncaregivers. There was no increased CHD risk among those providing care for an ill parent (Lee et al., 2003). The Caregiver Health Effects Study (CHES) study categorized approximately 800 spouses on the basis of their level of caregiving demand: those with disabled spouses for whom they do not provide care; those who provide care to a disabled spouse but report no caregiver strain; and those who provide care for a disabled spouse and report either physical or emotional strain. These groups were compared with spouses whose partners were not disabled, reporting no difficulty with activities of daily living. After controlling for the presence of illness and subclinical cardiovascular disease in the spouse, those spouses who provided care for a disabled partner and reported caregiver strain had 63 percent higher 4-year mortality than those whose spouses were not disabled (Schulz and Beach, 1999).

Caregivers also report increased symptoms of psychological distress. A meta-analysis of differences between caregivers of older adults with various illnesses and noncaregivers found the largest differences were in depression, stress, self-efficacy, and subjective well-being (Pinquart and Sörensen, 2003). For example, depression among caregivers was higher than in comparable groups of noncaregivers. Depression was higher among caregivers of people with dementia and more common in women than men, spouses than other family caregivers, and caregivers for whom both the perceived and the actual workload are greater (Pinquart and Sörensen, 2003; Schoenmakers et al., 2010). More time spent in caregiving is associated with higher levels of depressive symptoms (Cannuscio et al., 2004).

Caregiving can have an economic impact as well. Caregivers have a lower labor force participation rate than do adults not involved in caregiving. Effects seem particularly pronounced among women, caregivers who are in poor health themselves, older caregivers, those with more caregiving involvement, immediate family members, caregivers with young children at home, those who cared for people with more limitations, caregivers with lower incomes, and those with less education (Lilly et al., 2007). In all, 58 percent of caregivers of adults are currently employed, with 48 percent working full-time and 10 percent working part-time. And 69 percent report making work changes to accommodate caregiving, such as going in late or leaving early (65 percent), taking a leave of absence (18 percent), turning down a promotion (5 percent), losing job benefits (4 percent), giving up work entirely (7 percent), or retiring early (3 percent) (NAC and AARP, 2009). Caregiving can affect productivity through both absenteeism and presenteeim (decreased productivity while at work) (Giovannetti et al., 2009). Time spent in the physical care of the ill person or in helping them access health care may increase absenteeism at work. Even when the caregiver is at work, he or she may be distracted by worries about the family member or by spending time dealing with insurance companies, health care records, etc. Furthermore, caregivers may be locked into jobs or prevented from advances or job transfers because of fear of loss of insurance and the need to stay in geographic proximity to the person for whom they provide care.

Economic Consequences of Chronic Illness on the Individual

Chronic illness can wreak havoc on the socioeconomic standing of an individual and his or her family (Jeon et al., 2009). Overwhelming evidence connects lower socioeconomic status with poorer health, putting a large portion of the worldwide population at risk for developing one or more chronic illnesses and further financial hardship (Jeon et al., 2009). The prevalence of chronic illness increases with age, increasing the likelihood of developing a health-related financial and economic burden as an individual gets older (Woo et al., 1997). This burden includes both direct (e.g., out-of-pocket costs of health care) and indirect (e.g., loss of work income) consequences for the individual and/or his or her caregiver or families. In terms of direct consequences, taking a microeconomic approach, a strong association exists between financial stress, disability, and poor physical and mental health and between poverty rates and chronic illness (Jeon et al., 2009). The estimated costs of addressing disability consumed approximately 29 percent of household income and 49 percent for those with severe restrictions (Jeon et al., 2009). Based on these estimates, those with one or more chronic illnesses are six times more likely to sink down to the poverty line than are those without one (Jeon et al., 2009). One Australian study interviewed 52 patients with one or more chronic illnesses and 14 caregivers (or spouses or offspring) of those patients and found that 60 percent of the patients and 79 percent of the caregivers reported experiencing financial difficulties associated with the patients' chronic illness (Jeon et al., 2009). In all, 84 percent of both groups identified the basic cost of disease management as a primary financial challenge, and 64 percent of both groups reported experiencing financial difficulty related to addressing the patients' chronic illness and believing that it negatively affected their quality of life (Jeon et al., 2009). Overall, both groups reported financial stress related to affordability of treatment, including out-of-pocket expenses for medications, regular check-ups, and lack of support resources, and affordability of other things, including healthy food, exercise and gym membership, and partaking in social activities (Jeon et al., 2009). In another study, conducted by Teo et al. (2011), 42 percent of the estimated cost burden of COPD was attributed to medical management alone, an expense put in different weights on the shoulders of the patients and their caregivers. For every dollar spent on fibromyalgia-related health care expenses for its employees, certain employers spent an additional $57 to $143 on direct and indirect costs, masking any evidence of successful treatment (Robinson et al., 2003). For indirect costs alone, Ivanova et al. (2010) compared a group of employees with treatment-resistant depression (TRD) and nontreatment-resistant major depressive disorder and found TRD-likely employees were more likely to have a disability and go through more disability days. Furthermore, although TRD-likely employees had lower rates of medical-related absenteeism, they did go through a higher number of medical-related absenteeism days (Ivanova et al., 2010). From that, TRD-likely employees have more days away from work, creating a loss in productivity for the employee and extra cost for the employer (Ivanova et al., 2010). The indirect consequences of chronic illness, like missing multiple days from work and reduced productivity, increases the risk of losing employment, an event that reinforces financial pressures. Without substantial caregiver, family, or employer support, individuals with one or more chronic illnesses may sink into financial hardship beyond repair.

Effects of Comorbidity

The burden of chronic illness is often compounded by multiple chronic conditions, a situation that is often referred to as multimorbidity or comorbidity. Typically, the term *comorbidity* is used in the context of an index condition (e.g., cancer) to reflect the impact of other (comorbid) conditions (e.g., heart failure) on prognosis, quality of life, and treatment. Multimorbidity is used to describe MCCs that in aggregate may affect prognosis, quality of life, and treatment. Although most important conditions begin as single diagnostic entities, they may vary in their rate of progression for many reasons other than the primary pathological process. For example, prior conditions may already be present at the time of the occurrence of the new condition, leading to an increased burden for these "new" index conditions. Multimorbidities can contribute to worse outcomes because of complications that affect multiple organ systems, either individually (e.g., macular degeneration may affect vision and osteoarthritis may affect mobility in the same person) or synergistically (e.g., diabetes and hypertension together may accelerate atherosclerotic coronary, cerebrovascular, and peripheral vascular disease). Multimorbidities can also complicate treatment regimens, including competing guidelines for care that may confuse people, decreasing adherence or leading to conflicting therapeutic regimens (Boyd et al., 2005; Tinetti et al., 2004). One condition can also interfere with the ability to adhere to treatment for another condition, such as osteoarthritis occurring in individuals with diabetes or cardiovascular disease inhibiting

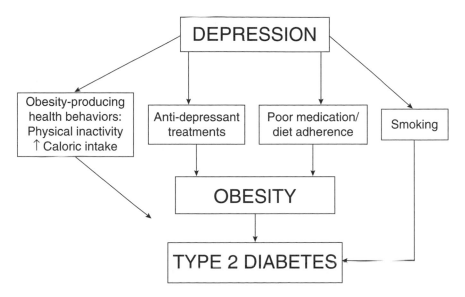

FIGURE 2-4 Depression and the risk of diabetes.

participation in physical activity (Bolen et al., 2009). Primary mental illnesses, such as depression, can increase the risk for medical conditions and the adverse outcomes associated with them (Figure 2-4).

In addition, comorbid depression or anxiety is associated with higher numbers of medical symptoms across a wide variety of illnesses (Katon et al., 2007), in part because of their association with poor adherence to self-care regimens (Lin et al., 2004) and heightened awareness of symptoms (Katon et al., 2001).

Finally, secondary conditions of varying importance and impact can occur because of the debilitating effects of the primary illness. These secondary conditions can take various forms depending on the primary condition and the nature of care, including falls, fractures, depression and other mental consequences, constipation, bedsores, anemia, obesity, sleep disorders, social dysfunction, spasticity, and injuries from various medical devices. These are important not only for their health impact but also because many can be prevented or mitigated with optimal care. Thus, they are also important objects of surveillance in order to define the population burden of chronic disease. This understanding that functional limitation due to one chronic condition may lead to disability through the development of other chronic illnesses provides an opportunity for the prevention of disability. If prevention approaches for people with chronic illness can reduce the risk of developing additional ones, the risk of disability may be reduced as well.

Illness-Environment Interactions

The interaction between persons with chronic illness and their environments can also contribute to the burden and consequences they may experience. For example, a person with late-stage Alzheimer's disease who has a family caregiver or has the resources to hire a paid caregiver may be able to remain at home, whereas a similar person without this support system is likely to be institutionalized. Similarly, a person with severe rheumatoid arthritis who works in the service industry may be able to continue working by use of voice recognition technology and telecommuting from home, whereas someone who works in construction would be unable to work.

Adverse Effects of Clinical Treatment

Another reason for variation in the rate of development of disability is adverse effects of treatment. Some illnesses may lead to less physical fitness, as with fatigue and muscle atrophy. Moreover, it is well described that patients undergoing varying kinds of clinical care are subject to the adverse effects of that care (IOM, 1999). Adverse effects occur in all elements of care, including medications (Kongkaew et al., 2008); institutionalization, such as hospitalizations and surgical procedures (Michel et al., 2004); and long-term care in various settings (Dhalla et al., 2002). Patients with chronic illnesses, because of extensive and often intensive care experiences, are thus particularly likely to experience adverse effects, even if, in general, their health is better off with the care than without it. Although the severity of adverse effects is sometimes difficult to characterize in detail, care surveillance systems and quality improvement programs clearly demonstrate the general scope of the problem and the need for remediation whenever possible. It is very difficult to identify studies that summarize the net health impact of adverse effects across common chronic illnesses. In complex illnesses, it may be difficult to distinguish between an effect of the illness and the effect of the treatment. Nonetheless, there is an important need to understand the role of adverse effects in affecting the health trajectories of those with chronic illness.

EXEMPLAR CHRONIC ILLNESSES

One of the charges to the committee was to suggest a new set of diseases for which to provide increased emphasis in terms of surveillance and chronic disease control efforts. As always, such programmatic emphases may change over time, in part because of the advent of new community or clinical interventions that can improve the lives of individuals with chronic illness. There are many illnesses from which to choose—in many ways, almost an endless menu of conditions that can lead to suffering and disability.

In addressing the challenges of living well with chronic illness, priorities must be established. Although priority setting in public health and health care is not a new concept, it is a matter of growing importance (Ham, 1997). The combination of constrained resources and increasing demands has led policy makers to address priority setting more directly than in the past. In particular, an explicit part of the committee's task asked "Which chronic diseases should be the focus of public health efforts to reduce disability and improve functioning and quality of life?"

Fundamentally, the determination of priorities for public health intervention begins with the burden of disease and preventability (Sainfort and Remington, 1995). Other considerations include size of the chronic disease problem, perceptions of urgency, severity of the problem, potential for economic loss, impact on others, effectiveness, propriety, economics, acceptability, legality of solutions, and availability of resources (Vilnius and Dandoy, 1990).

Although there is no correct approach to setting priorities, it is beneficial to have a common planning framework. The framework should

- include multiple perspectives, including patients, providers, employers, and community members;
- use clear and consistent criteria for selecting priorities, whenever possible;
- result in aims and objectives that are clear and feasible;
- consider at what level the decisions are being made (e.g., federal, state, local); and
- include the values of these involved in the decisions.

Despite the challenges involved in setting programmatic priorities, a number of organizations have used these measures and approaches to set health priorities. The Oxford Health Alliance based in the United Kingdom convened a group from around the world of academics, nongovernmental organizations, activists, corporate and industry executives, patients' rights advocates, health professionals, and others to focus on preventing the worldwide epidemic of chronic diseases (http://www.oxha.org). In 2006, they launched the "3four50" effort (http://www.3four50.com/). This "open space for health" promotes chronic disease prevention by focusing on the three risk factors (poor diet, lack of physical activity, and tobacco use) that lead to four chronic diseases (cardiovascular disease, diabetes, chronic lung diseases, and some cancers) contributing to more than 50 percent of deaths worldwide.

CDC has not set priorities explicitly but has developed the approach called Winnable Battles to describe public health priorities with large-scale impact on health and with known, effective strategies to intervene (CDC, [d]). The charge under Winnable Battles is to identify optimal strategies and to rally resources and partnerships to accelerate a measurable impact on health. The priority areas for CDC include some that relate directly to chronic disease, including physical activity promotion, obesity elimination, and tobacco control.

Although the federal *Healthy People 2010* did not explicitly set national priorities, it established leading health indicators to reflect major public health concerns in the United States (CDC, [b]). These leading health indicators were selected on the basis of their capacity to motivate action, the availability of data to measure progress, and their importance as public health issues. The Institute of Medicine (IOM) published a report recommending leading health indicators for *Healthy People 2020* (2011a). These also include several that pertain to living well with chronic illness. In this chapter, we have explained the additional framework used to select paradigm diseases based on the great variation in their causes, onset, clinical patterns, and outcomes (see Table 2-1). These highlight some of the important dimensions and variations in chronic illnesses that are relevant to patients, the health care system, and the nation, including

a. time course, chronicity, and downstream consequences;
b. enormous variation in etiology and pathogenesis;
c. late-stage manifestations;
d. symptom patterns;
e. functional impairment and disability;
f. secondary consequences, such as falls, sleep disorders, pressure sores;
g. multimorbidity associated with several coexisting chronic illnesses;
h. management burden, both to the patient, the family, and other caregivers and to the health care system;
i. social consequences, such as isolation;
j. economic consequences to the patient and society;
k. impact on the environment; and
l. important adverse effects of therapy.

Given such great diversity and a real absence of population data for these dimensions (except possibly in some instances for the most common diseases), the committee took the exemplar approach to highlight disease complexity, diversity, cross-cutting commonalities, and the implications for multidimensional approaches to chronic disease surveillance and control.

The multidimensional approach to selecting the exemplars was derived from the committee's view that an additional approach to chronic disease was needed to supplement current approaches for selecting the most common, high-mortality diseases for public health control efforts. The committee's approach, while appreciating the wisdom and practicality of current approaches, is grounded in other considerations:

1. Current approaches to selecting diseases for control activity based on such criteria as prevalence, mortality, disability, and economic cost to the care system are useful, but these criteria are often orthogonal to each other, and thus the selection algorithm is in several ways arbitrary.
2. Current approaches to selecting diseases for public health focus inadequately address the great variation in clinical manifestations and trajectories that make public health approaches complex and challenging.
3. Current approaches are not inclusive of the large number of less common illnesses that impact individuals and communities in important ways.
4. The recognized problem of MCCs has not been adequately addressed in current disease control activities.

For these reasons, the committee recommended an "exemplar" approach to address some of these perceived inadequacies. This approach starts with a framework, presented in this chapter, that begins not with a specific set of conditions or criteria for them but with a broad set of clinical manifestations and other consequences experienced by individuals with chronic illness. The committee thinks that this framework highlights a new and alternative approach to public health chronic disease control. The exemplars did not come from a list. Rather, they come from the clinical and research experience of committee members and were chosen to highlight some important features of chronic diseases that have received less emphasis in the past, including

1. Great diversity in clinical manifestations within and among chronic diseases and the great variation in their manifestations as illnesses continue their natural histories.
2. The inclusion of illnesses that can be manifest across the life course, raising the possibility of public health interventions that may be effective at various life stages of disease. The life course approach also more effectively deals with the occurrence of recurrent or additional different conditions (MCCs).
3. The highlighting of important psychological and social consequences that come with many chronic illnesses, including individu-

als with primary mental illnesses and those that are secondary to other conditions.

4. The highlighting of the chronic, multiple, degenerative age-related conditions, for which public health approaches are perhaps less well developed.

In addition, the committee endorses CDC's emphasis on "winnable battles" and thinks that the exemplar approach will help identify new types of battles and population-based interventions in the management and control of chronic diseases. Accordingly, the committee has selected nine emblematic diseases, health conditions, and impairments, because together they encompass and flesh out the range of key issues that affect the quality of life of patients with the full spectrum of chronic illnesses. More importantly, if interventions, policies, and surveillance were developed to address these nine diseases, they would also address diseases similar to them. The exemplar approach also avoids the trap of pitting one disease against another in competing for resources and attention. Rather, it conceptualizes the commonalities across diseases with the intent of developing strategies that benefit all affected by the vast array of chronic diseases.

Thus, we have sampled from the different patterns (clinical manifestations and trajectories) of chronic diseases in order to represent the important dimensions of varying chronic disease manifestations. The nine clinical clusters—not all specific and individual diseases and conditions in the literal sense—are described below, with brief comments on their epidemiology and community impact. Each represents an important challenge to public health, in addition to those diseases that have received more attention, namely, the diseases responsible for much of morbidity and mortality and significantly add to health care cost in the United States and other developed countries. The nine are arthritis, cancer survivorship, chronic pain, dementia, depression, diabetes mellitus type 2, posttraumatic disabling conditions, schizophrenia, and vision and hearing loss.

Arthritis

Arthritis is the term used to describe more than 100 rheumatic diseases and conditions that affect joints, tissues surrounding the joints, and other connective tissue.

Arthritis is a highly prevalent condition. It is estimated that 50 million adults in the United States (approximately one in five) report doctor-diagnosed arthritis (CDC, 2011a). Arthritis is more prevalent in older age groups, women, individuals who are overweight, and individuals with lower socioeconomic status. It affects members of all racial and ethnic groups (AAOS, 2008; CDC, 2011a; Dalstra et al., 2005). Although arthritis is more prevalent in older age groups, with half of adults age 65 and older reporting arthritis, nearly two-thirds of the adults reporting doctor-diagnosed arthritis are younger than age 65 (AAOS, 2008). As the U.S. population ages, the prevalence of arthritis is projected to increase over current levels to 67 million by 2030 (CDC, 2011a; Hootman and Helmick, 2006).

In addition to being one of the most prevalent chronic illnesses, arthritis is the leading cause of disability (McNeil and Binette, 2001) and one of the leading causes of work limitations (Stoddard et al., 1998). In 2008, 29 million persons over age 18, 13 percent of all adults in the United States, had self-reported activity limitations attributable to arthritis (AAOS, 2008). As with the frequency of arthritis, the prevalence of arthritis-attributable activity limitations increases as people age. Among adults age 65 and older, 28 percent reported activity limitations attributed to arthritis in 2008 (AAOS, 2008). In terms of work disability, 5.3 percent of all U.S. working-age adults (age 18 to 64) reported work limitations due to arthritis (CDC, 2011a).

Significant personal and societal burdens result from the high prevalence of arthritis and limitations and disability associated with it. In 2004, the estimated annual cost of medical care for arthritis and joint pain was $281.5 billion (AAOS, 2008). Of this amount, $37.3 billion is estimated to be incremental cost that can be directly attributed to arthritis and joint pain (AAOS, 2008). The indirect cost of arthritis and related rheumatic conditions due to lost earnings was estimated to be $54.3 billion in 2004 (AAOS, 2008). This includes an estimated $22 billion as a result of OA, $17.1 billion from RA, and $15.2 billion from gout (AAOS, 2008). These costs do not include the intangible costs of an individual forgoing the activities that they and society value.

Arthritis, in particular, is often comorbid with other conditions. A total of 24 percent of adults with arthritis have heart disease, 19 percent have chronic respiratory illnesses, and 16 percent have diabetes (CDC, [a]). Conversely, 57 percent of people with heart disease and 52 percent of people with diabetes have arthritis.

The most commonly occurring type of arthritis is osteoarthritis (OA), characterized by progressive damage to the cartilage and other joint tissues (AAOS, 2008). OA frequently affects the hands, knees, and hips. Other forms of arthritis that occur frequently include rheumatoid arthritis (RA), systemic lupus erythematosus (SLE), fibromyalgia, and gout (CDC, 2011a). Pain, stiffness, and swelling are common symptoms for these conditions, and some forms of arthritis, such as RA and SLE, also have a systemic component whereby multiple organs can be affected (Arthritis Foundation, 2008). The prevalence of OA can be estimated in terms of either radiographic changes related to the presence of OA or as symptomatic

OA, which includes having pain, aching, or stiffness in the same joint that shows radiographic OA (AAOS, 2008). More than 27 million U.S. adults have OA, and it is estimated that half of all adults will develop symptomatic OA of the knee at some point their lives (Arthritis Foundation and CDC, 2010; Murphy et al., 2008). In addition to being more common in women and obese individuals, OA is more common in certain occupations, including mining, construction, agriculture, and certain segments of the service industry (Arthritis Foundation and CDC, 2010). Approximately 25 percent of people with knee OA have difficulty performing activities of daily living and also have pain on ambulation (Arthritis Foundation and CDC, 2010). OA interferes with working adults' (age 18 to 64) work productivity, and their employment rates are lower than among adults without arthritis (Arthritis Foundation and CDC, 2010). It is estimated that $3.4 to 13.2 billion is spent on job-related OA costs per year (Arthritis Foundation and CDC, 2010). In terms of direct medical costs, in 2004, OA resulted in more than 11 million physician and outpatient visits, 662,000 hospitalizations, and more than 632,000 total joint replacements (Arthritis Foundation and CDC, 2010).

RA, the second most common type of arthritis, is a chronic autoimmune disease that causes pain, stiffness, swelling, and limitation in the motion and function of multiple joints. The prevalence of RA is estimated to be around 0.6 percent of the population over the age of 17, approximately 1.3 million adults in 2005 (AAOS, 2008). RA is twice as common in women as in men. In 2006, RA accounted for 2.9 million ambulatory care visits and 15,400 short-stay hospitalizations (AAOS, 2008). This estimate does not account for hospitalizations related to arthritis treatment complications, such as gastrointestinal bleeding related to the use of nonsteroidal anti-inflammatory drugs, and it does not account for hospitalizations related to orthopedic procedures (AAOS, 2008).

In summary, arthritis and related rheumatic conditions have a significant impact on the quality of life of affected individuals, with substantial physical, psychosocial, and economic consequences.

Cancer Survivorship

The number of cancer survivors in the United States is on the rise; in 2007 there were nearly 12 million people alive in the United States with a previous cancer diagnosis, up from approximately 3.5 million in 1971 (NCI, 2011; Rowland et al., 2004). Survivors older than 65 comprise 7 million of the 12 million survivors, the largest survivor age group (NCI, 2011). With the aging of the U.S. population, this group of cancer survivors 65 is projected to grow faster than other age groups (Smith et al., 2009). In addition, cancer is expected to increase more rapidly in all nonwhite racial and ethnic groups; between 2000 and 2030, cancer cases are expected to increase by 31 percent in whites, and by 99 percent in nonwhite racial and ethnic groups (Smith et al., 2009).

Cancer is a serious and often life-threatening disease, requiring difficult and intensive treatments that may leave survivors with lasting negative health consequences, despite a stabilization or elimination of their cancer. Cancer treatment can affect the health, functioning, and well-being of survivors. These can be divided into long-term effects (side effects/complications that begin during treatment and persist beyond the end of treatment) or late effects (side effects/treatment toxicities that are unrecognized or subclinical at the end of treatment but emerge later because of developmental processes), decreased ability to compensate as the survivor ages, or organ senescence (IOM and NRC, 2006). Nearly every organ system and tissue has the potential to be affected by cancer treatment, including cardiovascular, pulmonary, neurological, lymphatic, bone, endocrine, gastrointestinal, hematologic, hepatic, immune, ophthalmologic, and renal systems. A thorough description of the medical and psychosocial effects of cancer can be found in the IOM report *From Cancer Patient to Cancer Survivor: Lost in Transition* (IOM and NRC, 2006), but some examples of lasting and late effects are described below.

Highly effective and frequently used anthracycline chemotherapy can cause left ventricular dysfunction and heart failure (Pinder et al., 2007; Towns et al., 2008). For example, Pinder et al. (2007) found a 26 percent increased risk of congestive heart failure in breast cancer survivors between the ages of 66 and 70 who received anthracycline-based chemotherapy, compared with those who did not receive adjuvant chemotherapy. Newer targeted therapies, such as trastuzumab (Herceptin), bevacizumab, and sunitinib, also can have detrimental effects on the heart (Chu et al., 2007; Floyd et al., 2005).

Cancer surgery that removes lymph nodes (as well as radiation therapy to the nodes) can lead to lymphedema, the collection of fluid in a limb or other body part due to impedance of the flow of fluid in the lymphatic system, leading to swelling, pain, and loss of function. Lymphedema is frequently a concern for breast cancer survivors (NCI, [a]); it can also affect survivors of melanoma, gynecologic, genitourinary, and head and neck cancers (Cormier et al., 2010).

Radiation therapy can damage healthy tissue as well as tumor cells; effects on healthy tissue may involve cell killing through DNA double-strand breaks but also increased risk of fibrosis and impaired function in blood and lymph vessels. The effects of the damage depend on the area that was irradiated; for example, survivors who have radiation treatment for gynecologic cancers report 12 times the risk of bowel incontinence compared with controls who have not had cancer (Lind et al., 2011).

Other aftereffects of cancer are prevalent but are more difficult to tie to specific treatment toxicities. Nevertheless, cancer survivors report persistent problems with fatigue, sleep difficulties, and psychological distress, particularly anxiety about recurrence (Bower et al., 2008). Furthermore, survivors are at increased risk of second primary tumors, either because of host susceptibility or treatment effects, necessitating careful surveillance for cancer recurrence and detection of new cancer (IOM and NRC, 2006).

More than ever before, cancer is being managed like a chronic disease. In part this is due to the late effects described above. However, it is also because the treatment of cancer has been extended for many cancer sites. For example, women with estrogen-receptor positive breast cancer receive the recommendation to take estrogen-suppressing therapy for 5 years, and in some cases survivors experience troublesome side effects, such as joint and muscle pain (Mao et al., 2009). The treatment of chronic myelogenous leukemia has been revolutionized by the use of imatinib, a targeted agent that has relative low toxicity but is taken for an indefinite period of time to keep the disease at bay. Even metastatic disease, which has historically resulted in a rapid decline and death, has more treatment options, so that for certain disease sites, such as breast and colon, survivors with metastatic disease are living longer. Survivors with metastatic illness often stay on a therapy until it stops working or the side effect burden becomes too great, when they may switch to another therapy.

Lasting and late effects, as well as side effects from continuous treatment, have negative repercussions for health and functioning in a range of areas. Results from analyses of the National Health Interview Survey show that cancer survivors are more likely to rate their health as fair or poor (31 percent) than the noncancer controls (17.9 percent). They also are more likely than controls to report functional limitations, including needing help with ADL (cancer survivors, 4.9 percent; controls, 3 percent), instrumental activities of daily living (cancer survivors, 11.4 percent; controls, 6.5 percent), and any limitation (cancer survivors, 36.2 percent; controls, 23.8 percent). Survivors are more likely to report being unable to work and being more limited in the amount of type of work they can do because of health (Yabroff et al., 2004).

These functional limitations persist long after diagnosis; one study found that the odds of having a functional limitation in cancer survivors versus controls was similar for survivors within 5 years of diagnosis and more than 5 years after diagnosis; in an analysis of data from the National Health and Nutrition Examination Survey, Ness et al. (2006) found that the odds of physical performance limitations were 85 percent higher in survivors within 5 years of diagnosis compared with adults who had not had cancer, and by 49 percent among those who were 5 or more years from diagnosis after controlling for sex, age, race/ethnicity, and annual household income. Age and comorbid health problems also complicate the health status of cancer survivors.

Because age is one of the strongest risk factors for cancer, most cancer survivors are older (60 percent are age 65 or older; NCI, 2011), and 42.1 percent have one or more chronic illnesses other than their cancer (compared with 19.7 percent among those who have not had cancer (Hewitt et al., 2003). Approaches to living well need to take into account issues of aging and MCCs.

Chronic Pain

Pain varies in severity and locale. It can be mild or acute, but in many cases it can be chronic. Some of the most commonly occurring chronic pain originates from headaches, the lower back, cancer, arthritis, peripheral nerve damage, and an unknown source (NINDS, [a]). Approximately 100 million adults within the United States suffer from chronic pain (IOM, 2011b). The different forms and origins of pain vary in prevalence. As various studies have shown, however, chronic pain is on the rise, continuing to affect both men and women and individuals of all races and ethnicities. The level of chronic pain experienced worldwide is expected to continue to increase as the population ages and rates of obesity and physical inactivity leading to pain-related conditions soar (Phillips and Harper, 2011). For example, a survey of North Carolina residents found that the prevalence of chronic low back pain increased from 3.9 to 10.2 percent between 1992 and 2006 (Freburger et al., 2009). Similarly, the number of cancer diagnoses continues to rise, with 50 to 90 percent of patients suffering from cancer- and treatment-related pain (WHO, 2008; Zaza and Baine, 2002). Recent literature suggests that racial and ethnic minorities, including African Americans and Hispanics, have greater chances of going undertreated for pain than white Americans (Green et al., 2003).

Chronic pain may result from a previous injury or medical condition, or it may have no known cause (NINDS, [a]). It can be considered a disease, as it has the potential to increasingly damage the nervous system over time (IOM, 2011b). Chronic pain often occurs with a variety of comorbidities. In many instances, it occurs in conjunction with other pain-inducing conditions, such as chronic fatigue syndrome, fibromyalgia, and vulvodynia (NINDS, [a]). Furthermore, it often occurs in conjunction with other mental conditions, such as depression and multiple mood and anxiety disorders, including panic disorder and posttraumatic stress disorder (Bair et al., 2003; McWilliams et al., 2003).

Chronic pain and musculoskeletal disorders typically score lowest in terms of quality of life (Phillips and Harper, 2011). Depending on the type and severity of pain experienced, chronic pain can cause a substantial amount of disablement. Even differing levels of pain with the same origin, such as the low back, can lead to differing levels of disablement. Low back pain symptoms range from being specific and part of a specific pathology to being localized or part of a widespread, unknown pathology (Wormgoor et al., 2006). As pain decreases in specificity, patients often focus on it more, resulting in greater distress and dissatisfaction with life factors (Wormgoor et al., 2006). It has also been found, however, that as pain increases in specificity, loss of function and activity limitations increase (Wormgoor et al., 2006). In either form, the studied group illustrates that pain leads to negative consequences in functioning. In another study, individuals who suffer from chronic daily headaches demonstrated significant decreases in all health-related markers on the SF-36 health survey compared with healthy individuals, with the highest decreases found in role, physical, bodily pain, vitality, and social functioning (Guitera et al., 2002). In the population studied, chronicity of pain had greater influence than intensity of pain on quality of life (Guitera et al., 2002). A review of 52 studies conducted by Jensen and colleagues (2007) found solid evidence that the presence and severity of chronic neuropathic pain is associated with impairments in physical, emotional, role, and social functioning.

The burden associated with chronic pain reaches far beyond the individual suffering from it (Phillips and Harper, 2011). Significant functional disablement translates into substantial financial outcomes, reaching beyond the individual to the individual's caretaker and family, community, and country. Evidence shows that chronic pain has a substantial impact on productivity levels, as it results in higher rates of absenteeism and the likelihood of leaving the workforce (Phillips and Harper, 2011). One study showed that, among spouses of individuals suffering from chronic pain, 35 percent had to take on extra work to support the family, 43 percent had to take time off to care for the pain sufferer, 37 percent had to assume greater financial-related task responsibility, and 89 percent had to assume greater household responsibility (Hahn et al., 2001). Mechanical low back pain ranks fourth out of the top 10 most costly physical health conditions affecting American businesses today in terms of total medical expenses, medical-related absences, and short-term disability payments (Goetzel et al., 2003). Ricci and colleagues (2005) estimated the annual lost productive work time cost due to arthritis in the U.S. workforce at around $7.11 billion, with 65.7 percent attributable to the 38 percent of workers with pain exacerbations. In a previous IOM report, it was estimated that the annual cost of chronic pain in the United States runs anywhere from $560 to $635 billion (IOM, 2011b).

In the battle against the development of chronic pain, a myriad of primary preventive interventions have been tested. Psychological factors are tightly connected to the development of costly disability (Linton and

---

BOX 2-1
Findings from *Relieving Pain in America*

- **Need for interdisciplinary approaches.** Given chronic pain's diverse effects, interdisciplinary assessment and treatment may produce the best results for people with the most severe and persistent pain problems.
- **Importance of prevention.** Chronic pain has such severe impacts on all aspects of the lives of its sufferers that every effort should be made to achieve both primary prevention (e.g., in surgery for broken hip) and secondary prevention (of the transition from the acute to the chronic state) through early intervention.
- **Wider use of existing knowledge.** While there is much more to be learned about pain and its treatment, even existing knowledge is not always used effectively, and thus substantial numbers of people suffer unnecessarily.

SOURCE: IOM, 2011b.

Ryberg, 2001). Because of this, cognitive-behavioral interventions often have positive results in preventing further disability (Linton and Ryberg, 2001). Linton (2002) showed that it is possible to identify patients who suffer from musculoskeletal pain at high risk for developing pain-related disability and to successfully lower their risk of work disability through cognitive-behavioral intervention. Once disability appears, however, similar therapy methods still appear successful. Linton and Ryberg (2001) provided evidence of this as study participants suffering from chronic neck and back pain undergoing cognitive-behavioral group intervention showed significantly better results in terms of fear-avoidance beliefs, number of pain-free days, and use of sick leave.

Relevant findings from the IOM's report *Relieving Pain in America* are presented in Box 2-1.

Dementia

Dementia affects 13 percent of persons age 65 and older and up to 43 percent of persons age 85 and older (Alzheimer's Association, 2011a). In the United States, an estimated 5.4 million persons are affected by Alzheimer's disease (Alzheimer's Association, 2011b). Moreover, the burden of dementia is even higher, as Alzheimer's disease accounts for only 60 to 80 percent of cases of dementia. Although dementia is commonly thought of as a condition of the elderly, an estimated 220,000 to 640,000 persons under age 65 are also affected (Alzheimer's Association, 2006). Studies in nursing homes indicate that 26 to 48 percent of residents have dementia (Magaziner et al., 2000; O'Brien and Caro, 2001).

These patients and their families have needs far beyond those of healthier older persons and those who have chronic illnesses that do not affect memory. In many respects, dementia is a prototypic chronic disease that requires both medical and social services to provide a high quality of care and to prevent complications, including repeated hospitalizations (Chodosh et al., 2004) and high care costs. In 2011, Medicare and Medicaid programs for people with Alzheimer's disease were estimated at $130 billion (Okie, 2011). The clinical manifestations of dementia are protean and devastating and include cognitive impairment, immobility and falls, swallowing disorders and aspiration pneumonia, urinary and fecal incontinence, and behavioral disturbances (e.g., agitation, aggression, depression, hallucinations), which lead to caregiver stress and burnout.

Most cases of dementia start insidiously, often beginning with mild memory symptoms and progressing to mild cognitive impairment when deficits can be demonstrated on clinical examination. By the time of diagnosis of dementia, there are deficits in other dimensions of cognition (e.g., language, visual-spatial, executive function) in addition to memory that interfere with functioning. As the illness progresses, patients progressively lose memory and function and, at the late stages, may have no or unintelligible speech. Patients spend more years with severe dementia than in earlier stages (Arrighi et al., 2010). Almost all patients with dementia have at least one coexisting medical illness, especially coronary heart disease (26 percent), diabetes (23 percent), congestive heart failure (16 percent), and cancer (13 percent). Persons with dementia and these illnesses have more hospital stays than those with the same illnesses without dementia (Alzheimer's Association, 2011a). Although dementia has variable rates of progression and lengths of survival after diagnosis, the median is 4 to 8 years (Brookmeyer et al., 2002; Ganguli et al., 2005; Helzner et al., 2008; Larson et al., 2004).

Dementia is a particularly devastating illness because the clinical manifestations affect the ability to maintain function and manage other chronic illnesses. Moreover, as dementia progresses, its complications often result in caregiving needs that may overwhelm the care of other preexisting and new chronic illnesses.

Nationwide in 2010, an estimated 15 million caregivers provided 17 billion hours of care worth $202 billion (Alzheimer's Association, 2011a). And 80 percent of care provided in the home for patients with dementia is delivered by family caregivers who provide ADL and IADL functions, manage safety issues and behavioral symptoms, and coordinate medical and supportive care. Although these caregivers report positive feelings about this role, 61 percent rated the emotional stress of caregiving as high or very high (Alzheimer's Association, 2011a), and approximately one-third report symptoms of depression (Taylor et al., 2008; Yaffe et al., 2002). The physical health of caregivers may also be affected. For example, caregivers of dementia patients have increased rates of coronary heart disease (Vitaliano et al., 2002).

Current medications can sometimes slow the course of decline of Alzheimer's disease and some other dementias, but they do not cure the disorder. The addition of a dementia care manager to primary care practices can improve quality of care, reduce complications of aggression and agitation, and prevent caregiver depression (Callahan et al., 2006). Similarly, a disease management program led by care managers has been shown to improve patient health-related quality of life, overall quality of patient care, caregiving quality, social support, and level of unmet caregiving assistance needs (Vickrey et al., 2006). In addition, partnering with local Alzheimer's Association chapters can improve the quality of dementia care (Reuben et al., 2010).

Research is needed on models of care that link health care systems with community-based organizations to provide the wide range of services needed by patients with dementia. This research needs to include developing payment structures for community-based social services that are necessary to provide comprehensive care for persons with dementia. As stated in the IOM report *Retooling for an Aging America: Building the Health Care Workforce* (2009), "research is needed for the development and promulgation of technological advancements that could enhance an individual's capacity to provide care for older adults including the use of ADL technologies and information technologies that increase the efficiency and safety of care and caregiving."

Depression

Major depression is a common chronic illness that causes a substantial degree of impairment and disability (Michaud et al., 2006). National studies in the United States found a point prevalence of about 7 percent in 2001 and 2002 (Compton et al., 2006). Cohort studies found that the lifetime prevalence of major depression is 17 percent (National Comorbidity Survey Replication, 2007). The prevalence among women is about twice that among men (Murphy et al., 2000), and the lifetime prevalence is higher for whites than for African Americans (Williams et al., 2007). Both point prevalence and lifetime prevalence of major depression is higher for younger than for older persons (Kessler et al., 2010). However, depression is more common in older persons with a greater number of chronic illnesses, including those with disabilities (Charney et al., 2003; Lebowitz et al., 1997; Lyness et al., 2006).

Major depression causes a large burden of suffering on both individuals and society. One extensive study of the burden of chronic illnesses in the United States for 1996 found that major depression was the leading cause of lost disability-adjusted life-years (DALYs) for people age 25 to 44 (Michaud et al., 2006). Another study of a nationally representative sample of people age 18 and older investigated the association between life role disability in the previous 30 days and 30 different chronic illnesses. Musculoskeletal illnesses and depression had the largest effects on disability of any of the other illnesses (Merikangas et al., 2007). Depression is also a frequent complicating factor for many other chronic illnesses. It frequently accompanies such illnesses as diabetes, disabling osteoarthritis, and cognitive impairment. One study found that 71 percent of Medicare recipients with depression have four or more other chronic illnesses (Wolff and Boult, 2005).

Multiple studies and meta-analyses have found that collaborative care—including depression screening, assessment, enhanced patient education, use of allied health professionals to provide close follow-up, a consultant psychiatrist as backup, and stepped-care treatment approaches with incremental increases in treatment for people with persistent symptoms—is effective in reducing depression and increasing function (Gilbody et al., 2006; Katon et al., 2010). Screening for depression is recommended by the U.S. Preventive Services Task Force (USPSTF, 2009).

Despite effective management options, few physician organizations use evidence-based programs for patients with depression. One study of 1,040 physician organizations found that only 29 (3.2 percent) used four effective organized care management processes for patients with depression (Casalino et al., 2003).

Given the overlap between depression and MCCs, other interventions that are complex approaches to integrating community and clinical resources may be considered. One systematic review and meta-analysis of 89 randomized controlled trials of community-based complex interventions found reductions in nursing home admissions (RR 0.87; 95 percent CI 0.83–0.90), risk of hospital admission (0.94; 0.91–0.97), and falls (0.90; 0.86–0.95) (Beswick et al., 2008). One randomized controlled trial, for example, examined the effect of geriatric care management, which included home-based care by a nurse practitioner and a social worker collaborating with a primary care physician and a geriatrics interdisciplinary team, on low-income people age 65 and older with MCCs. After 2 years, the study found significant improvements for patients receiving the intervention in four of eight SF-36 quality of life scales, including general health, vitality, social functioning, and mental health (Counsell et al., 2007).

The CDC's National Center for Chronic Disease Preventions and Health Promotion, Division of Adult and Community Health recently published a *Public Health Action Plan to Integrate Mental Health Promotion and Mental Illness Prevention with Chronic Disease Prevention, 2011–2015* (CDC, 2011c). This plan recognizes the interconnection between chronic disease and mental health, including major depression, and outlines the goal to include the promotion of mental health as part of efforts to prevent chronic disease. The committee commissioned a paper by Wayne J. Katon on improving recognition and depression care in individuals with common chronic illnesses (see Appendix A).

Type 2 Diabetes

Diabetes mellitus is defined as a group of metabolic diseases character-ized by hyperglycemia resulting from defects in insulin secretion from the pancreatic beta (β) cells; insulin action at the level of skeletal muscle, liver, and fat; or both (American Diabetes Association, 2010). It is estimated that 25.6 million, or 11.3 percent of adults age 20 and older in the United States, have diagnosed and undiagnosed diabetes, and 90 to 95 percent of diagnosed cases involve type 2 diabetes (CDC, 2011b). The prevalence of diabetes is similar in men and women (CDC, 2011b). Diabetes is a par-ticular public health burden among the elderly: 26.9 percent of adults age 65 and older have diabetes (10.9 million individuals) (CDC, 2011b). And non-Hispanic blacks and Mexican Americans have twice the age- and sex-standardized prevalence of diagnosed diabetes compared with non-Hispanic whites (Cowie et al., 2009). Risk factors for type 2 diabetes include increas-ing age, obesity, physical inactivity, having a prior history of gestational diabetes, having hypertension or dyslipidemia, being a member of a high-risk racial/ethnic group (i.e., African, Hispanic, Asian, Native American, or Pacific Islander), or having a family history of type 2 diabetes, particularly in first-degree relatives (American Diabetes Association, 2010, 2011).

The onset of type 2 diabetes is often insidious and asymptomatic; a pre-clinical stage of prediabetes is defined as having impaired fasting glucose, impaired glucose tolerance, or a high risk hemoglobin A1c (HbA1c) value of 5.7 to 6.4 percent (American Diabetes Association, 2010). Approxi-mately 35 percent of U.S. adults over age 20 have prediabetes, and 50 per-cent of elderly individuals have prediabetes (CDC, 2011b). Type 2 diabetes often develops with obesity, which induces insulin resistance. Although the β cell attempts to compensate for insulin resistance by secreting increasing amounts of insulin, this compensatory mechanism eventually fails with progressive β cell dysfunction, resulting in hyperglycemia and development of type 2 diabetes (American Diabetes Association, 2010). There is quite a bit of variability in the degree of β cell dysfunction along the spectrum of insulin resistance, which is why some patients with type 2 diabetes require more aggressive pharmacological intervention earlier than others. The resultant hyperglycemia, if untreated, can lead to long-term complications, including microvascular complications (i.e., retinopathy, nephropathy, and peripheral and autonomic neuropathy) and macrovascular complications (i.e., coronary heart disease, cerebrovascular disease, and peripheral arterial disease). Diabetes is the leading cause of incident blindness in adults age 20 to 74 and the leading cause of end-stage renal disease (CDC, 2011b). Mild to severe nervous system damage occurs in 60 to 70 percent of individuals with diabetes and includes peripheral neuropathy, gastroparesis, and erectile dysfunction, among others (CDC, 2011b). Peripheral neuropathy is a major contributor to lower extremity amputation. Other complications include periodontal disease, increase in susceptibility to infectious diseases, decrease in functional status, and depression (CDC, 2011b).

There are several evidence-based therapies that can prevent development of complications. Intensive control of hyperglycemia, with a target HbA1c of 7 percent, has been shown to reduce the risk of microvascular complications for individuals with type 2 diabetes (UK Prospective Diabetes Study Group, 1998). Interventions to reduce hypertension have been shown to reduce the risk of both cardiovascular disease and retinopathy for people with type 2 diabetes; aggressive lowering of LDL cholesterol with HMG-CoA reductase inhibitors reduces the risk of cardiovascular disease, the leading cause of death among those with diabetes (American Diabetes Association, 2011). Angiotensin-converting enzyme inhibitors and angiotensin receptor blockers have been shown to reduce the risk of incident nephropathy and progression to end-stage renal disease in type 2 diabetes (American Diabetes Association, 2011). For individuals with diabetes and macular edema or severe nonproliferative or high-risk proliferative diabetic retinopathy, laser photocoagulation therapy reduces the risk of vision loss (American Diabetes Association, 2011).

Diabetes is associated with limitations in physical functioning and the ability to perform ADLs (De Rekeneire et al., 2003; Gregg et al., 2000; Maty et al., 2004; Ryerson et al., 2003; Volpato et al., 2002). Potential mediators of this association include diabetes complications and comorbidities (Kalyani et al., 2010; Volpato et al., 2002), hyperglycemia (De Rekeneire et al., 2003; Kalyani et al., 2010), and depression (Egede, 2004; Volpato et al., 2002); however, in some populations, diabetes remains associated with functional disability even after accounting for these factors (Maty et al., 2004). Diabetes also carries a high patient self-management burden due to the need for daily self-monitoring of blood glucoses by patients on insulin therapy and/or oral diabetes medications, carbohydrate intake, medication administration, avoidance of hypoglycemia, and maintenance of an exercise routine.

Diabetes is also associated with reduced quality of life, particularly among individuals with multiple and/or severe complications (Rubin and

Peyrot, 1999). Patients with type 2 diabetes who are diet-controlled or whose hyperglycemia is managed with oral antidiabetic agents report better quality of life than those managed with insulin (Bradley et al., 2011; Rubin and Peyrot, 1999); however, individuals with type 2 diabetes poorly controlled on oral agents report improved quality of life following transition to insulin therapy (Bradley et al., 2011; Jennings et al., 1991; Wilson et al., 2004), a result probably related to improved glycemic control. Quality of life can also be influenced by the type of insulin used to treat hyperglycemia (Bradley and Gilbride, 2008; Bradley and Speight, 2002). However, the majority of pharmacological intervention studies that included clinical outcomes for type 2 diabetes have not concurrently measured quality of life outcomes. The United Kingdom Prospective Diabetes Study assessed a measure of health status rather than quality of life, so it remains unclear if quality of life was different between the intensive and conventional therapy treatment groups at the end of the study (Bradley et al., 2011). The PANORAMA Study in Europe will shed further light on the impact of various diabetes treatment regimens and glycemic control on patient-reported outcomes, including quality of life (Bradley et al., 2011). This observational study will recruit 5,000 individuals with type 2 diabetes in nine European countries and investigate the association between treatment regimens, levels of glycemia, quality of life, treatment satisfaction, fear of hypoglycemia, and health status (Bradley et al., 2011). Because pharmacological therapies that prevent diabetes complications are administered within the clinical health care system, future studies are needed to determine whether the interface between the health care and public health systems and community-based organizations can improve adherence to these treatments while also improving patient-reported outcomes.

Posttraumatic Disabling Conditions

Posttraumatic disabling conditions (PTDCs) are a diverse group of conditions with heterogeneous causes and outcomes that cumulatively can yield a substantial amount of short- and long-term morbidity, mortality, and permanent disability. It is very difficult to define the population rates of such conditions because they are not easy to define or detect in population surveys. Outcome studies generally come from institutional registries and may underestimate the total community burden of PTCDs, which have always been considered a group from a public health perspective. Although primary injury prevention for some types of community-acquired trauma has been a public health priority for many years, individual PTCDs are not as common as naturally occurring conditions. With a few general policy exceptions, such as the Americans with Disabilities Act, ameliorating the chronic disability and reducing the secondary conditions associated with these disabilities has never been a public health priority.

As noted, PTCDs are extremely diverse. Knee meniscus injuries from many causes can lead to chronic degenerative arthritis years or decades after the injury or repair, although some early interventions can mitigate some of this adverse long-term outcome (Zafagnini et al., 2011). It is estimated that about 235,000 Americans are admitted to hospitals each year with nonfatal traumatic brain injuries (TBIs) (Corrigan et al., 2010). Long-term improvement with rehabilitation can be obtained for TBI patients with disordered consciousness, but this process can be prolonged over many years (Nakase-Richardson et al., 2011). Late deaths more than 30 days after hospital discharge from a variety of causes occur commonly among trauma patients (Claridge et al., 2010), suggesting substantial community experiences with posttraumatic states. Trauma patients who survive surgical intensive care units for more than 3 years have substantial long-term disability rates (Livingston et al., 2009). Severe burn injuries may lead to substantial disability and disfigurement, restricted movement, and long-term metabolic abnormalities (Jeschke et al., 2011). Falls and fractures are very common among older adults, leading to increased disability and joint replacement. For example, on the basis of emergency room visits, it was estimated that in excess of 1 million fall-related wrist and forearm injuries occurred over a 7-year period in the United States (Orces and Martinez, 2011). Taken together, a substantial segment of the U.S. population is living with the varying but sometimes severe consequences of a variety of traumatic events. There are many other important sources of trauma with long-term consequences, such as work and home implements and firearms. As other patient groups have done, posttrauma patients have organized to improve their circumstances (Bradford et al., 2011).

A clear public health recognition of the cumulative importance of posttrauma patients is worthy of consideration. There is an important need to create a public health taxonomy of PTDCs that encompasses commonalities and assesses long-term health outcomes, allowing for more precise population surveys and more effective population surveillance of the burdens of trauma. Also, as with other chronic illnesses, monitoring for secondary disease and dysfunctions associated with PTDCs and for a community-oriented research program that attempts to minimize long-term adverse outcomes and promote improved prevention could be valuable.

Schizophrenia

Schizophrenia is a severe, chronic, and disabling mental disorder. Individuals with schizophrenia often experience terrifying symptoms, such as auditory and visual hallucinations and illusions, or believing that other people are reading their minds, controlling their thoughts, or plotting to harm them. These symptoms may leave them fearful and withdrawn. "Their speech and behavior can be so disorganized that they may be incomprehensible or frightening to others" (http://www.schizophrenia.com/family/sz.overview.htm).

About 1 percent of the Americans develop schizophrenia over their lifetime, affecting more than 2 million Americans in a given year. Although schizophrenia appears equally frequently among men and women, the onset of the illness is earlier in men, usually in the late teens or early twenties; women typically experience the onset of illness in their twenties to early thirties (http://www.schizophrenia.com/family/szfacts.htm).

Available treatments can relieve many symptoms, but most people with schizophrenia continue to experience some symptoms throughout their lives. Medication compliance with this population is difficult, and it has been estimated that no more than one in five individuals fully recovers (http://www.schizophrenia.com/family/sz.overview.htm). Homelessness also makes it difficult to provide consistent and effective treatment to many individuals with schizophrenia. It is estimated that 6 percent of homeless individuals have schizophrenia. Homeless individuals with schizophrenia may experience a worsening of their symptoms caused by the stress of living on the streets. Poor hygiene, lack of sleep, and the threat of violence may accelerate a person's decline into psychosis (http://www.health.am/psy/more/homelessness-schizophrenia/).

Schizophrenia is considered the most chronic, disabling, and costly mental illness. The indirect excess cost due to unemployment is the chief contributor to overall schizophrenia excess annual costs. In 2002, the cost of schizophrenia in the United States was about $62.7 billion, including $22.8 billion in excess direct health care costs: $7.0 billion for outpatient services, $5.0 billion for drugs, $2.8 billion for inpatient services, and $8.0 billion for long-term care. The total direct non–health care excess costs, including living cost offsets, were estimated at about $7.6 billion, and the total indirect excess costs were estimated at about $32.4 billion (Wu et al., 2005).

The management and consequences of living with schizophrenia are numerous and difficult. For example, people who have schizophrenia abuse alcohol, illicit drugs, and nicotine more than the general population does (http://www.schizophrenia.com/family/sz.overview.htm). In addition to reducing the effect of antipsychotic treatment, substance abuse is a health hazard that places the schizophrenic person at increased risk for MCCs over time. About one-third of the excess mortality in schizophrenics is due to unnatural causes, such as suicide, whereas two-thirds is due to natural causes (Lawrence et al., 2010). The largest number of deaths is due to cardiovascular disease (Lawrence et al., 2010). Research has also shown that persons with schizophrenia and substance abuse are also at an increased risk for committing a violent crime (Fazel et al., 2009).

The burden of schizophrenia on families and caregivers is significant. A shift toward a community-based approach to mental illness management and the increased role of family in the daily care of mentally ill persons has also had a psychosocial, physical, and financial impact on families. Caregiver burden associated with mental illness refers to the "negative responses that occur when caregivers assume unpaid and unanticipated responsibility for the person for whom they are caring who has a disabling mental health problem" (Schulze and Rössler, 2005). In addition, the concept of "burdens of care" involves "subtle but distressing notions such as shame, embarrassment, feelings of guilt and self-blame" (Awad and Voruganti, 2008). In the United States, 40 to 80 percent of persons with schizophrenia, depending on the subgroup, live with a relative or spouse (UNC Center for Excellence in Community Mental Health, [a]).

Vision and Hearing Loss

Visual and hearing losses are common disorders, especially among the elderly. In 2008, 15 percent of Americans age 18 and older were estimated to have hearing difficulty (without a hearing aid) and 11 percent had visual impairment (defined as trouble seeing, even with glasses or contact lenses) (NCHS, 2009). The rates of both hearing and vision problems increase with age, rising to 43 and 21 percent, respectively, among those age 75 and older (NCHS, 2009). Moreover, each of the four major eye diseases that cause visual impairment (cataract, age-related macular degeneration, glaucoma, and diabetic retinopathy) is more common with advancing age. Women are more likely to have vision problems than are men, but men are more likely than are women to have hearing problems (NCHS, 2009). Asian adults and black adults are less likely to have hearing difficulty than are white adults (NCHS, 2009). Poorer adults and those with Medicaid coverage are also more likely to have sensory problems than those who are wealthier or have private insurance or Medicare-only coverage (NCHS, 2009).

Subjectively reported or objectively measured visual impairment is predictive of decline in ADL and IADL function at 10 years and over 10 years (Reuben et al., 1999). Bilateral noncorrectable vision loss leads to dependence, nursing home placement, and worse emotional well-being (Horowitz, 2003; Vu et al., 2005). Noncorrectable unilateral visual loss is associated with increased risk of falling (Vu et al., 2005). Hearing loss has been associated with anxiety, social isolation, and depressive symptoms (NCOA, 1999). Self-reported or objectively measured hearing impairment predicts impairment in walking a quarter-mile, climbing up and down steps, and performing heavy chores (e.g., yard work, washing windows)

(Reuben et al., 1999). Combined objectively measured hearing and visual impairment has the highest risk (relative risk 8.03) for subsequent ADL impairment (Reuben et al., 1999).

Sensory impairment also results in a high economic burden. The annual cost of visual impairment and blindness was estimated in 2002 at $5.5 billion (Frick et al., 2007), and a cohort-survival study estimated that $4.6 billion will be spent over the lifetime of persons who acquired their impairment in 1998 (Mohr et al., 2000).

The treatment of sensory impairment depends on the cause. For visual impairment, cataracts can be cured by surgery with intraocular lens implantation. The other eye disorders are managed with a variety of medications and surgical procedures aimed at preventing further visual impairment. In addition, visual assistive devices, including eyeglasses, electronic video magnifiers, spectacle-mounted telescopes for distance vision, and closed-circuit television to enlarge text, are useful, as well as technologies like talking books. Community-based organizations (e.g., Braille Institute, the Lighthouse) provide direct services in addition to counseling and adaptive equipment. Insurance coverage for these services and equipment is variable.

For hearing impairment, the primary treatment approach is amplification, either by hearing aids or assistive listening devices (e.g., devices that have a microphone and headphones that facilitate hearing). In addition, text telephones (TTY) and telephone devices for the deaf (TDD) are often available at no cost to hearing-impaired persons. Other technology, such as FM loop systems, can be used for groups of people who have FM receivers or telecoil switches in their hearing aids. Infrared group listening devices can also be useful. Medicare does not cover amplification devices, including hearing aids. Selected groups of hearing-impaired persons may benefit from cochlear implants. A major barrier to treatment for persons with hearing impairment is denial of the problem or its importance by affected persons (NCOA, 1999).

A North Carolina study identified the common barriers to hearing-impaired persons accessing basic services as lack of access to communication, lack of understanding of the indicators and consequences of hearing loss, insufficient resources to effectively advocate for themselves in obtaining services, and lack of knowledge of existing resources available (North Carolina Department of Health and Human Services, 2009). There are community-based organizations and groups that facilitate living with hearing loss (e.g., Better Hearing Institute, Association of Late-Deafened Adults, Hearing Loss Association of America). Many states sponsor programs for hearing loss that offer various type of counseling and educational services (North Carolina Department of Health and Human Services, 2009).

Vision impairment is associated with considerable caregiver burden. A French study found that a quarter of caregivers of persons with blindness could not go out for an entire day and better than half reported that the caregiving burden affected their physical and emotional health and mental welfare and that they needed to modify their work (Brézin et al., 2005). A Japanese study found hearing impairment to be associated with increased caregiver burden (Kuzuya and Hirakawa, 2009).

WHO ARE THE PEOPLE WITH CHRONIC ILLNESSES?

Age and Chronic Illnesses

The relationship between aging and chronic illness is complex and variable. Differences between older and younger persons must be recognized and considered in a population-based approach to living well with chronic illness.

First, with aging, chronic diseases become more prevalent: 43 percent of Medicare beneficiaries have three or more illnesses (IOM, 2009) and 23 percent have more than five (Anderson, 2005). Moreover, the percentage of persons with MCCs rises with age. These multiple illnesses often require different and sometimes conflicting treatments (Boyd et al., 2005; Tinetti et al., 2004). As the number of medications used to treat multiple illnesses increases, the risk of adverse effects also increases (Agostini et al., 2004).

Second, the type, severity, number, and particular combination of chronic illnesses among the elderly vary. Older persons may accumulate conditions that have become inactive. For example, an 85-year-old woman with breast cancer, coronary artery disease, and chronic kidney disease may have had a mastectomy 20 years ago, had a coronary artery bypass 15 years ago, and have no restrictions from kidney disease other than dose adjustment for kidney function. Conversely, another woman with the same diagnoses may be receiving chemotherapy, taking six cardiac medications for her heart disease, and receiving dialysis. Some chronic illnesses (e.g., dementia, osteoarthritis, hypertension, sensory impairments) occur almost exclusively or at much higher prevalence among older persons. Dementia, which may affect up to 43 percent of persons age 85 and older (Alzheimer's Association, 2011a), is a particularly devastating disease because the protean manifestations affect the ability to maintain function and manage other chronic illnesses. As this disorder progresses, it predominates with needs that often overwhelm other preexisting and new chronic illnesses.

Third, the interaction of aging and chronic illness must be considered. The physiological functional reserve decreases with aging, often referred to as "homeostenosis." As a result, the ability to compensate for illness processes is usually lower than for younger persons. A construct termed "allostatic load" has been used to describe the burden of multiple chronic subclinical disturbances that are more common in older persons yet have prognostic importance (Seeman et al., 2001). At a clinical level, some normal aspects of aging (e.g., changes in vision, dexterity) may affect the ability to manage chronic illnesses. Consider the elderly person with diabetes and presbyopia and impaired visual contrast sensitivity who must measure and administer variable doses of insulin. Similarly, the age-related decrease in renal function and increase in the percentage of body fat affect the dosing, toxicity, and distribution of medications.

Fourth, the interaction among socioeconomic factors and chronic illness must be recognized. With aging, a variety of social supports change. For example, older persons may retire, become widowed, cease driving, move to different housing. Any of these may affect the ability to live independently or cope with chronic illness. Many of the functional capabilities that younger persons, even with those with chronic illness, take for granted, are gone or are in jeopardy of being lost. For example, persons with post-polio syndrome who have adapted to their impairments may find that, with aging, these adaptive responses are no longer sufficient to maintain function. Similarly, the loss of a spouse who has been a caregiver for a person with Alzheimer's disease may precipitate a crisis, even though the person's clinical status has not changed.

Fifth, prognosis and personal goals change with aging. Even in the absence of chronic illness and disability, life expectancy declines with aging (Keeler et al., 2010). Limited life expectancy may affect choices in managing chronic illness as well as the goals of care. These goals may differ considerably from those of younger persons with chronic illnesses, who may have a much longer life expectancy. Older persons' goals may relate to a functional or health state (e.g., being able to walk independently), symptom control (e.g., control of pain or dyspnea), living situation (e.g., remaining in one's home), or short-term survival (e.g., living long enough to reach a personal milestone, such as a family member's wedding) rather than long-term survival. Sometimes an older person's physician believes that a better outcome is possible but the patient declines to follow the recommended route (e.g., physical therapy to regain mobility). In addition, patient preferences for specific treatments may lead to care that is not the best evidence-based option "(e.g., using pads to manage urinary incontinence even though effective behavioral and pharmacological therapy is available)" (Reuben, 2009).

Demographic Disparities

Health Disparities and Living Well with Chronic Illness

As noted in Chapter 1, the health of Americans is better now than at any other time in history. As compared with those living in 1900, Americans today are "healthier, live longer, and enjoy lives that are less likely to be marked by injuries, ill health, or premature death," according to an earlier IOM report (IOM, 2003a). However, these gains are not shared with all members of society. Health disparities exist and persist. Race, as well as income, account for the pronounced disparities in care and therefore the disparities in health status between white and minority Americans (Watson, 2003). Recent reports on health disparities document the relatively poor health of African Americans, American Indians, Native Hawaiians, and Latinos, and other underrepresented groups when compared with white Americans (IOM, 2003b). Not only are racial and ethnic groups often less healthy; they also tend to have shorter life expectancies, higher rates of chronic illnessess, worse outcomes when diagnosed with an illness, and less access to quality health care (IOM, 2003b). In 2003 the IOM produced the report entitled *Unequal Treatment: Confronting Racial and Ethnic Disparities in Health Care*, which highlighted how within racial and ethnic groups in the United States there are remarkably consistent racial and ethnic disparities across a range of illnesses and health care services (IOM, 2003b).

CDC defines health disparities as significant differences between one population and another that can occur by gender, race or ethnicity, education or income, disability, geographic location, or sexual orientation (CDC's Office of Minority Health and Health Disparities, [a]). For racial and ethnic minorities, these disparities exist in a number of illnesses, including cardiovascular disease, HIV/AIDS, hypertension, diabetes, and mental illness (CDC's Office of Minority Health and Health Disparities, [a]). The severity of health disparities among specific groups becomes stark when the total U.S. population is segmented by race and ethnicity and about a third of the U.S. population consists of minorities impacted by disparate health (CDC's Office of Minority Health and Health Disparities, [a]; Center for Prevention and Health Services, 2009).

Health behaviors and lifestyles greatly contribute to chronic illness and health disparities. Research has demonstrated that a myriad of sources and complexities account for these disparities. However, socioeconomic status (SES), class status, lack of health insurance, and the quality of care different racial and ethnic groups receive are also powerful factors that impact the ability for people to make healthy decisions and live full and engaged lives, living well despite their chronic illness.

Specifically, SES is highly related to the presence and persistence of health disparities. Individuals with "lower socioeconomic status [SES] die earlier and have more disabilities than those with higher [SES]" (Schroeder, 2007). And the most extreme disparities in health occur among the impoverished, including individuals who are impoverished because of their health-related problems, as well as individuals whose health has suffered as a result of poverty. Environmental factors, such as lead paint, water and air pollution, dangerous neighborhoods, lack of outlets for physical activity, as well as other health-compromising factors, contribute to single and MCCs for individuals with lower SES (Schroeder, 2007).

Class is also highly related to the prevalence of chronic illness among in racial and ethnic groups. Similar to SES in a stepwise pattern from lowest to highest, class is defined by income, total wealth, education, employment, and residential neighborhood (Schroeder, 2007). The class gradient in health means that people in the lower class gradient are more likely to practice unhealthy behaviors, partly due to inadequate grocery stores, constrained conditions to exercise (Schroeder, 2007), and the inability to secure the resources needed to support healthy living or manage chronic illnesses. Class is a determinant of the nation's health and an important factor for public health leaders to consider in population-based efforts to help individuals living with chronic illnesses.

Lack of health insurance is a barrier to access to quality care, is a serious determinant of health, and contributes to disparities in health. As Box 2-2 shows, racial and ethnic minorities are much more likely to be uninsured than white Americans.

Inequalities in quality of care also exist and also contribute to poor health outcomes. A large body of published research revealed that racial and ethnic minorities and/or poor disadvantaged patients receive inadequate quality care (IOM, 2003b). And the differences in health care quality do not disappear when controlled for SES differences or health insurance, which means that disparities across the range of chronic illnesses and health care services cannot be attributed to economic status or access to care alone.

The concept of living well adopted by the committee in this report—the best achievable state of health that encompasses all dimensions of physical, mental, and social well-being—may be heavily clouded in the minds of individuals with single or MCCs who live in communities where complex and social inequities are deeply rooted. The committee thinks that public health action to lead and enhance efforts to help racial and ethnic groups

---

BOX 2-2
Access to Care: Uninsured in 2010

- 11.7 percent of Whites, not Hispanic
- 18.1 percent of Asian Americans
- 20.8 percent of African American
- 30.7 percent of Latinos

SOURCE: U.S. Census Bureau, 2011.

with chronic illness live better with better health outcomes is important and achievable.

Health Literacy

Health literacy includes general comprehension of the human body, healthy behaviors, and the workings of the health care system (HHS, 2010). It is a complex construct that measures an individual's ability to function effectively in the health care system (Berkman et al., 2011). Today's health care system requires a particularly sophisticated level of understanding from individuals to receive needed care, and lower health literacy is commonly found among minorities, the elderly, and patients with chronic illnesses (Schillinger et al., 2002).

The National Assessment of Adult Literacy from 2003 categorized 14 percent of adults as "below basic" in health literacy (NCES, 2006). Between socioeconomic and racial and ethnic groups, only 9 percent of white respondents were categorized as below basic compared with 24 percent of African Americans and 41 percent of Hispanics (NCES, 2006). In addition, 3 percent of respondents with a college degree and some graduate study and 49 percent of respondents with less than a high school education placed at the below-basic level (NCES, 2006). A systematic review conducted by Berkman et al. (2011) found that "low health literacy was consistently associated with more hospitalizations; greater use of emergency care; lower receipt of mammography screening and influenza vaccine; poorer ability to demonstrate taking medications appropriately; poorer ability to interpret labels and health messages; and, among elderly persons, poorer overall health status and higher mortality rates." Previous studies among indigent and Medicare patient populations have shown that older individuals have lower health literacy (Gazmararian et al., 2003). One study found that an estimated 81 percent of English-speaking patients over age 60 treated at a public hospital had inadequate levels of health literacy (Gazmararian et al., 2003). A separate study found that all low-income, community-dwelling with adults between the ages of 60 and 94 possessed reading skills averaging at the fifth-grade level and one-fourth of the adults admitted having trouble comprehending written information from physicians (Gazmararian et al., 2003).

Individuals with poor health literacy are more likely to report having a chronic illness. In a population-based cross-sectional study of 2,923 Medicare managed care enrollees in four U.S. cities, about 22.2 percent had "inadequate" health literacy and about 11.3 percent had "marginal" health literacy (Wolf et al., 2005). In statistically significant unadjusted analyses, people with inadequate health literacy had more self-reported cases of diabetes (18.7 versus 12.8 percent, p < 0.001), heart failure (6.1 versus

3.8 percent, p = 0.05), and arthritis (57.3 versus 50.1 percent, p = 0.01) than people with adequate health literacy had. Furthermore, individuals with inadequate health literacy were more likely to report greater difficulty in completing daily activities and fewer accomplishments due to worse physical health and higher levels of pain (Wolf et al., 2005). Even after adjusting for higher prevalence of chronic illness, individuals with inadequate health literacy had worse physical and mental health (Wolf et al., 2005).

Although those with poor health literacy are more likely to report having a chronic illness, the reverse is also true. Individuals with poor health literacy often know less about any chronic illness they might have (Gazmararian et al., 2003). Previous studies have documented a weaker base of chronic illness knowledge among those with asthma, diabetes, and hypertension (Gazmararian et al., 2003). In a more recent study, Gazmararian et al. (2003) surveyed 653 newly enrolled Medicare patients age 65 and older with one or more chronic illnesses to see how much these patients knew about their own chronic illness(es). Of those surveyed, 24 percent had inadequate and 12 percent had marginal health literacy. Analysis reinforced previous study findings of higher chronic illness knowledge among those with higher health literacy (Gazmararian et al., 2003).

Studies such as the one conducted by Gazmarmarian et al. (2003) point to serious repercussions among those with chronic illnesses and lower health literacy. For example, congestive heart failure (CHF) is a common reason for hospitalizations among those age 65 and older; however, many cases for rehospitalization are preventable with proper CHF management, knowledge, and skills, which are possessed by those with higher levels of health literacy (Baker et al., 2002). Similarly, patients with type 2 diabetes and inadequate health literacy report weaker glycemic control and higher prevalence of retinopathy (Schillinger et al., 2002). Findings like this suggest that inadequate health literacy disproportionately contributes to the burden experienced by those with type 2 diabetes from disadvantaged populations (Schillinger et al., 2002).

With the passage of the Affordable Care Act, millions of new patients will gradually flood the health care system, receiving treatment for previously unaddressed or undiagnosed chronic illnesses. However, with many patients possessing weak health literacy, most health efforts will be in vain, as health literacy has a proven record with poorer health outcomes. To reverse poor health literacy and improve health outcomes among patients throughout the United States, and particularly disadvantaged populations, the 2010 National Action Plan to Improve Health Literacy was developed. It has seven goals: (1) "develop and disseminate health and safety information that is accurate, accessible, and actionable"; (2) "promote changes in the health care system that improve health information, communication, informed decision-making, and access to health services"; (3) "incorporate accurate, standards-based, and developmentally appropriate health and science information and curricula in child care and education through the university level"; (4) "support and expand local efforts to provide adult education, English language instruction, and culturally and linguistically appropriate health information services in the community"; (5) "build partnerships, develop guidance, and change policies"; (6) "increase basic research and the development, implementation, and evaluation of practices and interventions to improve health literacy"; and (7) "increase the dissemination and use of evidence-based health literacy practices and interventions." To translate these goals and strategies into action and effectively promote higher levels of health literacy, these actions need to be multidisciplinary, evidence-based, and evaluated, and to involve the communities and individuals most affected.

Primary and Secondary Prevention

Elsewhere in the chapter the problems of MCCs (comorbidity) are well characterized in terms of their impact and importance. Although some secondary conditions are related to progressive primary illnesses (e.g., falls and fractures associated with disabling progressive neurological illnesses), persons with chronic illnesses are also subject to additional, unrelated illnesses by virtue of aging, personal risk profiles, and perhaps other biological vulnerabilities associated with the original illness (e.g., genetic risks of multiple cancer syndromes, tobacco exposures). Although there are authoritative sources of effective primary and secondary preventive interventions for persons in clinical practice (U.S. Preventive Services Task Force) and in the community (The Community Guide), neither of these resources systematically or comprehensively addresses these important interventions for persons with overt chronic illnesses. In fact, there is good evidence that quality primary care, including preventive services, may be deficient among those with mental and disabling illnesses (Havercamp et al., 2004; Mitchell et al., 2009; Reichard et al., 2011).

Indeed, one can find expert opinion, clinical recommendations or a true evidence base related to certain primary preventive interventions (e.g., influenza vaccine for certain risk groups) for primary prevention and screening and screening in the disease-specific literature, but, after thorough literature review, the committee thinks that there are major gaps in research-based recommendations for routine preventive activities for those with common and important chronic diseases. Although there may be an abiding logic in many instances to extend preventive recommendations intended for healthy persons to those with chronic illnesses (e.g., smoking cessation, hypertension control), an enhanced research and systematic review approach to this problem is clearly indicated.

BOX 2-3
Primary Preventive Interventions

- Vaccines for adults with chronic illnesses, as recommended by the Advisory Committee on Immunization Practices, including tetanus, diphtheria, and acellular pertussis vaccine; pneumonia vaccine; zoster vaccine; and the newly developed high-dose influenza vaccine, as clinically indicated (Chen et al., 2011).
- Special food safety and food preparation instructions for persons with any conditions associated with immune-compromised states or treatments, such as occur in cancer patients (USDA, 2006).
- Education to recognize and seek care immediately when the symptoms of stroke appear in an individual (American Stroke Association, [a]).
- Personal and family monitoring of environmental alerts, such as extreme heat, cold, or air pollution conditions, all associated with increased morbidity and mortality risk among those with chronic illnesses (Wen et al., 2009).
- Preparedness education for persons with chronic illnesses when natural disasters occur. For example, maintaining electrical devices that are needed for illness management when power outages occur (Khan, 2011).

Emphasis on Primary Preventive Interventions

In addition to the need to determine the needs and outcomes of general preventive interventions for persons with chronic illnesses, there are several such interventions that may require special emphasis—interventions that have been given little attention. The level of evidence for most of these varies, but in general there have been enough studies to raise these interventions to the level of consideration for public health policy. Some of them have been assessed only in outbreak situations, and some are not subject to experimental trial interventions per se, except in the situation in which techniques for behavior modification are indicated. The list in Box 2-3 is not exhaustive, but the committee thinks these preventive efforts need some further consideration for dissemination activities that target persons with chronic illness.

RECOMMENDATIONS 1–5

Recommendations 1–4 are the result of the committee's efforts to answer statement of task question 2—which chronic diseases should be the focus of public health efforts to reduce disability and improve functioning and quality of life?

Recommendation 1

The committee recommends that CDC select a variety of illnesses for special consideration based on a planning process that first and foremost emphasizes the inclusion of chronic illnesses with cross-cutting clinical, functional, and social implications that impact the individuals who live with them. In addition, the committee suggests that other important criteria for illness selection include

- nonduplication with major illnesses for which public health programs have already been developed (e.g. cardiovascular disease, stroke);
- those with important implications for various models of chronic illness care, such as public health, health system, and self-care programs, especially when effective health service interventions are possible;
- variation in organ systems and long-term clinical manifestations and outcomes; and
- those for which the effective public health preventive interventions are either most feasible or at least the subject of promising research.

Recommendation 2

Although research has attempted to characterize MCCs, the complexity of single chronic illnesses over time has not allowed for MCC taxonomies that will be easily applicable to public health control of chronic diseases. Thus, the committee recommends that CDC:

1. Continue to review the scientific literature to monitor for potential MCC taxonomies that are useful for planning, executing, and evaluating disease control programs of MCC occurrences.
2. Explore surveillance techniques that are more likely to capture MCCs effectively. This should include counting not merely the co-occurrence of diseases and conditions but also the order of occurrence and the impact on quality of life and personal function.
3. Emphasize MCC prevention by selecting for execution and evaluation one or more exploratory public health interventions aimed at preventing or altering the course of new disease occurrences in patients with MCCs or who are at risk for them. This might include established approaches, such as tobacco control or experimental approaches, such as metabolic or genetic screening.

4. Increase demonstration programs for chronic disease control that cut across specific diseases or MCCs and emphasize mitigating the secondary consequences of a variety of chronic conditions, such as falls, immobility, sleep disorders, and depression.

Recommendation 3

The committee recommends that the secretary of HHS support the states in developing comprehensive population-based strategic plans with specific goals, objectives, actions, time frames, and resources that focus on the management of chronic illness among their residents, including community-based efforts to address the health and social needs of people living with chronic illness and experiencing disparities in health outcomes. Such strategic plans should also include steps to collaborate with community-based organizations, the health care delivery system, employers and businesses, the media, and the academic community to improve living well for all residents with chronic illness, including those experiencing disparities in health outcomes.

Recommendation 4

The committee recommends that, in addition to addressing individual illnesses in the community, all relevant federal and state agencies charged with public health and community approaches to control chronic illness, to the extent feasible, extend surveillance, evaluation, and mitigation programs to the widest possible range of chronic illnesses. This approach recognizes the commonality of important health, functional, and social outcomes for the population of individuals who live with different chronic illnesses.

Finally, the committee offers a fifth recommendation to answer the question what is the role of primary prevention (for those at highest risk) secondary, and tertiary prevention of chronic disease in reducing or minimizing life impacts?

Recommendation 5

The committee recommends that the federal health and related agencies that create and promulgate guidelines for general and community and clinical preventive services evaluate the effectiveness of these services for persons with chronic illness, and specifically catalog and disseminate these guidelines to the public health and health care organizations that implement them.

CHRONIC ILLNESS AND THE NATION'S
HEALTH AND ECONOMIC WELL-BEING

Chronic illness imposes very considerable costs on society. This is due to many factors, including their high—and, in many cases, apparently increasing—prevalence; the aging of the population; advances in treatment that help maintain many individuals; their occurrence across the life course, despite being somewhat stereotypically associated with older ages; and the highly disabling nature of many chronic illnessess, especially when inadequately treated.

In Chapter 1, the committee mentions a number of different methods for quantifying the consequences of chronic illness at a population level, including methods for assessing disability and premature mortality; "direct" costs of medical care and other services provided to prevent and/or treat chronic illness; and "indirect" costs of chronic illness, such as reduced labor output and other consequences that lie beyond the health care system. Such methods can and in many cases have been used to estimate the consequences associated with particular illnesses or categories of illness. Thus, it might be natural to ask what such methods explain in terms of which consequences of chronic illness—or even which specific chronic illnesses—are most important for the nation's health and economic well-being. In this section, we provide some conceptual discussion of this issue, from a national population perspective. Earlier in this chapter, the committee provides additional details on the health, economic, and other consequences of chronic illnesses at a more "micro" level, from the perspective of the people who have such illnessess and others in their communities.

Most fundamentally, chronic illnesses can reduce the quality of life of the people who live with them, via the symptoms and dysfunctions they cause. In economic terms, one manifestation of this is that chronic illness degrades society's productive capacity by reducing people's labor output, with people withdrawing from the labor market entirely due to poor health, shifting from full-time to part-time work and/or missing work periodically, accumulating less "human capital" (i.e., knowledge and skills), and being less effective at work ("presenteeism"). At the individual level, this may be reflected in lower earnings and other negative consequences among the people who have the chronic illness(es). At the societal level, a given person's reduced productivity may also reduce the productivity of others, such as in teamwork settings, and—very importantly for many chronic illnesses—via informal caregiving. The disease burden borne by people who would be outside the formal labor force in any case, such as retired people, is also important to consider. While lost labor earnings are irrelevant, retirees' potential contributions to society are potentially large and not limited to their labor market participation. Indeed, most generally, a person's suffering—or premature mortality—has negative consequences for the person's family, friends, and others. In all these ways, potentially preventable negative consequences of illness represent an opportunity cost to society.

These costs related to work and retirement described above generally fall in the category of "indirect" costs of illness. There are, of course, also very considerable "direct" costs associated with chronic illness—that is, the costs of health care per se—outpatient and inpatient treatment, diagnostic tests and other ancillary services, prescription and nonprescription pharmaceuticals, medical devices, therapy/rehabilitation services, and so on, as well as public health initiatives focused on primary or secondary prevention. Direct costs represent an opportunity cost for the people or institutions (e.g., insurers, employers, taxpayers) who pay for the services, in the sense that most health care is an "intermediate good" that is consumed not for its own sake but because of its (expected) effect on health; without a particular disease burden, these resources could be used for other purposes. However, direct costs also represent income/earnings for the people or institutions providing the care and are thus not entirely a deadweight loss. Despite general skepticism about the sustainability of the nation's direct health care spending—which has risen in absolute terms and as a percentage of national income throughout recent decades (Kaiser Family Foundation, 2010)—there is no objective standard for how much health care spending is too much. Still, the direct costs associated with chronic illness have many adverse societal consequences, including that they undermine public and private health insurance programs.

It is important to recognize that there is a kind of reciprocal relationship between direct and indirect costs. For example, public health investments are specifically intended to prevent illness, which both promotes well-being and reduces the need for health care services. Thus, up-front costs of effective public health interventions can raise direct costs while being implemented but decrease indirect costs via successful disease prevention. At the same time, clinical health care services are, in no small part, intended to preserve or restore well-being, including work and social functioning and the ability to live independently. Health care can also raise the direct costs of an illness while decreasing the indirect costs. In contrast, poor or restricted access to effective preventive or curative services can lower—or increase—direct costs while increasing indirect costs, sometimes drastically. As a result, one can't simply add direct and indirect costs for particular diseases to generate a "total" cost to society of those diseases, and the methods for determining the costs of illness are thus extremely complex. The relevant question is what would happen to the disease burden associated with a given condition if direct costs for that condition were higher, lower, or had a different composition than under the status quo.

In this sense, the most important consequences of chronic illness are those that could be prevented efficiently. Information on current disease burden—whether in the form of direct and/or indirect costs—is not by itself sufficient information to prioritize new investments in prevention or treatment, nor in research and development. At an economic level, new spending should be relatively cost-effective, in terms of yielding as large a benefit as possible for a given cost (or, for research and development, as large an expected benefit as possible, since the outcome of such efforts is uncertain in general). There may also be ethical or other reasons to prioritize prevention and treatment of particular diseases, or for particular population subgroups, beyond their cumulative burden of illness or even the cost-effectiveness of intervention.

In Chapter 1, the committee referenced a body of research that has estimated direct health care costs in the United States overall (i.e., the national health accounts [CMS, 2009]) and for certain chronic diseases or disease categories, as well as a complementary literature that has examined indirect costs attributed to certain diseases or disease categories. In principle, such evidence could support identifying diseases with the largest economic burden in particular categories, and/or the categories of cost that are most salient across chronic diseases overall. In practice, however, we think that the available evidence is currently inadequate to support this in any robust way.

For example, while the U.S. national health accounts apply a consistent methodology across the spectrum of health and health care, these accounts cannot currently be broken out by diseases or disease category (with the exception of mental and substance use disorders), as noted in Chapter 1. Also, of particular relevance for this report, the U.S. national health accounts do not fully capture public health interventions that may be relevant for preventing or otherwise mitigating chronic disease. They do count direct costs of "publicly provided health services such as epidemiological surveillance, inoculations, immunization/vaccination services, disease prevention programs, the operation of public health laboratories, and other such functions" (CMS, 2009, p. 26). However, the committee could not determine to what extent the national health accounts capture spending on health promotion and disease prevention initiatives that are not delivered directly to individuals, such as disability-friendly urban design. Also, they specifically exclude "government spending for public works, environmental functions (air and water pollution abatement, sanitation and sewage treatment, water supplies, and so on)" (CMS, 2009, p. 26), although this includes some core aspects of public health that are intended to—and in practice do—mitigate the societal burden of many chronic diseases.

In terms of assessing the costs of specific diseases or disease categories, the cost of illness literature consists of many distinct studies of direct and—in our estimation, less commonly—indirect costs. With important exceptions, such as the Milken Institute study mentioned in Chapter 1 that assessed costs in five major categories of illness, most condition-specific studies have been conducted independently of each other. In practice, the studies in this literature have generally been different in terms of their data sources, scope of assessed costs, period of assessment, and other aspects of methodology. This makes it difficult or impossible to compare findings across different diseases in a consistent way, even for those diseases for which data are available. The committee also notes that some studies in this literature have been sponsored and/or conducted by entities with a stake in the outcome.

Another issue with the available literature on direct and indirect costs of particular chronic diseases is that a given cost may be counted multiple times across different studies, for example, because of difficulty attributing particular direct or indirect costs to a given disease. This is a risk even across studies that have used approximately equivalent methodology. Such double-counting may particularly affect accounting for the direct costs of public health interventions, which may target multiple diseases simultaneously, or even target no condition per se but affect rates and outcomes for multiple conditions. Finally, as is generally true of all health indicators, data on direct and indirect costs at a national level may mask considerable variation across subnational areas and/or population subgroups.

There are a number of ways to improve the quality and utility of information on the economic burdens of chronic disease, and—importantly—on opportunities to prevent or reduce them. For example, disease-specific national health accounts, as proposed by Rosen and Cutler (2009), could provide useful new information by illuminating not only the total direct costs attributable to particular diseases but also the current composition of those costs across types of service. More comprehensive capture of public health programs that encompass estimates of direct costs, including such programs that focus on communities and interventions that address varied diseases as well as individuals with MCCs rather than individuals, including those that may affect many different chronic (and acute) illnesses, would also be valuable. This seems relatively straightforward in the overall national health accounts, in which attribution to specific diseases is not required, but even disease-specific estimates should explicitly address the role of general/broad public health and other interventions that affect the disease(s) of interest.

Improving population health surveillance systems at the national and the subnational level would contribute substantially to the ability to assess direct and especially indirect costs of illness along with other measures of disease burden and health status. It would also be likely to inform the development and targeting of new disease prevention and treatment programs and aid in assessing the potential costs and benefits of investments in such programs. Perhaps most valuable, however, would be a systematic effort to assess not only the burdens associated with particular diseases but also the opportunity—and opportunity costs—of potential investments in their prevention and treatment. In this context, we endorse the concept—if not necessarily the specific methods or substantive findings—of efforts of this type conducted in other settings. For instance, the Disease Control Priorities Project (DCPP, [a]) examined a wide range of health problems affecting developing countries (including some consideration of chronic diseases). The Copenhagen Consensus Center (Copenhagen Consensus Center, [a]) has conducted analogous research on a wide range of health and non-health issues, including a recent program to identify investment priorities in HIV/AIDS prevention. And the new Center for Medicare and Medicaid Innovation (Center for Medicare and Medicaid Innovation, [a]) created as part of the Affordable Care Act of 2010, is specifically seeking to identify interventions to address the so-called triple aim of improving the health of the population; enhancing the patient experience of care (including quality, access, and reliability); and reducing, or at least controlling, the per capita cost of care (Institute for Healthcare Improvement, [a]). The committee thinks that a similar approach could be applied to identify high-priority opportunities to improve the lives of people living with chronic illness.

RECOMMENDATION 6

The statement of task asks the committee to consider what consequences of chronic disease are most important to the nation's health and well-being.

Recommendation 6

The committee recommends that CDC support the greater use of new and emerging economic methods, as well as those currently in use, in making policy decisions that will promote living well with chronic illnesses, including

1. those with greater use of cost-effectiveness techniques;
2. more exploitation of methods used in determining national health accounts, but for specific and important chronic illnesses with long-term outcomes;
3. enhanced consideration of opportunity costs for various program decisions; and
4. those with a greater focus on economic evaluation of interventions that involve MCCs and cut across a variety of community settings.

REFERENCES

AAOS (American Academy of Orthopaedic Surgeons). 2008. Chapter 4. Arthritis and related conditions. In *The Burden of Musculoskeletal Diseases in the United States: Prevalence, Societal and Economic Cost.* Pp. 75–102. http://www.boneandjointburden.org/pdfs/BMUS_chpt4_arthritis.pdf (accessed October 20, 2011).

Agostini, J.V., L. Han, and M.E. Tinetti. 2004. The relationship between number of medications and weight loss or impaired balance in older adults. *Journal of the American Geriatrics Society* 52(10):1719–1723.

Alzheimer's Association. 2006. *Early-Onset Dementia. A National Challenge, a Future Crisis.* Washington, DC: Alzheimer's Association. http://www.alz.org/national/documents/report_earlyonset_summary.pdf (accessed October 5, 2011).

Alzheimer's Association. 2011a. Alzheimer's disease facts and figures. *Alzheimer's and Dementia* 7(2). http://www.alz.org/downloads/Facts_Figures_2011.pdf (accessed October 5, 2011).

Alzheimer's Association. 2011b. *California's Alzheimer's Statistics.* http://www.alz.org/documents_custom/Facts_2011/ALZ_CA.pdf?type=interior_map&facts=undefined&facts=facts (accessed October 5, 2011).

American Diabetes Association. 2010. Diagnosis and classification of diabetes mellitus. *Diabetes Care* 33(Supplemental 1):S62-S69.

American Diabetes Association. 2011. Standards of medical care in diabetes. *Diabetes Care.* 34(Suppl 1):S11-S61.

American Stroke Association (a). *Warning Signs.* http://www.strokeassociation.org/STROKE ORG/WarningSigns/Warning-Signs_UCM_308528_SubHomePage.jsp (accessed September 2, 2011).

Anderson, G.F. 2005. Medicare and chronic conditions. *New England Journal of Medicine* 353(3):305–309.

Arrighi, H.M., P.J. Neumann, I.M. Lieberburg, and R.J. Townsend. 2010. Lethality of Alzheimer's disease and its impact on nursing home placement. *Alzheimer Disease and Associated Disorders* 24(1):90–95.

Arthritis Foundation. 2008. *Primer on Rheumatic Disease,* 13th ed. Edited by J.H. Klippel, J.H. Stone, L.J. Crofford, and P.H. White. New York: Springer and Arthritis Foundation.

Arthritis Foundation and CDC (Centers for Disease Control and Prevention). 2010. *A National Public Health Agenda for Osteoarthritis.* http://www.cdc.gov/arthritis/docs/oaagenda.pdf (accessed October 15, 2011).

Awad, A.G., and L.N. Voruganti. 2008. The burden of schizophrenia on caregivers: A review. *Pharmoeconomics* 26(2):149–162.

Bair, M.J., R.L. Robinson, W. Katon, and K. Kroenke. 2003. Depression and pain comorbidity: A literature review. *Archives of Internal Medicine* 163(20):2433–2445.

Baker, D.W., J.A. Gazmararian, M.V. Williams, T. Scott, R.M. Parker, D. Green, J. Ren, and J. Peel. 2002. Functional health literacy and the risk of hospital admission among Medicare managed care enrollees. *American Journal of Public Health* 92(8):1278–1283.

Bayliss, E.A., J.F. Steiner, D.H. Fernald, L.A. Crane, and D.S. Main. 2003. Descriptions of barriers to self-care by persons with comorbid chronic diseases. *Annals of Family Medicine* 1(1):15–21.

Berkman, N.D., S.L. Sheridan, K.E. Donahue, D.J. Halpern, and K. Crotty. 2011. Low health literacy and health outcomes: An updated systematic review. *Annals of Internal Medicine* 155(2):97–107.

Beswick, A.D., K. Rees, P. Dieppe, S. Ayis, R. Gooberman-Hill, J. Horwood, and S. Ebrahim. 2008. Complex interventions to improve physical function and maintain independent living in elderly people: A systematic review and meta-analysis. *Lancet* 371(9614):725–735.

Biessels, G.J., I.J. Deary, and C.M. Ryan. 2008. Cognition and diabetes: A lifespan perspective. *Lancet Neurology* 7:184–190.

Bolen, J., L. Murphy, K. Greenlund, C.G. Helmick, J. Hootman, T.J. Brady, G. Langmaid, and N. Keenan. 2009. Arthritis as a potential barrier to physical activity among adults with heart disease—United States, 2005 and 2007. *MMWR* 58(7):165–169. http://www.cdc.gov/mmwr/PDF/wk/mm5807.pdf (accessed November 16, 2011).

Bower, J.E. 2008. Behavioral symptoms in patients with breast cancer and survivors. *Journal of Clinical Oncology* 26(5):768–777.

Boyd, C.M., J. Darer, C. Boult, L.P. Fried, L. Boult, and A.W. Wu. 2005. Clinical practice guidelines and quality of care for older patients with multiple comorbid diseases: implications for pay for performance. *Journal of the American Medical Association* 294(6):716–724.

Bradford, A.N., R.C. Castillo, A.R. Carlini, S.T. Wegener, H. Teter, Jr., and E.J. Mackenzie. 2011. The trauma survivors network: Survive. Connect. Rebuild. *The Journal of Trauma* 70:1557–1560.

Bradley, C., and C.J. Gilbride. 2008. Improving treatment satisfaction and other patient-reported outcomes in people with type 2 diabetes: The role of once-daily insulin glargine. *Diabetes, Obesity, and Metabolism* 10(Suppl 2):50–65.

Bradley, C., and J. Speight. 2002. Patient perceptions of diabetes and diabetes therapy: Assessing quality of life. *Diabetes/Metabolism Research and Reviews* 18(Suppl 3):S64–S69.

Bradley, C., P. de Pablos-Velasco, K.G. Parhofer, E. Eschwège, L. Gönder-Frederick, and D. Simon. 2011. PANORAMA: A European study to evaluate quality of life and treatment satisfaction in patients with type 2 diabetes mellitus—Study design. *Primary Care Diabetes*. 2011 Jul 11 [Epub ahead of print].

Brézin, A.P., A. Lafuma, F. Fagnani, M. Mesbah, and G. Berdeaux. 2005. Prevalence and burden of self-reported blindness, low vision, and visual impairment in the French community: A nationwide survey. *Archives of Ophthalmology* 123(8):1117–1124.

Brookmeyer, R., M.M. Corrada, F.C. Curriero, and C. Kawas. 2002. Survival following a diagnosis of Alzheimer's disease. *Archives of Neurology* 59(11):1764–1767.

Callahan, C.M., M.A. Boustani, F.W. Unverzagt, M.G. Austrom, T.M. Damush, A.J. Perkins, B.A. Fultz, S.L. Hui, S.R. Counsell, and H.C. Hendrie. 2006. Effectiveness of collaborative care for older adults with Alzheimer disease in primary care: A randomized controlled trial. *Journal of the American Medical Association* 295(18):2148–2157.

Cannuscio, C.C., G.A. Colditz, E.B. Rimm, L.F. Berkman, C.P. Jones, and I. Kawachi. 2004. Employment status, social ties, and caregivers' mental health. *Social Science and Medicine* 58(7):1247–1256.

Casalino, L., R.R. Gillies, S.M. Shortell, J.A. Schmittdiel, T. Bodenheimer, J.C. Robinson, T. Rundall, N. Oswald, H. Schauffler, and M.C. Wang. 2003. External incentives, information technology, and organized processes to improve health care quality for patients with chronic diseases. *Journal of the American Medical Association* 289(4):434–441.

Cassell, E.J. 1983. The relief of suffering. *Archives of Internal Medicine* 143(3):522–523.

CDC (Centers for Disease Control and Prevention) (a). *Arthritis—Data and Statistics—Comorbidities*. http://www.cdc.gov/arthritis/data_statistics/comorbidities.htm (accessed October 5, 2011).

CDC (b). *Healthy People 2010 Leading Health Indicators at a Glance*. http://www.cdc.gov/nchs/healthy_people/hp2010/hp2010_indicators.htm (accessed October 5, 2011).

CDC (c). *Osteoarthritis*. http://www.cdc.gov/arthritis/basics/osteoarthritis.htm (accessed February 14, 2012).

CDC (d). *Winnable Battles*. http://www.cdc.gov/winnablebattles/ (accessed July 4, 2011).

CDC. 2011a. *Arthritis. Meeting the Challenge. At a Glance 2011.* Atlanta, GA. http://www.cdc.gov/chronicdisease/resources/publications/aag/pdf/2011/Arthritis-AAG-2011-508.pdf (accessed October 5, 2011).

CDC. 2011b. *National Diabetes Fact Sheet: National Estimates and General Information on Diabetes and Pre-diabetes in the United States, 2011.* Atlanta, GA. http://www.cdc.gov/diabetes/pubs/pdf/ndfs_2011.pdf (accessed November 16, 2011).

CDC. 2011c. *Public Health Action Plan to Integrate Mental Health Promotion and Mental Illness Prevention with Chronic Disease Prevention.* Atlanta, GA. http://www.cdc.gov/mentalhealth/docs/11_220990_Sturgis_MHMIActionPlan_FINAL-Web_tag508.pdf (accessed October 15, 2011).

CDC's Office of Minority Health and Health Disparities (a). *Fact Sheet—CDC Health Disparities and Inequalities Report—U.S., 2001.* http://www.cdc.gov/minorityhealth/reports/CHDIR11/FactSheet.pdf (accessed December 19, 2011).

Cella, D., W. Riley, A. Stone, N. Rothrock, B. Reeve, S. Yount, D. Amtmann, R. Bode, D. Buysse, S. Choi, K. Cook, R. Devellis, D. DeWalt, J.F. Fries, R. Gershon, E.A. Hahn, J.S. Lai, P. Pilkonis, D. Revicki, M. Rose, K. Weinfurt, R. Hays, and PROMIS Cooperative Group. 2010. The Patient-Reported Outcomes Measurement Information System (PROMIS) developed and tested its first wave of adult self-reported health outcome item banks: 2005-2008. *Journal of Clinical Epidemiology* 63(11):1179–1194.

Center for Medicare and Medicaid Innovation (a). *The CMS Innovation Center.* http://innovations.cms.gov/ (accessed December 19, 2011).

Center for Prevention and Health Services. 2009. *Eliminating Racial and Ethnic Health Disparities; A Business Case Update for Employers.* Washington, DC: Center for Prevention and Health Services. http://minorityhealth.hhs.gov/Assets/pdf/checked/1/Eliminating_Racial_Ethnic_Health_Disparities_A_Business_Case_Update_for_Employers.pdf (accessed December 19, 2011).

Charney, D.S., C.F. Reynolds, III, L. Lewis, B.D. Lebowitz, T. Sunderland, G.S. Alexopoulos, D.G. Blazer, I.R. Katz, B.S. Meyers, P.A. Arean, S. Borson, C. Brown, M.L. Bruce, C.M. Callahan, M.E. Charlson, Y. Conwell, B.N. Cuthbert, D.P. Devanand, M.J. Gibson, G.L. Gottlieb, K.R. Krishnan, S.K. Laden, C.G. Lyketsos, B.H. Mulsant, G. Niederehe, J.T. Olin, D.W. Oslin, J. Pearson, T. Persky, B.G. Pollock, S. Raetzman, M. Reynolds, C. Salzman, R. Schulz, T.L. Schwenk, E. Scolnick, J. Unützer, M.M. Weissman, R.C. Young, and Depression and Bipolar Support Alliance. 2003. Depression and Bipolar Support Alliance consensus statement on the unmet needs in diagnosis and treatment of mood disorders in late life. *Archives of General Psychiatry* 60(7):664–672.

Chen, W.H., A.S. Cross, R. Edelman, M.B. Sztein, W.C. Blackwelder, and M.F. Pasetti. 2011. Antibody and Th1-type cell-mediated immune responses in elderly and young adults immunized with the standard or a high dose influenza vaccine. *Vaccine* 29(16):2865–2873.

Chodosh, J., T.E. Seeman, E. Keeler, A. Sewall, S.H. Hirsch, J.M. Guralnik, and D.B. Reuben. 2004. Cognitive decline in high-functioning older persons is associated with an increased risk of hospitalization. *Journal of the American Geriatrics Society* 52(9):1456–1462.

Chu, T.F., M.A. Rupnick, R. Kerkela, S.M. Dallabrida, D. Zurakowski, L. Nguyen, K. Woulfe, E. Pravda, F. Cassiola, J. Desai, S. George, J.A. Morgan, D.M. Harris, N.S. Ismail, J.H. Chen, F.J. Schoen, A.D. Van den Abbeele, G.D. Demetri, T. Force, and M.H. Chen. 2007. Cardiotoxicity associated with tyrosine kinase inhibitor sunitinib. *Lancet* 370(9604):2011–2019.

Claridge, J.A., W.H. Leukhardt, J.F. Golob, A.M. McCoy, and M.A. Malangoni. 2010. Moving beyond traditional measurement of mortality after injury: Evaluation of risk factors for late death. *Journal of the American College of Surgeons* 210(5):788–796.

CMS (Centers for Medicare and Medicaid Services). 2009. *National Health Expenditures Accounts: Definitions, Sources, and Methods, 2009*. https://www.cms.gov/national healthexpenddata/downloads/dsm-09.pdf (accessed December 19, 2011).

Compton, W.M., K.P. Conway, F.S. Stinson, and B.F. Grant. 2006. Changes in the prevalence of major depression and comorbid substance use disorders in the United States between 1991-1992 and 2001-2002. *American Journal of Psychiatry* 163(12):2141–2147.

Copenhagen Consensus Center (a). http://www.copenhagenconsensus.com (accessed December 19, 2011).

Cormier, J.N., R.L. Askew, K.S. Mungovan, Y. Xing, M.I. Ross, and J.M. Armer. 2010. Lymphedema beyond breast cancer: A systematic review and meta-analysis of cancer-related secondary lymphedema. *Cancer* 6(22):5138–5149.

Corrigan, J.D., A.W. Selassie, and J.A. Orman. 2010. The epidemiology of traumatic brain injury. *Journal of Head Trauma Rehabilitation* 25(2):72–80.

Counsell, S.R., C.M. Callahan, D.O. Clark, W. Tu, A.B. Buttar, T.E. Stump, and G.D. Ricketts. 2007. Geriatric care management for low-income seniors: A randomized controlled trial. *Journal of the American Medical Association* 298(22):2623–2633.

Cowie, C.C., K.F. Rust, E.S. Ford, M.S. Eberhardt, D.D. Byrd-Holt, C. Li, D.E. Williams, E.W. Gregg, K.E. Bainbridge, S.H. Saydah, and L.S. Geiss. 2009. Full accounting of diabetes and pre-diabetes in the U.S. population in 1988-1994 and 2005-2006. *Diabetes Care* 32(2):287–294.

Cukierman, T., H.C. Gerstein, and J.D. Williamson. 2005. Cognitive decline and dementia in diabetes—systematic overview of prospective observational studies. *Diabetologia* 48(12):2460–2469.

Dalstra, J.A., A.E. Kunst, C. Borrell, E. Breeze, E. Cambois, G. Costa, J.M. Geurts, E. Lahelma, H. Van Oyen, N.K. Rasmussen, E. Regidor, T. Spadea, and J.P. Mackenbach. 2005. Socioeconomic differences in the prevalence of common chronic diseases: An overview of eight European countries. *International Journal of Epidemiology* 34(2):316–326.

DCPP (The Disease Control Priorities Project) (a). *About DCPP*. http://www.dcp2.org/page/main/Home.html (accessed December 19, 2011).

De Groot, M., R. Anderson, K.E. Freedland, R.E. Clouse, and P.J. Lustman. 2001. Association of depression and diabetes complications: A meta-analysis. *Psychosomatic Medicine* 63(4):619–630.

De Rekeneire, N., H.E. Resnick, A.V. Schwartz, R.I. Shorr, L.H. Kuller, E.M. Simonsick, B. Vellas, T.B. Harris, and Health, Aging, and Body Composition study. 2003. Diabetes is associated with subclinical functional limitation in nondisabled older individuals: The Health, Aging, and Body Composition study. *Diabetes Care* 26(12):3257–3263.

Dhalla, I.A., G.M. Anderson, M.M. Mamdani, S.E. Bronskill, K. Sykora, and P.A. Rochon. 2002. Inappropriate prescribing before and after nursing home admission. *Journal of American Geriatrics Society* 50(6):995–1000.

Egede, L.E. 2004. Diabetes, major depression, and functional disability among U.S. adults. *Diabetes Care* 27(2):421–428.

Fazel, S., N. Långström, A. Hjern, M. Grann, and P. Lichtenstein. 2009. Schizophrenia, substance abuse, and violent crime. *Journal of the American Medical Association* 301(19):2016–2023.

Floyd, J.D., D.T. Nguyen, R.L. Lobins, Q. Bashir, D.C. Doll, and M.C. Perry. 2005. Cardiotoxicity of cancer therapy. *Journal of Clinical Oncology* 23(30):7685–7696.

Freburger, J.K., G.M. Holmes, R.P. Agans, A.M. Jackman, J.D. Darter, A.S. Wallace, L.D. Castel, W.D. Kalsbeek, and T.S. Carey. 2009. The rising prevalence of chronic low back pain. *Archives of Internal Medicine* 169(3):251–258.

Frick, K.D., E.W. Gowe, J.H. Kempen, and J.L. Wolff. 2007. Economic impact of visual impairment and blindness in the United States. *Archives of Ophthalmology* 125(4):544–550.

Ganguli, M., H.H. Dodge, C. Shen, R.S. Pandav, S.T. DeKosky. 2005. Alzheimer's disease and mortality: A 15-year epidemiological study. *Archives of Neurology* 62(5):779–784.

Gardetto, N.J. 2011. Self-management in heart failure: Where have we been and where should we go? *Journal of Multidisciplinary Healthcare* 4:39–51.

Gazmararian, J.A., M.V. Williams, J. Peel, and D.W. Baker. 2003. Health literacy and knowledge of chronic disease. *Patient Education and Counseling* 51(3):267–275.

Gilbody, S., P. Bower, J. Fletcher, D. Richards, and A.J. Sutton. 2006. Collaborative care for depression: A cumulative meta-analysis and review of longer-term outcomes. *Archives of Internal Medicine* 166(21):2314–2321.

Giovannetti, E.R., J.L. Wolff, K.D. Frick, and C. Boult. 2009. Construct validity of the Work Productivity and Activity Impairment questionnaire across informal caregivers of chronically ill older patients. *Value Health* 12(6):1011–1017.

Goetzel, R.Z., K. Hawkins, R.J. Ozminkowski, and S. Wang. 2003. The health and productivity cost burden of the "top 10" physical and mental health conditions affecting six large U.S. employers in 1999. *Journal of Occupational and Environmental Medicine* 45(1):5–14.

Gonzalez, J.S., M. Peyrot, L.A. McCarl, E.M. Collins, L. Serpa, M.J. Mimaga, and S.A. Safren. 2008. Depression and diabetes treatment nonadherence: A meta-analysis. *Diabetes Care* 31(12):2398–2403.

Green, C.R., K.O. Anderson, T.A. Baker, L.C. Campbell, S. Decker, R.B. Fillingim, D.A. Kaloukalani, K.E. Lasch, C. Myers, R.C. Tait, K.H. Todd, and A.H. Vallerand. 2003. The unequal burden of pain: Confronting racial and ethnic disparities in pain. *Pain Medicine* 4(3):277–294.

Gregg, E.W., G.L. Beckles, D.F. Williamson, S.G. Leveille, J.A. Langlois, M.M. Engelgau, and K.M. Narayan. 2000. Diabetes and physical disability among older U.S. adults. *Diabetes Care* 23(9):1272–1277.

Guitera, V., P. Muñoz, J. Castillo, and J. Pascual. 2002. Quality of life in chronic daily headache: A study in a general population. *Neurology* 58(7):1062–1065.

Hahn, B., S. Dogra, and S. King-Zeller. 2001. Impact of chronic pain on health care resource use, daily activities and family burden. *Pain Medicine* 1(2):195–196.

Ham, C. 1997. Priority setting in health care: Learning from international experience. *Health Policy* 42(1):49–66.

Havercamp, S.M., D. Scandlin, and M. Roth. 2004. Health disparities among adults with developmental disabilities, adults with other disabilities, and adults not reporting disability in North Carolina. *Public Health Reports* 119(4):418–426.

Helzner, E.P., N. Scarmeas, S. Cosentino, M.X. Tang, N. Schupf, and Y. Stern. 2008. Survival in Alzheimer's disease: A multiethnic, population-based study of incident cases. *Neurology* 71(19):1489–1495.

Hewitt, M., J.H. Rowland, and R. Yancik. 2003. Cancer survivors in the United States: Age, health, and disability. *Journals of Gerontology: Series A, Biological Sciences and Medical Sciences* 58(1):82–91.

HHS (U.S. Department of Health and Human Services), Office of Disease Prevention and Health Promotion. 2010. *National Action Plan to Improve Health Literacy*. Washington, DC. http://www.health.gov/communication/hlactionplan/pdf/Health_Literacy_Action_Plan.pdf (accessed October 6, 2011).

Hootman, J.M., and C.G. Helmick. 2006: Projections of U.S. prevalence of arthritis and associated activity limitations. *Arthritis Rheumatology* 54(1):226–229.

Horowitz, A. 2003. Depression and vision and hearing impairments in later life. *Generations* 27:32–38.

Institute for Healthcare Improvement (a). *The IHI Triple Aim*. http://www.ihi.org/offerings/Initiatives/TripleAim/Pages/default.aspx (accessed December 19, 2011).

IOM (Institute of Medicine). 1999. *To Err Is Human: Building a Safer Health System*. Washington, DC: National Academy Press.

IOM. 2003a. *The Future of the Public's Health in the 21st Century*. Washington, DC: The National Academies Press.

IOM. 2003b. *Unequal Treatment: Confronting Racial and Ethnic Disparities in Health Care*. Washington, DC: The National Academies Press. [OU—PUB DATE IS 2003]

IOM. 2009. *Retooling for an Aging America: Building the Health Care Workforce*. Washington, DC: The National Academies Press.

IOM. 2011a. *Leading Health Indicators for Healthy People 2020 Letter Report*. Washington, DC: The National Academies Press.

IOM. 2011b. *Relieving Pain in America: A Blueprint for Transforming Prevention, Care, Education, and Research*. Washington, DC: The National Academies Press.

IOM and NRC (National Research Council). 2006. *From Cancer Patient to Cancer Survivor— Lost in Transition: An American Society of Clinical Oncology and Institute of Medicine Symposium*. Washington, DC: The National Academies Press.

Ivanova, J.I., H.G. Birnbaum, Y. Kidolezi, G. Subramanian, S.A. Khan, and M.D. Stensland. 2010. Direct and indirect costs of employees with treatment-resistant and non-treatment-resistant major depressive disorder. *Current Medical Research and Opinion* 26(10):2475–2484.

Jennings, A.M., K.S. Lewis, S. Murdoch, J.F. Talbot, C. Bradley, and J.D. Ward. 1991. Randomized trial comparing continuous subcutaneous insulin infusion and conventional insulin therapy in type II diabetic patients poorly controlled with sulfonylureas. *Diabetes Care* 14(8):738–744.

Jensen, M.P., M.J. Chernoff, and R.H. Dworkin. 2007. The impact of neuropathic pain on health-related quality of life: Review and implications. *Neurology* 68(15):1178–1182.

Jeon, Y., B. Essue, S. Jan, R. Wells, and J.A. Whitworth. 2009. Economic hardship associated with managing chronic illness: A qualitative inquiry. *BMC Health Services Research* 9:182. http://www.biomedcentral.com/1472-6963/9/182 (accessed November 17, 2011).

Jeschke, M.G., G.G. Gauglitz, G.A. Kulp, C.C. Finnerty, F.N. Williams, R. Kraft, O.E. Suman, R.P. Mlcak, and D.N. Herndon. 2011. Long-term persistence of the pathophysiological response to severe burn injury. *PLoS One* 6(7):e21245.

Kaiser Family Foundation. 2010. *U.S. Health Care Costs*. http://www.kaiseredu.org/Issue-Modules/US-Health-Care-Costs/Background-Brief.aspx (accessed October 12, 2011).

Kalyani, R.R., C.D. Saudek, F.L. Brancati, and E. Selvin. 2010. Association of diabetes, comorbidities, and A1C with functional disability in older adults: Results from the National Health and Nutrition Examination Survey (NHANES), 1999-2006. *Diabetes Care* 33(5):1055–1060.

Katon, W., M. Sullivan, and E. Walker. 2001. Medical symptoms without identified pathology: Relationship to psychiatric disorders, childhood and adult trauma, and personality traits. *Annals of Internal Medicine* 134(9, Part 2):917–925.

Katon, W., E.H. Lin, and K. Kroenke. 2007. The association of depression and anxiety with medical symptom burden in patients with chronic medical illness. *General Hospital Psychiatry* 29(2):147–155.

Katon, W., J. Unützer, K. Wells, and L. Jones. 2010. Collaborative depression care: History, evolution and ways to enhance dissemination and sustainability. *General Hospital Psychiatry* 32(5):456–464.

Keeler, E., J.M. Guralnik, H. Tian, R.B. Wallace, and D.B. Reuben. 2010. The impact of functional status on life expectancy in older persons. *Journals of Gerontology: Series A, Biological and Medical Sciences* 65(7):727–733.

Kessler, R.C., H. Birnbaum, E. Bromet, I. Hwang, N. Sampson, and V. Shahly. 2010. Age differences in major depression: Results from the National Comorbidity Survey Replication (NCS-R). *Psychological Medicine* 40(2):225–237.

Khan, A.S. 2011. Public health preparedness and response in the USA since 9/11: A national health security imperative. *Lancet* 378(9794):953–956.

Klein, R., B.E. Klein, S.E. Moss, M.D. Davis, and D.L. DeMets. 1989. The Wisconsin Epidemiologic Study of Diabetic Retinopathy. X. Four-year incidence and progression of diabetic retinopathy when age at diagnosis is 30 years or more. *Archives of Ophthalmology* 107(2):244–249.

Kongkaew, C., P.R. Noyce, and D.M. Ashcroft. 2008. Hospital admissions associated with adverse drug reactions: A systematic review of prospective observational studies. *Annals of Pharmacotherapy* 42(7):1017–1025.

Kuzuya, M., and Y. Hirakawa. 2009. Increased caregiver burden associated with hearing impairment but not vision impairment in disabled community-dwelling older people in Japan. *Journal of the American Geriatrics Society* 57(2):357–358.

Larson, E.B., M.F. Shadlen, L. Wang, W.C. McCormick, J.D. Bowen, L. Teri, and W.A. Kukull. 2004. Survival after initial diagnosis of Alzheimer disease. *Annals of Internal Medicine* 140(7):501–509.

Lawrence, D., S. Kisely, and J. Pais. 2010. The epidemiology of excess mortality in people with mental illness. *Canadian Journal of Psychiatry* 55(12):752–760.

Lebowitz, B.D., J.L. Pearson, L.S. Schneider, C.F. Reynolds, III, G.S. Alexopoulos, M.L. Bruce, Y. Conwell, I.R. Katz, B.S. Meyers, M.F. Morrison, J. Mossey, G. Niederehe, and P. Parmelee. 1997. Diagnosis and treatment of depression in late life. Consensus statement update. *Journal of the American Medical Association* 278(14):1186–1190.

Lee, S., G.A. Colditz, L.F. Berkman, and I. Kawachi. 2003. Caregiving and risk of coronary heart disease in U.S. women: A prospective study. *American Journal of Preventive Medicine* 24(2):113–119.

Lilly, M.B., A. LaPorte, and P.C. Coyte. 2007. Labor market work and home care's unpaid caregivers: A systematic review of labor force participation rates, predictors of labor market withdrawal, and hours of work. *The Milbank Quarterly* 85(4):641–690.

Lin, E.H., W. Katon, M. Von Korff, C. Rutter, G.E. Simon, M. Oliver, P. Ciechanowski, E.J. Ludman, T. Bush, and B. Young. 2004. Relationship of depression and diabetes self-care, medication adherence, and preventive care. *Diabetes Care* 27(9):2154–2160.

Lind, H., A.C. Waldenström, G. Dunberger, M. al-Abany, E. Alevronta, K.A. Johansson, C. Olsson, T. Nyberg, U. Wilderäng, G. Steineck, and E. Åvall-Lundqvist. 2011. Late symptoms in long-term gynaecological cancer survivors after radiation therapy: A population-based cohort study. *British Journal of Cancer* 105(6):737–745.

Linton, S.J. 2002. Early identification and intervention in the prevention of musculoskeletal pain. *American Journal of Industrial Medicine* 41(5):433–442.

Linton, S.J., and M. Ryberg. 2001. A cognitive-behavioral group intervention as prevention for persistent neck and back pain in a non-patient population: A randomized controlled trial. *Pain* 90(1–2):83–90.

Livingston, D.H., T. Tripp, C. Biggs, and R.F. Lavery. 2009. A fate worse than death? Long-term outcome of trauma patients admitted to the surgical intensive care unit. *Journal of Trauma* 67(2):341–348.

Lustman, P.J., R.J. Anderson, K.E. Freedland, M. De Groot, R.M. Carney, and R.E. Clouse. 2000. Depression and poor glycemic control: A meta-analytic review of the literature. *Diabetes Care* 23(7):934–942.

Lyness, J.M., A. Niculescu, X. Tu, C.F. Reynolds, III, and E.D. Caine. 2006. The relationship of medical comorbidity and depression in older, primary care patients. *Psychosomatics* 47(5):435–439.

Magaziner, J., P. German, S.I. Zimmerman, J.R. Hebel, L. Burton, A.L. Gruber-Baldini, C. May, and S. Kittner. 2000. The prevalence of dementia in a statewide sample of new nursing home admissions aged 65 and older: Diagnosis by expert panel. Epidemiology of Dementia in Nursing Homes Research Group. *Gerontologist* 40(6):663–672.

Mao, J.J., C. Stricker, D. Bruner, S. Xie, M.A. Bowman, J.T. Farrar, B.T. Greene, and A. DeMichele. 2009. Patterns and risk factors associated with aromatase inhibitor-related arthralgia among breast cancer survivors. *Cancer* 115(16):3631–3639.

Maty, S.C., L.P. Fried, S. Volpato, J. Williamson, F.L. Brancati, and C.S. Blaum. 2004. Patterns of disability related to diabetes mellitus in older women. *Journals of Gerontology: Series A, Biological and Medical Sciences* 59(2):148–153.

McNeil, J.M., and J. Binette. 2001. Prevalence of disabilities and associated health conditions among adults—United States, 1999. *MMWR* 50(7):120–125. http://www.cdc.gov/mmwr/ preview/mmwrhtml/mm5007a3.htm (accessed November 16, 2011).

McWilliams, L.A., B.J. Cox, and M.W. Enns. 2003. Mood and anxiety disorders associated with chronic pain: An examination in a nationally representative sample. *Pain* 106(1–2):127–133.

Merikangas, K.R., M. Ames, L. Cui, P.E. Stang, T.B. Ustun, M. Von Korff, and R.C. Kessler. 2007. The impact of comorbidity of mental and physical conditions on role disability in the U.S. adult household population. *Archives of General Psychiatry* 64(10):1180–1188.

Mezuk, B., W.W. Eaton, S. Albrecht, and S.H. Golden. 2008. Depression and type 2 diabetes over the lifespan: A meta-analysis. *Diabetes Care* 31(12):2383–2390.

Michaud, C.M., M.T. McKenna, S. Begg, N. Tomijima, M. Majmudar, M.T. Bulzacchelli, S. Ebrahim, M. Ezzati, J.A. Salomon, J.G. Kreiser, M. Hogan, and C.J. Murray. 2006. The burden of disease and injury in the United States 1996. *Population Health Metrics* 4(11). http://www.pophealthmetrics.com/content/4/1/11 (accessed November 16, 2011).

Michel, P., J.L. Quenon, A.M. de Sarasqueta, and O. Scemama. 2004. Comparison of three methods for estimating rates of adverse events and rates of preventable adverse events in acute care hospitals. *British Medical Journal* 328(7433):199. http://www.bmj.com/ content/328/7433/199.full (accessed November 17, 2011).

Mitchell, A.J., D. Malone, and C.C. Doebbeling. 2009. Quality of medical care for people with and without comorbid mental illness and substance misuse: Systematic review of comparative studies. *The British Journal of Psychiatry: The Journal of Mental Science* 194(6):491–499.

Mohr, P.E., J.J. Feldman, J.L. Dunbar, A. McConkey-Robbins, J.K. Niparko, R.K. Rittenhouse, and M.W. Skinner. 2000. The societal costs of severe to profound hearing loss in the United States. *International Journal of Technology Assessment in Health Care* 16(4): 1120–1135.

Mokdad, A.H., J.S. Marks, D.F. Stroup, and J.L. Gerberding. 2004. Actual causes of death in the United States, 2000. *Journal of the American Medical Association* 291(10):1238–1245.

Munshi, M., L. Grande, M. Hayes, D. Ayres, E. Suhl, R. Capelson, S. Lin, W. Milberg, and K. Weinger. 2006. Cognitive dysfunction is associated with poor diabetes control in older adults. *Diabetes Care* 29(8):1794–1799.

Murphy, J.M., N.M. Laird, R.R. Monson, A.M. Sobol, and A.H. Leighton. 2000. A 40-year perspective on the prevalence of depression: The Stirling County Study. *Archives of General Psychiatry* 57(3):209–215.

Murphy, L., T.A. Schwartz, C.G. Helmick, J.B. Renner, G. Tudor, G. Koch, A. Dragomir, W.D. Kalsbeek, G. Luta, and J.M. Jordan. 2008. Lifetime risk of symptomatic knee osteoarthritis. *Arthritis and Rheumatism* 59(9):1207–1213.

NAC (National Alliance for Caregiving) and AARP. 2009. *Caregiving in the U.S. 2009*. http:// www.caregiving.org/data/Caregiving_in_the_US_2009_full_report.pdf (accessed October 15, 2011).

Nagi, S.Z. 1976. An epidemiology of disability among adults in the United States. *The Milbank Memorial Fund Quarterly. Health and Society* 54(4):439–467.

Nakase-Richardson, R., J. Whyte, J.T. Giacino, S. Pavawalla, S.D. Barnett, S.A. Yablon, M. Sherer, K. Kalmar, F.M. Hammond, B. Greenwald, L.J. Horn, R. Seel, M. McCarthy, J. Tran, and W.C. Walker. 2011. Longitudinal outcomes of patients with disordered consciousness in the NIDRR TBI model systems program. *Journal of Neurotrauma* 2011, Aug 4 [Epub ahead of print].

National Comorbidity Survey Replication. 2007. *NCS-R Lifetime Prevalence Estimates*. http://www.hcp.med.harvard.edu/ncs/ (accessed October 17, 2011).

NCES (National Center for Education Statistics). 2006. *The Health Literacy of America's Adults: Results From the 2003 National Assessment of Adult Literacy (NCES 2006-483)*. Washington, DC. http://nces.ed.gov/pubs2006/2006483.pdf (accessed October 6, 2011).

NCHS (National Center for Health Statistics). 2009. Summary health statistics for U.S. adults: National Health Interview Survey, 2008. *Vital Health Statistics* 10(242). http://www.cdc.gov/nchs/data/series/sr_10/sr10_242.pdf (accessed November 17, 2011).

NCI (National Cancer Institute) (a). *Lymphedema (PDQ®)*. http://www.cancer.gov/cancertopics/pdq/supportivecare/lymphedema/healthprofessional/page1 (accessed February 14, 2012).

NCI. 2011. *News. U.S. Cancer Survivors Grows to Nearly 12 Million*. http://www.cancer.gov/newscenter/pressreleases/2011/survivorshipMMWR2011/print (accessed December 19, 2011).

NCOA (National Council on Aging). 1999. *The Consequences of Untreated Hearing Loss in Older Persons*. Washington, DC: National Council on Aging. http://www.hearingoffice.com/download/UntreatedHearingLossReport.pdf (accessed October 6, 2011).

Ness, K.K., M.M. Wall, J.M. Oakes, L.L. Robison, and J.G. Gurney. 2006. Physical performance limitations and participation restrictions among cancer survivors: A population-based study. *Annals of Epidemiology* 16(3):197–205.

Newman, S., L. Steed, and K. Mulligan. 2004. Self-management interventions for chronic illness. *Lancet* 364(9444):1523–1537.

NINDS (National Institute of Neurological Disorders and Stroke) (a). *NINDS Chronic Pain Information Page*. http://www.ninds.nih.gov/disorders/chronic_pain/chronic_pain.htm (accessed September 12, 2011).

North Carolina Department of Health and Human Services Division of Services for the Deaf and the Hard of Hearing. 2009. *The Impact of Hearing Loss on Older Adults in North Carolina*. Raleigh, NC: North Carolina Department of Health and Human Services Division of Services for the Deaf and the Hard of Hearing. http://www.ncdhhs.gov/dsdhh/leg_study.pdf (accessed October 6, 2011).

O'Brien, J.A., and J.J. Caro. 2001. Alzheimer's disease and other dementia in nursing homes: Levels of management and cost. *International Psychogeriatrics* 13(3):347–358.

Okie, S. 2011. Confronting Alzheimer's Disease. *New England Journal of Medicine* 365(12): 1069–1072.

Orces, C.H., and F.J. Martinez. 2011. Epidemiology of fall-related forearm and wrist fractures among adults treated in U.S. hospital emergency departments. *Injury Prevention* 17(1):33–36.

Phillips, C.J., and C. Harper. 2011. The economics associated with persistent pain. *Current Opinion in Supportive and Palliative Care* 5(2):127–130.

Pinder, M.C., Z. Duan, J.S. Goodwin, G.N. Hortobagyi, and S.H. Giordano. 2007. Congestive heart failure in older women treated with adjuvant anthracycline chemotherapy for breast cancer. *Journal of Clinical Oncology* 25(25):3808–3815.

Pinquart, M., and S. Sörensen. 2003. Differences between caregivers and noncaregivers in psychological and physical health: A meta-analysis. *Psychology and Aging* 18(2):250–267.

Reichard, A., H. Stolzle, and M.H. Fox. 2011. Health disparities among adults with physical disabilities or cognitive limitations compared to individuals with no disabilities in the United States. *Disability and Health Journal* 4(2):59–67.

Reuben, D.B. 2009. Medical care for the final years of life: "When you're 83, it's not going to be 20 years." *Journal of the American Medical Association* 302(24):2686–2694.

Reuben, D.B., S. Mui, M. Damesyn, A.A. Moore, and G.A. Greendale. 1999. The prognostic value of sensory impairment in older persons. *Journal of the American Geriatrics Society* 47(8):930–935.

Reuben, D.B., C.P. Roth, J.C. Frank, S.H. Hirsch, D. Katz, H. McCreath, J. Younger, M. Murawski, E. Edgerly, J. Maher, K. Maslow, and N.S. Wenger. 2010. Assessing care of vulnerable elders—Alzheimer's disease: A pilot study of a practice redesign intervention to improve the quality of dementia care. *Journal of the American Geriatrics Society* 58(2):324–329.

Ricci, J.A., W.F. Stewart, E. Chee, C. Leotta, K. Foley, and M.C. Hochberg. 2005. Pain exacerbation as a major source of lost productive time in U.S. workers with arthritis. *Arthritis and Rheumatism* 53(5):673–681.

Roberts, R.O., Y.E. Geda, D.S. Knopman, T.J. Christianson, V.S. Pankratz, B.F. Boeve, A. Vella, W.A. Rocca, and R.C. Peterson. 2008. Association of duration and severity of diabetes mellitus with mild cognitive impairment. *Archives of Neurology* 65(8):1066–1073.

Robinson, R.L., H.G. Birnbaum, M.A. Morley, T. Sisitsky, P.E. Greenberg, and A.J. Claxton. 2003. Economic cost and epidemiological characteristics of patients with fibromyalgia claims. *Journal of Rheumatology* 30(6):1318–1325.

Rosen, A.B., and D.M. Cutler. 2009. Challenges in building disease-based national health accounts. *Medical Care* 47(7 Suppl 1):S7–S13.

Rothrock, N.E., R.D. Hays, K. Spritzer, S.E. Yount, W. Riley, and D. Cella. 2010. Relative to the general U.S. population, chronic diseases are associated with poorer health-related quality of life as measured by the Patient-Reported Outcomes Measurement Information System (PROMIS). *Journal of Clinical Epidemiology* 63(11):1195–1204.

Rowland, J., A. Mariotto, N. Aziz, G. Tesauro, E.J. Feuer, D. Blackman, P. Thompson, and L.A. Pollack. 2004. Cancer survivorship—United States, 1971–2001. *Morbidity and Mortality Weekly Report* 53(24):526–529. http://www.cdc.gov/mmwr/preview/mmwrhtml/mm5324a3.htm (accessed December 19, 2011).

Royer, A. 1998. *Social Isolation: The Most Distressing Consequence of Chronic Illness*. http://research.allacademic.com/meta/p_mla_apa_research_citation/1/1/0/2/1/p110216_index.html?phpsessid=7fc502fc26e39b3c7a03341b5cc8d2b1 (accessed October 15, 2011).

Rubin, R.R., and M. Peyrot. 1999. Quality of Life and Diabetes. *Diabetes/Metabolism Research and Reviews* 15(3):205–218.

Rugulies, R. 2002. Depression as a predictor for coronary heart disease. A review and meta-analysis. *American Journal of Preventive Medicine* 23(1):51–61.

Ryerson, B., E.F. Tierney, T.J. Thompson, M.M. Engelgau, J. Wang, E.W. Gregg, and L.S. Geiss. 2003. Excess physical limitations among adults with diabetes in the U.S. population, 1997-1999. *Diabetes Care* 26(1):206–210.

Sainfort, F., and P.L. Remington. 1995. The Disease Impact Assessment System (DIAS). *Public Health Reports* 110(5):639–644.

Schillinger, D., K. Grumbach, J. Piette, F. Wang, D. Osmond, C. Daher, J. Palacios, G.D. Sullivan, and A.B. Bindman. 2002. Association of health literacy with diabetes outcomes. *Journal of the American Medical Association* 288(4):475–482.

Schoenmakers, B., F. Buntinx, and J. Delepeleire. 2010. Factors determining the impact of care-giving on caregivers of elderly patients with dementia. A systematic literature review. *Maturitas* 66(2):191–200.

Schroeder, S.A. 2007. We can do better—improving the health of the American people. *New England Journal of Medicine* 357:1221–1228.

Schulz, R., and S.R. Beach. 1999. Caregiving as a risk factor for mortality: The Caregiver Health Effects Study. *Journal of the American Medical Association* 282(23):2215–2219.

Schulze, B., and W. Rössler. 2005. Caregiver burden in mental illness: Review of measurement, findings and interventions in 2004-2005. *Current Opinion in Psychiatry* 18(6):684–691.

Seeman, T.E., B.S. McEwen, J.W. Rowe, and B.H. Singer. 2001. Allostatic load as a marker of cumulative biological risk: MacArthur studies of successful aging. *Proceedings of the National Academy of Sciences* 98(8):4770–4775.

Sinclair, A.J., A.J. Girling, and A.J. Bayer. 2000. Cognitive dysfunction in older subjects with diabetes mellitus: Impact on diabetes self-management and use of care services. All Wales Research into Elderly (AWARE) Study. *Diabetes Research and Clinical Practice* 50(3):203–212.

Smith, B.D., G.L. Smith, A. Hurria, G.N. Hortobagyi, and T.A. Buchholz. 2009. Future of cancer incidence in the United States: Burdens upon an aging, changing nation. *Journal of Clinical Oncology* 27(17):2758–2765.

Stoddard, S., L. Jans, J. Ripple, and L. Kraus. 1998. *Chartbook on work and disability.* Washington, DC: U.S. National Institute on Disability and Rehabilitation Research. http://www.infouse.com/disabilitydata/workdisability/ (accessed November 17, 2011).

Taylor, Jr., D.H., M. Ezell, M. Kuchibhatla, T. Ostbye, and E.C. Clipp. 2008. Identifying the trajectories of depressive symptoms for women caring for their husbands with dementia. *Journal of the American Geriatrics Society* 56(2):322–327.

Teo, W.S., W.S. Tan, W.F. Chong, J. Abisheganaden, Y.J. Lew, T.K. Lim, and B.H. Heng. 2011. The economic burden of chronic obstructive pulmonary disease. *Respirology* 2011, Sep 29 [Epub ahead of print].

Thabit, H., S.M. Kennelly, A. Bhagarva, M. Ogunlewe, P.M. McCormack, J.H. McDermott, and S. Sreenan. 2009. Utilization of Frontal Assessment Battery and Executive Interview 25 in assessing for dysexecutive syndrome and its association with diabetes self-care in elderly patients with type 2 diabetes mellitus. *Diabetes Research and Clinical Practice* 86(3):208–212.

Thacker, S.B., D.F. Stroup, V. Carande-Kulis, J.S. Marks, K. Roy, and J.L. Gerberding. 2006. Measuring the public's health. *Public Health Reports* 121(1):14–22. http://www.public healthreports.org/issueopen.cfm?articleID=1576 (accessed November 17, 2011).

Tinetti, M.E., S.T. Bogardus, Jr., and J.V. Agostini. 2004. Potential pitfalls of disease-specific guidelines for patients with multiple conditions. *New England Journal of Medicine* 351(27):2870–2874.

Towns, K., P.L. Bedard, and S. Verma. 2008. Matters of the heart: Cardiac toxicity of adjuvant systemic therapy for early-stage breast cancer. *Current Oncology* 15(Suppl 1):S16–S29.

Turkcapar, N., O. Demir, T. Atli, M. Kopuk, M. Turgay, G. Kinikli, and M. Duman. 2006. Late onset rheumatoid arthritis: Clinical and laboratory comparisons with younger onset patients. *Archives of Gerontology Geriatrics* 42(2):225–231.

UK Prospective Diabetes Study Group. 1998. Intensive blood-glucose control with sulpho-nylureas or insulin compared with conventional treatment and risk of complications in patients with type 2 diabetes (UKPDS 33). UK Prospective Diabetes Study (UKPDS) Group. *Lancet* 352(9131):837–853.

UNC Center for Excellence in Community Mental Health (a). *Myths, Half-truths, and Common Misconceptions about Schizophrenia and Severe and Persistent Mental Illness (SPMI).* http://www.unccmh.org/clients-and-families/learn-about-mental-illness/common-myths/ (accessed February 14, 2012).

U.S. Census Bureau. 2011. *Current Population Reports, P60-239, Income, Poverty, and Health Insurance Coverage in the United States: 2010.* Washington, DC. http://www.census.gov/prod/2011pubs/p60-239.pdf (accessed November 17, 2011).

USDA (U.S. Department of Agriculture). 2006. *Food Safety for People with Cancer.* http://www.fsis.usda.gov/PDF/Food_Safety_for_People_with_Cancer.pdf (accessed September 2, 2011).

USPSTF (U.S. Preventive Services Task Force). 2009. Screening for depression in adults: U.S. preventive services task force recommendation statement. *Annals of Internal Medicine* 151(11):784–792.

Vickrey, B.G., B.S. Mittman, K.I. Connor, M.L. Pearson, R.D. Della Penna, T.G. Ganiats, R.W. Demonte, Jr., J. Chodosh, X. Cui, S. Vassar, N. Duan, and M. Lee. 2006. The effect of a disease management intervention on quality and outcomes of dementia care: A randomized, controlled trial. *Annals of Internal Medicine* 145(10):713–726.

Vilnius, D., and S. Dandoy. 1990. A priority rating system for public health programs. *Public Health Reports* 105(5):463–470.

Vitaliano, P.P., J.M. Scanlan, J. Zhang, M.V. Savage, I.B. Hirsch, and I.C. Siegler. 2002. A path model of chronic stress, the metabolic syndrome, and coronary heart disease. *Psychosomatic Medicine* 64(3):418–435.

Volpato, S., C. Blaum, H. Resnick, L. Ferrucci, L.P. Fried, J.M. Guralnik, and Women's Health and Aging Study. 2002. Comorbidities and impairments explaining the association between diabetes and lower extremity disability: The Women's Health and Aging Study. *Diabetes Care* 25(4):678–683.

Vu, H.T.V., J.D. Keeffe, C.A. McCarty, and H.R. Taylor. 2005. Impact of unilateral and bilateral vision loss on quality of life. *British Journal of Ophthalmology* 89(3):360–363.

Warsi, A., P.S. Wang, M.P. LaValley, J. Avorn, and D.H. Solomon. 2004. Self-management education programs in chronic disease: A systematic review and methodological critique of the literature. *Archives of Internal Medicine* 164(15):1641–1649.

Watson, S.D. 2003. Forward. *St. Louis University Law Journal* 48(1).

Weijman, I., J.G. Ros Wynand, G. E.H.M. Rutten, W.B. Schaufeli, M.J. Schabracq, and J.A.M. Winnubst. 2005. Frequency and perceived burden of diabetes self-management activities in employees with insulin-treated diabetes: Relationships with health outcomes. *Diabetes Research and Clinical Practice* 68(1):56–64.

Wen, X.J., L. Balluz, and A. Mokdad. 2009. Association between media alerts of air quality index and change of outdoor activity among adult asthma in six states, BRFSS, 2005. *Journal of Community Health* 34(1):40–46.

WHO (World Health Organization) (a). *International Classification of Functioning, Disability and Health (ICF).* http://www.who.int/classifications/icf/en/ (accessed December 13, 2011).

WHO. 2008. *World Cancer Report.* Geneva, Switzerland: World Health Organization.

Williams, D.R., H.M. González, H. Neighbors, R. Nesse, J.M. Abelson, J. Sweetman, and J.S. Jackson. 2007. Prevalence and distribution of major depressive disorder in African Americans, Caribbean blacks, and non-Hispanic whites: Results from the National Survey of American Life. *Archives of General Psychiatry* 64(3):305–315.

Wilson, M., M.P. Moore, and H. Lunt. 2004. Treatment satisfaction after commencement of insulin in Type 2 diabetes. *Diabetes Research and Clinical Practice* 66(3):263–267.

Wolf, M.S., J.A. Gazmararian, and D.W. Baker. 2005. Health literacy and functional health status among older adults. *Archives of Internal Medicine* 165(17):1946–1952.

Wolff, J.L., and C. Boult. 2005. Moving beyond round pegs and square holes: Restructuring Medicare to improve chronic care. *Annals of Internal Medicine* 143(6):439–445.

Woo, J., S.C. Ho, S.G. Chan, A.L.M. Yu, Y.K. Yuen, and J. Lau. 1997. An estimate of chronic disease burden and some economic consequences among the elderly Hong Kong population. *Journal of Epidemiology and Community Health* 51(5):486–489.

Wormgoor, M.E.A., A. Indahl, M.W. van Tulder, and H.C.G. Kemper. 2006. Functioning description according to the ICF Model in chronic back pain: Disablement appears even more complex with decreasing symptom-specificity. *Journal of Rehabilitation Medicine* 38(2):93–99.

Wu, E.Q., H.G. Birnbaum, L. Shi, D.E. Ball, R.C. Kessler, M. Moulis, and J. Aggarwal. 2005. The economic burden of schizophrenia in the United States in 2002. *Journal of Clinical Psychiatry* 66(9):1122–1129.

Yabroff, K.R., W.F. Lawrence, S. Clauser, W.W. Davis, and M.L. Brown. 2004. Burden of illness in cancer survivors: Findings from a population-based national sample. *Journal of the National Cancer Institute* 96(17):1322–1330.

Yaffe, K., P. Fox, R. Newcomer, L. Sands, K. Lindquist, K. Dane, and K.E. Covinsky. 2002. Patient and caregiver characteristics and nursing home placement in patients with dementia. *Journal of the American Medical Association* 287(16):2090–2097.

Zafagnini, S., G.M. Marcheggiani Muccioli, N. Lopomo, D. Bruni, G. Giordano, G. Ravazzolo, M. Molinari, and M. Marcacci. 2011. Prospective long-term outcomes of the medial collagen mescus implant versus partial medial meniscectomy: A minimum 10-year follow-up study. *American Journal of Sports Medicine* 39(5):977–985.

Zaza, C., and N. Baine. 2002. Cancer pain and psychosocial factors: A critical review of the literature. *Journal of Pain and Symptom Management* 24(5):526–542.

3

Policy

INTRODUCTION

In the previous chapters, the committee framed the numerous challenges and opportunities for defining and measuring the determinants of living well with chronic illness. This chapter describes the associated challenges of designing and implementing effective public policies aimed at living well with chronic illnesses.

First, the chapter defines health policy, which is aimed at improving the delivery of health care (clinical medicine) and public health, and describes the need for better integration between the two fields. It includes a brief description about the barriers to developing effective health policy, including budgetary challenges, and the lack of systematic evidence-based policy assessment, evaluation, and surveillance.

Next, the chapter identifies the range of public policies that have an impact on living well with chronic illness. Using Frieden's pyramid of Factors that Impact Health (Frieden, 2010) as a framework, the chapter summarizes a continuum of policies ranging from structural (or distal) policies, which have the largest impact on the broad population of those who are chronically ill, to individual-level (or proximal) policy interventions, which have a more targeted impact on a smaller number of people.

Beginning with the base of Frieden's pyramid (Frieden, 2010), the chapter highlights numerous public policies that have an impact on the ability of high-risk populations with chronic illnesses to live well. Numerous social policies have proven critical in maintaining function and independence for chronically ill populations who are most disadvantaged in terms of income and/or disability. The recent Institute of Medicine (IOM) report *For the Public's Health: Revitalizing Law and Policy to Meet New Challenges* (2011) describes these policies and makes detailed recommendations about the need to review and revise various public health policies and laws in order to improve population health. Many of these policies and laws are designed to prevent illness in the general population and to help prevent further morbidity in those already chronically ill—for example, clean indoor air laws and smoking cessation interventions.

Extending through the tip of Frieden's pyramid, the chapter concludes with policies that impact health care delivery and self-care, also important in supporting those with chronic illness to live well. Recently passed federal health reform, the Affordable Care Act (ACA), represents the most significant changes to health care policy since the passage of Medicare and Medicaid in 1965. Given the numerous provisions targeted to improving health care delivery and population health, the chapter describes aspects of the ACA that are particularly relevant to the well-being of those with chronic illness.

Finally, in order to promote synergistic improvements in public policies that have the potential to impact health, the chapter describes a broad Health in All Policies (HIAP) strategy that seeks to assess the health implications from both health and nonhealth public- and private-sector policies.

Defining Health Care (Clinical Medicine) and Public Health Policy

In general, public policy refers to the "authoritative decisions made in the legislative, executive, or judicial branches of government that are intended to direct or influence the actions, behaviors, or decisions of others" (Longest and Huber, 2010). Health policy is the subset of public policies that impacts health care delivery (clinical medicine) and public health (population health).

Most health policy in the United States is health care (clinical medicine) policy, aimed at regulating or funding the loosely coordinated mechanisms for the financing, insurance, and delivery of individual-level health care services (Hardcastle et al., 2011; IOM, 2011; Shi and Singh, 2010). Whereas public health focuses on the health status of broad populations across generations, clinical care focuses on individuals. The committee discussed the need to expand beyond this fairly simplistic view of health and in Chapter 1 provides a framework (Figure 1-1) for considering the relationship among determinants of health, the spectrum of health, and policies and other interventions that help those with chronic illness to "live well."

To the extent that Americans often think in terms of their individual health status rather than in terms of population health, it may be understandable why policy makers focus on allocating resources and regulating policy in health care services. However, the health and well-being of the individual and the health of the population are interrelated and interdependent. Choucair (2011) suggests that "maintaining two disciplinary silos (public health and clinical medicine) is not the answer. Bridging the gap is critical if we are serious about improving the quality of life of our residents. . . . [W]e will not be successful unless we translate what we learn in research all the way into public policy." Many public policies that improve health, especially for those with chronic illness, could be provided more effectively and efficiently in a more integrated, better aligned health system (Hardcastle et al., 2011). The committee discusses the need for a more integrated health system in detail in Chapter 6 and provides several examples of partnerships among clinical care, public health, and community organizations that promote health for those with chronic illness.

Barriers to Effective Health Policy

As expressed in the recent IOM report (2011), "now is a critical time to examine the role and usefulness of the law and public policy more broadly, both in and outside the health sector, in efforts to improve population health." The report noted the need for improvements in public policy as a result of several factors, including but not limited to developments in the science of public health; the current economic crisis and severe budget cuts faced by local, state, and federal government; the lack of coordination of health policies and regulations; recent passage of federal health reform (the ACA); and increasing rates of obesity in the U.S. population.

Defining the appropriate role of government, however, is at the heart of public policy making in the United States. Although Americans value their health, many also value their ability to make individual choices about their health care, health behavior, and quality of life. Accordingly, many policy makers place high priority on individual liberties and, concomitantly, a limited role for government. Policy makers balance multiple competing public policy interests, made more challenging in the current economic climate in which competition for resources is high. For this reason, it is critical to integrate health care policy with public health policy and reframe them both to be consistent with other societal values, such as prosperity, economic development, long-term investment, and overall well-being. Reminding policy makers in all sectors of government that "businesses can rise and fall on the strength of their employees' physical and mental health, which influence[s] levels of productivity and, ultimately, the economic outlook of employers" (IOM, 2011) will help to emphasize the economic implications of population health. Given that two-thirds of U.S. health care spending is consumed by just 28 percent of people who have two or more chronic illnesses (Anderson, 2010), the country can avoid unnecessary costs and poor health by addressing the underlying cause of illness (Hardcastle et al., 2011).

The data and analytic methodology for assessing effective public policy is often lacking, and demonstrating causality between policy interventions and their intended outcome is difficult, especially for interventions that require longitudinal follow-up and assessment. The IOM report *For the Public's Health: Revitalizing Law and Policy to Meet New Challenges* (2011) outlined several important large-scale policy initiatives targeting childhood disadvantage to prevent poor health in adulthood. Examples include "home health visiting programs, early stimulation in child care programs, and preschool settings (i.e., Early Head Start and Head Start)" (IOM, 2011). Yet questions about the long-term efficacy of many of these types of interventions remain (The Brookings Center on Children and Families and National Institute for Early Education Research, 2010). Chapter 4 provides a detailed description of a number of community-based initiatives aimed at improving the health and well-being of those with chronic illness.

An added challenge to developing effective health policy, which is in itself an iterative cyclical process, is the fact that tracking and evaluating policy implementation and efficacy are not done in a systematic fashion at the state or federal level. Instead, surveillance of various public policies occurs across government, foundations, the private sector, and various nonprofit organizations. The Kaiser Family Foundation, the Robert Wood Johnson Foundation, the National Association for State Health Policy, and the Commonwealth Fund provide an abundance of information about current federal and state laws as they relate to chronic illness. In addition, such organizations as the Trust for America's Health and the County Health Rankings help to inform local, state, and national policy across the determinants of multiple chronic conditions (MCCs). Yet, generally speaking, these organizations do not systematically assess how well specific state and federal laws are being implemented or how well they are working to achieve their stated goals. Alternatively, organizations focused on specific illnesses, such as the Arthritis Foundation, can effectively advocate for state and federal policies that impact their constituencies. What is missing is widespread collaboration between these two extremes, as well as a focus on policies that pertain directly to well-being and quality of life. Many organizations are only beginning to work in a collective fashion to achieve similar policy goals, such as living well with chronic illness.

Other nonprofit organizations, such as the National Council for State Legislatures (NCSL), track state policies that pertain to such chronic illnesses as diabetes. NCSL provides information about diabetes minimum coverage requirements for state-regulated health insurance policies, state Medicaid diabetes coverage terms and conditions, and an overview of federal funding from the Centers for Disease Control and Prevention (CDC) to state-sponsored diabetes prevention and control programs (NCSL, 2011). In addition, NCSL, the National Governors Association, the National Academy for State Health Policy, and other groups also track other state-level health policy issues, such as state implementation of federal health reform. According to NCSL, at least 32 states have enacted and signed laws specific to ACA health insurance implementation as of July 2011. These laws cover a wide variety of issues in at least 15 categories.

In addition to the need for better surveillance of public policy, research on the relationship between law and legal practices and population health and well-being is still developing (Burris et al., 2010). Moreover, questions about the cost-effectiveness of various health policies are paramount. Policy makers require evidence about effectiveness, projected outcomes, and value in order to judge the merits of proposed policies. However, concerns about using science to measure cost-effectiveness in health care delivery have led some policy makers to raise concerns about the rationing of health care services by the government (California Healthline, 2010). *For the Public's Health: Revitalizing Law and Policy to Meet New Challenges* (IOM, 2011) extensively evaluated how research could be used to improve public policy surveillance. The committee suggested that "research on the comparative effectiveness and health impact of public health laws and policies could be conducted by documenting geographic variation and temporal change in population exposure to specific policy and legal interventions." The committee recommended that an interdisciplinary team of experts be given appropriate resources to evaluate evidence for outcome assessments of policies and regulations and derive new guidelines for setting evidence-based policy. Chapter 5 provides a detailed description and framework for chronic disease surveillance that will be required to adequately evaluate policies aimed at helping those with chronic illness to live well.

American Values in Public Policy

Even as new research establishes that social and environmental factors significantly influence health status, Americans often question this worldview (IOM, 2011). *For the Public's Health: Revitalizing Law and Policy to Meet New Challenges* (IOM, 2011) describes four "imperatives"—rescue, technology, visibility, and individualism—that influence American policy making. These imperatives tend to focus policy makers' attention on crises or novel events that have a compelling narrative, and away from concepts more commonplace, such as "living well":

1. *Rescue imperative*: people are more likely to feel emotionally connected to individual misfortune and circumstances, but less inclined to react to negative information conveyed in statistical terms.

2. *Technology imperative*: people find more appeal in cutting-edge biomedical technologies than in population-based interventions.
3. *Visibility imperative*: people take for granted public health activities that occur "behind the scenes" unless a crisis arises, such as influenza.
4. *Individualism imperative*: Americans generally value individualism, favoring personal rights over public goods.

CONTEXTUALIZING HEALTH POLICY
INTERVENTIONS: FRIEDEN'S PYRAMID

Although most interventions aimed to help people with chronic illness live well focus on the individual, the Health Impact Pyramid (Figure 3-1) illustrates why interventions focused more on public health may be beneficial as well (Frieden, 2010). The base of Frieden's pyramid includes health-related socioeconomic factors, with interventions aimed at reducing poverty and increasing educational levels. The next level of the pyramid

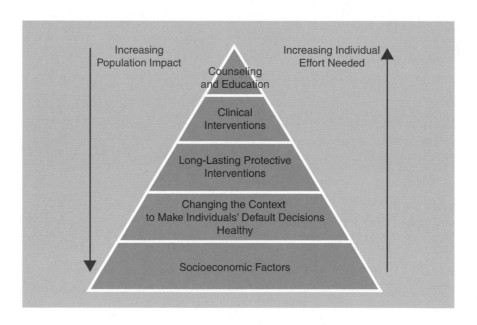

FIGURE 3-1 Health Impact Pyramid.
SOURCE: Frieden, T.R. 2010. A framework for public health action: The health impact pyramid. *American Journal of Public Health* 100(4):590–595. The Sheriden Press.

recommends changing the environmental context to prevent illness, using such interventions as water fluoridation and environmental changes to encourage physical activity. The third level involves one-time, or infrequent, protective interventions, such as vaccines to prevent infectious disease. The fourth and fifth levels of the pyramid include clinical interventions and counseling/educational interventions. The intervention levels differ in both the individual effort needed for the intervention to be successful and their potential impact. Moving down the pyramid, there is an inverse relationship: individual effort required decreases as the population impact increases. Although more individual approaches may be appropriate for helping those with chronic illness manage illness-specific aspects of their health (e.g., counseling and reminder systems to encourage diabetic patients to adhere to medication regimens), interventions further down will be of benefit as well (e.g., increasing access to facilities for physical activity can help those with arthritis be more physically active and improve their physical functioning). Each of these interventions can, and often does, have an impact on an individual's overall well-being.

Policies Aimed at Socioeconomic Factors

Frieden's pyramid (Figure 3-1) begins with a focus on socioeconomic factors. Persons with chronic illnesses need protection of their rights to accessibility of services, programs, public facilities, transportation, housing, and other necessities for independent living and having a high quality of life in addition to their public health and health care needs. Federal policies, such as the Ticket to Work and Self-Sufficiency program within the Medicaid system (Stapleton et al., 2008), or paid medical leave for employees and caregivers (Earle and Heymann, 2011) have proven instrumental in helping those with chronic illness live well.

These policies range from providing income support to low-income and disabled individuals—such as the Social Security Amendments of 1956, which created the Social Security Disability Insurance (SSDI) program—to transportation policies that require all new American mass transit vehicles to come equipped with wheelchair lifts (for example, the Urban Mass Transportation Act, 1970), to tax policies that preclude fringe benefits, such as health insurance, from being counted as taxable income, to community supports such as those provided through the Older Americans Act, such as nutrition assistance, home- and community-based services, as well as caregiver supports. The context of public law generally creates this environment. Although many of these broad social policies are expensive to implement and increasingly difficult to expand when resources are scarce, research suggests that there are associated cost savings as well as increased quality of life. Full description of the numerous policies that impact quality

---

BOX 3-1
Additional Examples of Public Policies That Impact Living Well with Chronic Illness

Independent living support policy

- 1965—The (American) Vocational Rehabilitation Amendment authorizes federal funds for construction of rehabilitation centers, expansion of existing vocational rehabilitation programs, and creation of the National Commission on Architectural Barriers to Rehabilitation of the Handicapped.
- 1965—The Older Americans Act provides funding based primarily on the percentage of an area's population 60 and older for nutrition and supportive home- and community-based services, disease prevention/health promotion services, elder rights programs, the National Family Caregiver Support Program, and the Native American Caregiver Support Program.
- 1978—Title VII of the Rehabilitation Act Amendments established the first federal funding for consumer-controlled independent living centers and the National Council of the Handicapped under the U.S. Department of Education.
- 1990—The Ryan White Comprehensive AIDS Resource Emergency Act was meant to help communities cope with the HIV/AIDS epidemic.

Transportation policies

- 1970—The Urban Mass Transportation Act requires all new American mass transit vehicles to come equipped with wheelchair lifts. Although the American Public Transportation Association delayed implementation, regulations were issued in 1990.

---

of life is beyond the scope of this report. However, a number of significant policies that are critical to helping those with chronic illness and disability are provided (see Box 3-1).

The Americans with Disabilities Act (ADA) of 1990 and the ADA Amendments Act of 2008 were considered national civil rights bills for people with disabilities. The scope of these laws includes the public sector (federal, state, and local governments) and the private sector (businesses with 15 or more employees), mandating "reasonable accommodations" for workers with disabilities. The ADA contains four mandate areas: employment protection; public service, including transportation and accessibility; nondiscrimination in public accommodations and services offered by most private entities; and telecommunication services. Given the committee's definition of "living well" as a self-perceived level of comfort, function,

Privacy policies

- 1996—The Health Insurance Portability and Accountability Act provided the first federal protections against genetic discrimination in health insurance. The act prohibited health insurers from excluding individuals from group coverage because of past or current medical problems, including genetic predisposition to certain diseases.
- 2008—The Genetic Information Nondiscrimination Act was designed to prohibit the improper use of genetic information in health insurance and employment. The act prohibits group health plans and health insurers from denying coverage to a healthy individual or charging that person higher premiums based solely on a genetic predisposition to developing a disease in the future. The legislation also bars employers from using individuals' genetic information when making hiring, firing, job placement, or promotion decisions.

Access to health care policies

- 1965—Medicare and Medicaid, established through passage of the Social Security Amendments of 1965, provides federally subsidized health care to disabled and elderly Americans covered by the Social Security program. These amendments changed the definition of disability under the Social Security Disability Insurance program from "of long continued and indefinite duration" to "expected to last for not less than 12 months."

and contentment with life, the role that the ADA has played in the lives of those with disability is immeasurable.

Although the ADA has proven essential for those with chronic illness, its implementation has significant disparities by condition. More specifically, analyses suggest that provisions of the ADA disproportionately underprotect people with psychiatric disabilities (Campbell, 1994). Research also has found that people with visual impairments rate the ADA lower than do people with hearing and mobility impairments (Hinton, 2003; Tucker, 1997). Furthermore, the "doubly disadvantaged," those with poor education and job skills plus a disability, do not appear to benefit in the long term from the ADA (Daly, 1997). Overall, the ADA has narrowed the gaps among those with and without disabilities in the areas of education and political participation. However, the similar gap in employment has not narrowed. The employment rate for those of working age with a disability is 75 percent of those with a nonsevere disability and 31 percent of those with a severe disability. For those without a disability, the employment rate is 84 percent (U.S. Census Bureau, 2010).

Other major concerns that impact the ability of those with chronic illness to live well are income and housing: 27.9 percent of those of working age with disabilities live below the poverty level compared with 12.5 percent of the general population (U.S. Census Bureau, 2011). SSDI is available to those who have worked long enough to pay taxes and are deemed disabled, and Social Security Income (SSI) is available for those deemed disabled and poor. Both programs require that (1) the recipient be deemed unable to complete work done previously or able to adjust to other work and (2) the disability persists for at least one year in duration. In 2008, the average SSDI payment was $12,048 per year, or 116 percent of the federal poverty level (FPL) for one person. Recent data suggest that for those on SSI income, housing costs consume somewhere between 60 and 140 percent of income (NAMI, 2010). Many with disabilities struggle to find affordable and accessible housing, despite the existence of disability-specific housing legislation and other U.S. Housing and Urban Development programs to provide affordable housing.

Caregivers of those with chronic illness often struggle with maintaining their own health and well-being as they care for their loved one. The Family and Medical Leave Act entitles eligible covered employees up to 12 weeks of job-protected, unpaid leave during any 12-month period in order to care for family members with a serious health illness or their own serious health illness; the employee maintains group health benefits during this leave. Even for those with the ability to maintain a job, recent data suggest that one of the largest causes of home foreclosures is a medical crisis. Specifically, a study of those going through home foreclosure in four states found that medical crises contributed to half of all home foreclosure filings (Robertson et al., 2008).

Public policies that address the next level of Frieden's pyramid, changing the context in order to make individuals' default decisions healthy, include state and local clean indoor air and smoke-free laws and ordinances as well as state tobacco taxes. Although the role of government in U.S. health care delivery has long been a contentious one (Starr, 1982), the case of tobacco control illustrates that a chronic disease risk factor can be amenable to U.S. public policy intervention. Data from the CDC celebrate "the 58.2 percent decrease in the prevalence of smoking among adults since 1964 [which] ranks among the 10 great public health achievements of the 20th century" (IOM, 2011). As described in *For the Public's Health: Revitalizing Law and Policy to Meet New Challenges* (IOM, 2011), "the tobacco story also provides a rich example of a suite of public health interventions (including the power to tax and spend, indirect regulation through litigation, and intervening on the information environment), several of them public policies, to improve population health, specifically by reducing mortality and morbidity due to its use." As outlined in the 2000 Surgeon General's *Reducing Tobacco Use* report (HHS, 2000), beginning in 1950, "the series of Surgeon General's reports began meticulous documentation of the biologic, epidemiologic, behavioral, pharmacologic, and cultural aspects of tobacco use. . . . The past several years have witnessed major initiatives in the legislative, regulatory, and legal arenas, with a complex set of results still not entirely resolved." The strides made in tobacco control have a direct impact on improving the well-being of those both with and without chronic illness.

Indeed, despite significant political obstacles, public health advocates have successfully developed and implemented public policy to prevent tobacco use at multiple levels of government. Halpin et al. (2010) outline a broad set of policies aimed at reducing demand for/restricting the supply of tobacco products that range from individual level interventions to broad societal interventions. Although the public health effort to lower tobacco use continues, the public policy lessons are generalizable to other areas in which policy action is needed in order to improve health outcomes. Specific policies include raising excise taxes on tobacco; lowering the cost of treatments for tobacco addiction; regulating exposure to environmental tobacco smoke; regulating the contents of tobacco products; regulating packaging and labeling; banning tobacco advertising, promotion, and sponsorship; prohibiting tobacco sales to minors; regulating physical access to tobacco products; and eliminating illicit tobacco trade (Halpin et al., 2010).

Public policies that address the third level of Frieden's pyramid and target long-lasting protective interventions include insurance mandates that require coverage of preventive services, like colonoscopies and immunizations. Those with functional impairment or disability are particularly susceptible to poor health behaviors given their mental, social, and economic burden as well as their family and caregiver stress. Growing evidence indicates that a comprehensive approach to prevention can save long-term health care costs, mitigate needless suffering, and improve overall well-being, but more evidence is needed to understand how these policies impact people with MCCs.

Examples of public policies that prevent chronic disease in the general population and reduce morbidity in those already living with a chronic illness are highlighted in Box 3-2. Chapter 4 on community-based intervention provides additional details on policies and interventions that affect lifestyle behaviors, screening and vaccination, and other inventions such as self-help and disease management.

BOX 3-2
Examples of Public Policies Aimed at
Preventing Chronic Disease

Increase physical activity

• Increased access to places for physical activity (e.g., walking trails in parks) (infrastructure)
• Enhanced school-based physical education classes (institutional policy)
• Urban design of neighborhoods with proximity to retail, schools, and recreation areas (zoning regulation)
• Point-of-service signs to increase stair walking (institutional policy)
• Street closures (institutional policy)
• Widening sidewalks (building codes)
• Bicycle paths (urban design, transportation, regulations)
• Creation of bicycle parking (institutional policy, building codes)
• Bicycle racks on trains and buses (institutional policy, transportation, regulations)
• Car, road, and fuel taxes (tax)

Improve diet

• Ban on use of trans fatty acids in restaurants (law)
• Menu labeling in restaurants (law)
• Removal of vending machines in schools (institutional policy)
• Adding salad bars at schools (institutional policy)
• Incentives for putting supermarkets in neighborhoods (zoning regulation)
• Creation of farmers' markets (institutional policy)
• Limitation on advertising of high-caloric, low-nutrition foods directed at children (law)
• Tax on high-caloric, low-nutrition foods (tax)

Policies Aimed at Clinical Interventions

The burden of chronic disease is staggering. Chapter 2 summarizes the burdens experienced by those affected, which range from a number of debilitating medical illnesses to disease self-management challenges, accompanying psychological health issues, and frequent social consequences for employment, education, parenting, etc. Families of the chronically ill are also impacted. Hardships for family members often include caregiver stress and economic consequences. Some of these issues can be addressed by appropriate evidence-based public policies aimed at individuals, communities, and populations. However, meeting the multiple needs of these individuals and their families remains an expensive proposition, and there is limited knowledge of which public policies are most instrumental in helping those with chronic illness to live well.

In terms of effective health care delivery, the Chronic Care Model (CCM) (Wagner et al., 1996) has long been a useful framework for attending to the multiple issues for managing chronic disease, ranging from self-management support to delivery system designs, decision support, information technology, community linkages, and health care organizations. The CCM model and its limitations are outlined in detail in Chapter 1. Five of the six elements in this model fall within the health care system, highlighting the need for better coordination among the elements of the CCM in a global care or support process and for more use of health information technology. Chapter 6 identifies particular ways in which community linkages can be used as part of a more comprehensive plan for self-management support (Ackermann, 2010).

Separate from limited models like the CCM, the current health system does not incentivize care coordination for those with chronic illness. Chapter 6 highlights aspects of the ACA aimed at government public health agencies, many of which currently provide health care services to the uninsured; with full implementation of the ACA anticipated in 2014, the law will provide access to health insurance for most Americans. However, the ACA does not mandate major changes in how the United States delivers and pays for most health care services but instead tests new and innovative models of reimbursement; this is described in more detail later in this chapter.

The current method of paying for most health care services in the United States continues to be fee-for-service (FFS), which creates financial incentives for doctors and hospitals to focus on the volume and intensity of services delivered rather than the quality, cost, or efficiency of care delivery (Council of Economic Advisers, 2009). Moreover, FFS does very little to support models like the CCM or the patient-centered medical home model (PCMH), which are centered on strong primary care. Starfield and others (Starfield, 2010; Starfield et al., 2005) have demonstrated that a strong primary care foundation can reduce costs and improve quality of care, prevent disease and death, and provide a more equitable distribution of health care services. In order to promote the delivery of high-value primary care and preventive services and reward improved outcomes, new models of provider payment that align incentives to support those with chronic illness while stabilizing and/or reducing total health care costs should be more broadly implemented (Bailit et al., 2010).

A crucial component of health system reform is fixing the current provider payment reimbursement system (Landon et al., 2010). There are a number of reimbursement models designed to better support and coordinate care for those with chronic illness, many of which will be pilot-tested as part of federal health reform, outlined below. These include enhancing FFS payments to provide support for care coordination; comprehensive global payment models that share reimbursement across providers (Goroll et al., 2007); and hybrid reimbursement models that incorporate FFS, adjusted prospective payment, and performance-based compensation (Baker and Doherty, 2009). Many of the PCMH demonstration projects include a hybrid payment model (Bitton et al., 2010). Peer-reviewed evaluations of the various reimbursement models are provided in more detail in Chapter 6. Landon et al. (2010) point to the reality of monetary incentives, stating that "economic theory suggests that implementing appropriate incentives through payment reform will result in primary care practices evolving over time toward the medical home ideal." The increased reimbursement can be used for a myriad of purposes: hiring care coordinators to support those with chronic illness; extending office hours to include evening and weekend availability; and purchasing or upgrading electronic health record (EHR) systems that support enhanced patient-provider communication and self-management.

THE AFFORDABLE CARE ACT

As briefly described above, the Patient Protection and Affordable Care Act (P.L. 111-148) and the Health Care and Education Reconciliation Act (P.L. 111-152)—together referred to as the Affordable Care Act or ACA—provide a number of reforms and opportunities that have the potential to improve the lives of individuals with chronic illness. In addition, the law gives new rights to those who have previously faced difficulties obtaining health insurance—a problem often faced by those living with chronic illness. For example, the law allows young adults under 26 to maintain coverage through their parents' health insurance, ends lifetime and most annual limits on care, and gives patients access to recommended preventive services without cost sharing. Importantly for those with chronic illness, it also bans insurance companies from denying coverage because of a person's preexisting medical illness.

A number of specific provisions are discussed below, and Annex 3-1 (at the end of the chapter) details a number of additional provisions that impact those living with chronic illness. In addition to the detailed description of the law provided below, in Chapter 6 the committee evaluates how the ACA can be used to help align public health and clinical care services in order to promote living well for those with chronic illness.

New Coverage Options and Subsidies to Purchase Insurance

By January 1, 2014, the ACA will require most individuals in the United States to obtain health insurance. Coverage options for the currently uninsured include the creation of state-based health insurance exchanges and the expansion of the Medicaid program. The Congressional Budget Office projects that 32 million people will be made newly eligible for insurance coverage either through their state's exchange or through the Medicaid expansion. In addition, eligible individuals and families will receive tax credits to cover premiums and cost sharing for qualified health plans purchased in a state exchange.

The state insurance exchanges created through the ACA aim to create efficient and competitive health insurance markets through which individuals and small businesses can purchase health insurance coverage. All qualified health plans in the new exchanges will be required to offer the "essential health benefits package" as defined by the law and will include at least the following general categories (as well as the items and services covered within the categories): ambulatory patient services; emergency services; hospitalization; maternity and newborn care; mental health and substance use disorder services, including behavioral health treatment, prescription drugs, and rehabilitative and habilitative services and devices; laboratory services; preventive and wellness services and chronic disease management; and pediatric services, including oral and vision care.[1] For many living with chronic illness, this new coverage provides important opportunities to access affordable, quality health insurance.

In addition to the new exchanges, starting January 1, 2014, Medicaid will be expanded to cover all individuals below 133 percent of the federal poverty level. Under the new Medicaid eligibility criteria, an estimated 14 million uninsured nonelderly adults and children will be eligible for Medicaid in 2014 (Ku, 2010). New Medicaid enrollees who qualify for Medicaid under the expansion are entitled to "benchmark" or "benchmark-equivalent" coverage.[2] The U.S. Department of Health and Human Services (HHS) secretary will define benchmark coverage, but this coverage must include all essential health benefits (as defined for the state exchange), including prescription drug coverage and mental health services.

---

[1] Qualified health plans operating in the state exchange are subject to the Mental Health Parity and Addiction Equity Act of 2008. Generally, the act requires that the financial requirements and treatment limitations imposed on mental health and substance use disorder benefits not be more restrictive than the predominant financial requirements and treatment limitations that apply to substantially all medical and surgical benefits.

[2] Benchmark coverage is based on Federal Employees Health Benefits insurance coverage, state employee coverage, and coverage offered by the health maintenance organization in the state that provides coverage for the largest number of non-Medicaid enrollees.

New Care Options for Those Living with Chronic Illness

A number of provisions in the ACA are targeted specifically to those living with chronic illness. For example, the law gives states an opportunity to offer Medicaid enrollees home- and community-based services and supports before individuals need institutional care. As of October 1, 2011, the new Community First Choice Option now provides states with the option to offer, through a Medicaid state plan amendment, home- and community-based attendant services and supports for certain Medicaid enrollees with disabilities whose income is up to 150 percent of FPL. These services and supports are intended to assist disabled individuals in accomplishing activities of daily living (such as eating, toileting, grooming, dressing, bathing, and transferring), instrumental activities of daily living (such as meal planning and preparation; managing finances; shopping for food, clothing, and other essential items; and performing household chores), and health-related tasks.

In addition, the new Medicaid health home provision will provide a new care option for those living with chronic illness. Beginning January 1, 2011, states were allowed to amend their state Medicaid plan and to assign Medicaid enrollees with chronic illnesses to a "health home" selected by the beneficiary. Health home services, provided by a designated provider, a team of health care professionals, or a health team, include (1) comprehensive care management, (2) care coordination and health promotion, (3) comprehensive transitional care, (4) patient and family support, (5) referral to community and social support services, and (6) use of health information technology to link services. Medicaid enrollees eligible for these health home services must meet one of three categories: (1) have at least two chronic illnesses (including mental health illnesses and substance abuse disorders), or (2) have one chronic illness and be at risk of developing a second one, or (3) have a serious and persistent mental health illness.

Finally, the ACA made important new investments in community health centers, which predominantly serve individuals and families with low income, many of whom have chronic illnesses. Currently, there are approximately 1,100 community health centers nationwide, serving 19 million patients at 7,900 sites. The ACA provided an additional $11 billion over 5 years for community health centers, which provide preventive and primary care to patients of all ages regardless of ability to pay. The majority of these mandatory dollars—$9.5 billion—will go to create new centers and expand care at existing centers. Another $1.5 billion will support construction and renovation projects.

New Care Concepts

Because the delivery of care is often fragmented, the ACA authorizes a number of new care concepts that are designed to improve care coordination and delivery especially for those living with chronic illness. For example, the ACA established a new entity within Centers for Medicare and Medicaid Services (CMS), the Centers for Medicare and Medicaid Innovation (CMI). CMI will test various innovative payment and service delivery models to ascertain if and how these models could reduce program expenditures while preserving or enhancing the quality of care provided to individuals enrolled in Medicare, Medicaid, and the Children's Health Insurance Program (CHIP).

CMI intends to prioritize testing models that could significantly aid those with chronic illness, including models that

- use comprehensive care plans;
- promote care coordination between providers;
- support care coordination for chronically ill patients at high risk of hospitalization;
- use medication therapy management;
- establish community-based health teams;
- promote patient decision-support tools;
- fund home health providers who offer chronic care management;
- promote greater efficiency in inpatient and outpatient services; and
- use a diverse network of providers to improve care coordination for individuals with two or more chronic illnesses and a history of prior hospitalization.

As outlined by CMI, the focus falls under three major areas: (1) patient care models ("developing innovations that make care safer, more patient-centered, more efficient, more effective, more timely, and more equitable"); (2) seamless coordinated care models ("models that make it easier for doctors and clinicians in different care settings to work together to care for Medicare, Medicaid, and CHIP beneficiaries"); and (3) community and population health models ("steps to improve public health and make communities healthier and stronger"). CMI will test models that promote better clinical care and health outcomes as well as reduce costs.

In addition to the creation of CMI, the ACA creates a new Medicare Shared Savings Program to incentivize groups of providers and suppliers to work together through accountable care organizations (ACOs). The goal of the shared savings program is to promote accountability and better care coordination for Medicare FFS beneficiaries. Starting January 1, 2012, professionals who organize into certified ACOs are eligible to receive additional payments for shared savings if the ACO: (1) meets the quality performance standards set by the HHS secretary and (2) spends below the established benchmark amount for a given year. Chapter 6 provides detailed information about how ACOs could be used to incentivize care coordination among multiple types of providers, including governmental public health agencies (GPHAs) and community-based organizations.

ACA Prevention Policies

The ACA also includes provisions to prevent illness. Preventing disease is especially important for those living with chronic illness.

The ACA establishes a National Prevention, Health Promotion, and Public Health Council to prioritize prevention across the federal government. The council, composed of senior officials across government, is designed to evaluate and coordinate prevention activities and the focused strategy across departments of promoting the nation's health. As outlined in the IOM report *For the Public's Health: Revitalizing Law and Policy to Meet New Challenges* (IOM, 2011), the council:

1. Creates a structure that specifically crosses government lines and brings different sectors of government to the table to talk about health in a structured way.
2. Engages both the legislative and executive branches at very high levels in an ongoing fashion.
3. Focuses on creation and agreement on strategy to achieve outcomes, one of the key points in the committee's first report.
4. Enables engagement of a broader range of nongovernment interests and input through an advisory mechanism.

In addition, the ACA contains multiple provisions to strengthen coverage of preventive services, both inside and outside the new health insurance exchanges. As of January 1, 2011, all new private insurance plans are required to cover a range of preventive services with no cost sharing, including any services given an A or B recommendation by the U.S. Preventive Services Task Force (USPSTF); any vaccination recommended by CDC's Advisory Committee on Immunization Practices; and certain preventive services for children, adolescents, and women.[3]

As of January 1, 2011, Medicare will offer full coverage for an "annual

---

[3]These provisions do not apply to health plans that are grandfathered—meaning that existing health plans are exempt as long as they do not change specific factors detailed in regulation, such as cost sharing. As existing health plans make changes over the next several years, it is expected that eventually most plans will fall under the requirement.

wellness visit" that includes a health risk assessment and customized prevention plan. In addition, all USPSTF-recommended services covered under Medicare must be provided with no cost sharing. In the Medicaid program, in 2013 and later, states that cover USPSTF-recommended services will receive a 1 percent enhancement to their federal match for those services. In addition, in 2013 and 2014, the ACA requires state Medicaid programs to pay primary care physicians for primary care services at the same rate, or greater, as the Medicare payment rate for these services.

In addition to strengthening coverage of preventive services, the ACA created the Prevention and Public Health Fund (PPHF), which provides mandatory funding for public health. The PPHF was set at $500 million in fiscal year 2010 and will increase to an annual total of $2 billion for 2015 and all ensuing years. To date, the PPHF has been used to strengthen the health and public health workforce, expand existing Public Health Service Act programs, bolster public health infrastructure through grants to states, and create and maintain new health promotion programs. The most prominent of these is the Community Transformation Grant (CTG) program, which aims to support communities in creating comprehensive change in the factors that affect people's health across multiple environments.

The CTG program authorizes the HHS secretary to award competitive grants to state and local governmental agencies and community-based organizations for implementation, evaluation, and dissemination of evidence-based community preventive health activities. These community prevention activities will be aimed at reducing chronic disease rates, preventing the development of secondary illnesses, addressing health disparities, and developing a stronger evidence base of effective prevention programming. Not only is this investment in chronic disease prevention unprecedented; it also represents an opportunity to transform how communities and government work together to solve large complex problems, like preventing chronic disease, reducing health inequities, and (potentially) containing health care costs. In September 2011, HHS awarded $103 million in funding to 61 recipients through the CTG program, and a concerted effort is under way to extract early results from the program that demonstrate impact.

HEALTH IN ALL POLICIES AND HEALTH IMPACT ASSESSMENTS

The committee discussed the need to think broadly about how public policy can improve the lives of those with chronic illness. The health research community typically focuses its attention on traditional health agencies, such as HHS or state and local health agencies. However, there is a growing recognition that policy decisions across a broad range of government agencies can influence human health, positively or negatively. The concept of Health in All Policies (HIAP) reflects this recognition and underscores the importance of considering the links between health and a wide set of government policies.

In some fields, the link to health is well established. For example, environmental factors can influence human health and development in a myriad of ways. Accordingly, there is a robust field of environmental health research, and environmental policies are often developed in ways that take into account the potential impact on health. In other policy fields, understanding the intersection with health is a newer concept. For example, transportation policy has not traditionally been a major area of research interest for health researchers, despite the fact that transportation access and design can have profound impacts on the health of individuals and communities. For example, the availability of public transportation decreases harmful pollution, creating safe throughways for "active transportation," such as biking; walking can increase physical activity and improve health; providing affordable transportation options in low-income communities improves access to jobs and to healthful food outlets.

Key to the successful achievement of a HIAP approach is avoiding unidirectional benefits. That is, the goal is not simply to bend policy decisions in all areas to suit the demands of the health research and advocacy community. Rather, the interrelationships between health and other social goods mean that the same policies that promote health will, in many cases, also serve other policy goals. For example, improved physical fitness is broadly considered to be a necessary response to address the child obesity epidemic in America. At the same time, improved physical fitness has been linked to improved academic performance. Therefore, school-based programs that offer time and opportunity for safe physical exercise could potentially improve children's health as well as their academic performance.

In 2010, the World Health Organization (WHO) and the Government of South Australia convened an International Meeting on Health in All Policies. The meeting drew on more than two decades of WHO work developing the concept of intersectoral collaboration for health. The meeting resulted in the "Adelaide Statement on Health in All Policies," which urges leaders and policy makers to "integrate considerations of health, well-being, and equity during the development, implementation, and evaluation of policies and services" (Krech and Buckett, 2010).

Building on the work of WHO, several countries have taken broad action to shift policy making toward the HIAP approach. The European Union (EU), for example, adopted the HIAP framework as official policy in 2006, building on successful implementation of a robust HIAP agenda developed in Finland (Ministry of Social Affairs and Health and European Observatory on Health Systems and Policies, 2006; Puska and Ståhl, 2010). Europe now has an explicit policy that a health impact assessment will apply to all new key EU policies (Koivusalo, 2010). The HIAP approach has proven successful in several EU member states (Ministry of Social Affairs and Health and European Observatory on Health Systems and Policies, 2006). For example, concurrent changes in agricultural, food manufacturing, and commercial policy in Finland led to a greatly improved Finnish diet (e.g., reduced fat content, increased fruit and vegetable consumption), leading to a drastic reduction in blood cholesterol levels; this produced an 80 percent reduction in annual cardiovascular disease mortality rates, increasing life expectancy by 10 years (Puska and Ståhl, 2010).

In addition to European countries, several of the Canadian Provinces have adopted a HIAP framework. Québec, for example, enacted a law in 2001 that requires all agencies to consult the Minister of Health and Social Services when they are formulating laws or regulations that could have an impact on health (Chomik, 2007). Based on early successes in the provinces, the Health Council of Canada is in the process of bringing the HIAP strategy to the national level through a "Whole-of-Government" initiative (Health Council of Canada, 2010).

The concept of HIAP has not gained as much traction in the United States compared with Europe and Canada (Collins and Koplan, 2009). However, interest in the topic is slowly growing, and HIA work is under way at the University of California, Los Angeles, the San Francisco Department of Public Health, and CDC. In October 2004, the Robert Wood Johnson Foundation and CDC came together to host a workshop in Princeton including domestic and international HIA experts to determine the steps needed to push the HIA field forward in the United States (CDC, [h]).

California has recently begun to shift its focus toward the HIAP framework. In 2010, Governor Schwarzenegger established a Health in All Policies Task Force charged with "identifying priority actions and strategies for state agencies to improve community health while also advancing the other goals of the state's Strategic Growth Council" (California Health in All Policies Task Force, 2010). The task force has identified numerous opportunities for cross-sector policies to improve health and well-being, including incorporating safety considerations for pedestrians and bikers into street designs; ensuring access to smoke-free environments; and leveraging government spending to support healthy eating by using the state's procurement policy to incentivize healthier food concessions on state property. Furthermore, the task force has had success forming relationships and building links between various sectors, which will form the basis of their future work.

Throughout the European and Canadian governments that have adopted the HIAP approach, Health Impact Assessments (HIAs) have been used as a primary tool for evaluating how policies and actions outside the health sector will impact population health. According to WHO, a Health Impact Assessment is a "means of assessing the health impacts of policies, plans, and projects in diverse economic sectors using quantitative, qualitative and participatory techniques" (WHO, [a]). In addition, HHS recommends HIAs as a planning resource for implementing *Healthy People 2020*, recognizing that HIAs can provide recommendations to increase positive health outcomes and minimize adverse health outcomes (CDC, [a]).

As the definition suggests, an HIA can be applied to many different types of policy decisions. Doing an HIA of a policy may mean assessing the likely impacts of a federal, state, or local law; a regulation issued by an administrative agency at any of these levels; or the manner in which a law or regulation is implemented. An HIA of a plan could refer to any public- or private-sector plan, and an HIA of a project can refer to a wide range of construction, economic, or other projects.

In general, an HIA is performed before the policy, plan, or project is implemented. The goal is to identify any potential impact on health before it is too late to change course. Although the emphasis of an HIA is often on preventing or mitigating any potential negative consequences, an HIA can also be used to optimize health benefits or to identify potential missed opportunities to improve health.

A challenging but promising element of HIAs is the need to collaborate across sectors and disciplines. For example, an assessment of the potential health impact of a new highway project may require involvement of health, environmental, and transportation experts. The health experts alone may need to include epidemiologists, community health experts, and physicians. In addition, these experts must interact extensively with policy makers and community members in order to meaningfully assess potential impacts. This kind of interdisciplinary approach can lead to better decision making with regard to the current project. Furthermore, it can inform public health experts about a broad range of other policy areas, positioning them to better identify opportunities for health improvement in the future (Rajotte et al., 2011).

CONCLUSION

The challenge of living well with chronic illness is shared by individuals and families, communities, health care providers, workplaces, organizations, and communities. Numerous public policies are critical to maintaining function and independence for chronically ill populations who are most disadvantaged in terms of income and/or disability for living well with chronic illness. These include important social policies and programs like SSI, SSDI, and the ADA, as well as numerous other public policies that create healthy environments in which to live.

There are also a number of health care policies that directly impact those with chronic illness through better coordination of health care delivery, many of which were included in recently passed federal health reform, the ACA. However, a system of coordinated policies and supports to assist those with chronic illness to live well is rare and not broadly considered by many policy makers. Better integration of health care policy and public health policy and assessing which policies are most effective at improving the function and well-being of those with chronic illness can ultimately lead to better health and economic outcomes.

In order to assist those with chronic illness to live well, the model adopted by the committee for this report and outlined in Chapter 1 (Figure 1-1) highlights the need to understand the complicated relationship among myriad determinants of health, health policies and other interventions, and the spectrum of health status. Adopting a HIAP strategy provides an opportunity to apply this model. Given its interdisciplinary approach to policy making, the HIAP framework creates synergistic improvements in overall health status via the assessment of the health implications from both health and nonhealth public- and private-sector policies. As such, HIAP can help to integrate health care and public health policy and better coordinate with various social supports and programs that are critical in helping those with chronic illness to function independently and live well.

RECOMMENDATIONS 7–8

The statement of task question asks what policy priorities could advance efforts to improve life impacts of chronic disease. In response, the committee makes two recommendations, derived from the discussion above.

Recommendation 7

The committee recommends that CDC routinely examine and adjust relevant policies to ensure that its public health chronic disease management and control programs reflect the concepts and priorities embodied in the current health and insurance reform legislation that are aimed at improving the lives of individuals living with chronic illness.

Recommendation 8

The committee recommends that the secretary of HHS and CDC explore and test a HIAP approach with HIAs as a promising practice on a select set of major federal legislation, regulations, and policies, and evaluate its impact on health related quality of life, functional status, and relevant efficiencies over time.

ANNEX 3-1 The Affordable Care Act: Provisions Impacting Chronic Illness

Provision	Description
Title I	
Extension of Dependent Coverage Sec. 1001	Mandates all group health plans and health insurance issuers offering group or individual health insurance that also offers dependent coverage to allow dependents to remain on their parent's health insurance until they turns 26 years of age.
Appeals Process Sec. 1001	Group health plans and health insurance issuers offering group or individual health insurance coverage must implement an effective internal appeals process for coverage determinations and claims, including appropriate notice of the process and the availability of any consumer assistance to help enrollees navigate their appeals. The plan must allow enrollees to review their files, present evidence and testimony as part of the appeals process, and receive continued coverage pending the outcome of the appeal.
Health Insurance Consumer Information Sec. 1002	Grants to states or Health Benefit Exchanges to establish, expand, or offer support for offices of health-consumer assistance or health insurance ombudsmen programs.
National Diabetes Prevention Program Sec. 1050	Authorizes a national program focused on reducing preventable diabetes in at-risk, adult populations.
Immediate Access to Insurance for Uninsured Individuals with a Pre-existing Condition Sec. 1101	Temporary high-risk health insurance pools have been established for individuals who have preexisting conditions and have been uninsured for at least 6 months. Pools provide health insurance coverage to eligible individuals; cover at least 65 percent of the costs of benefits; ensure that the out-of-pocket expense limit is no greater than the limit for high-deductible plans; vary premiums only by family structure, geography, actuarial value of the benefit, age, and tobacco use; and include an appeals process to enable individuals to appeal decisions under this section.
Closing the Medicare Prescription Drug "Doughnut Hole" Sec. 1101	Medicare beneficiaries who reached the Medicare prescription drug coverage gap or "doughnut hole" in 2010 received a $250 rebate. To close the "doughnut hole," coinsurance for generic drugs in the coverage gap will be reduced beginning in 2011, and a reduction in coinsurance for brand-name drugs in the gap begins in 2013.

ANNEX 3-1 Continued

Provision	Description
Affordable Choices of Health Benefit Plans (Exchanges) Sec. 1311	Each state must establish an American Health Benefit Exchange and a Small Business Health Options Program (SHOP) Exchange to facilitate the purchase of qualified health plans.
Title II	
Medicaid Expansion: Coverage for the Lowest Income Populations Sec. 2001	New eligibility for Medicaid beginning on January 1, 2014, for individuals under age 65 earning an income that does not exceed 133 percent of the federal poverty level.
Community First Choice Option Sec. 2401	An optional Medicaid benefit through which states could offer home- and community-based attendant services and supports to Medicaid beneficiaries with disabilities and whose income does not exceed 150 percent of the federal poverty line for activities of daily living beginning October 1, 2011.
Removing Barriers to Home- and Community-Based Services Sec. 2402	This provision gives states the option to provide more types of services through a state plan amendment (rather than a Medicaid waiver) for qualified disabled Medicaid individuals. They can provide targeted services to specific populations and extend full Medicaid benefits to individuals receiving home- and community-based services, but they may not limit the number of individuals eligible for home- and community-based services.
Money Follows the Person Rebalancing Demonstration Program (MFP) Sec. 2403	Extends the "Money Follows the Person Rebalancing Demonstration" through September 30, 2016, and adjusts the time period of required institutional residence (individuals must reside in an inpatient facility for no less than 90 consecutive days).
Providing Federal Coverage and Payment Coordination for Dual Eligible Beneficiaries Sec. 2602	The Federal Coordinated Care Office, housed in CMS, will bring together officials of the Medicare and Medicaid programs to more effectively integrate benefits under these programs and to improve coordination between federal and state governments for individuals eligible for benefits under both Medicare and Medicaid (dual eligibles).
State Option to Provide Health Homes for Enrollees with Chronic Conditions Sec. 2703	States have the option to amend their Medicaid benefits to enroll Medicaid beneficiaries with chronic illnesses into a health home selected by the beneficiary (including services that are provided by a designated provider, a team of health care professionals, or a health team).

continued

ANNEX 3-1 Continued

Provision	Description
Title III	
Hospital Value-Based Purchasing Program Sec. 3001	Establishes a value-based purchasing (VBP) program for hospitals participating in Medicare starting in fiscal year 2013. Under this program, a percentage of the hospital payment is tied to hospital performance on quality measures related to common and high-cost conditions.
The National Strategy for Quality Improvement in Health Care ("National Quality Strategy") Sec. 3011	A national strategy to improve the delivery of health care services, patient health outcomes, and population health, including a comprehensive strategic plan to achieve priorities identified by the HHS secretary.
Center for Medicare & Medicaid Innovation Sec. 3021	This new center will test various innovative payment and service delivery models to determine how these models reduce program expenditures while preserving or enhancing the quality of care provided to individuals enrolled in Medicare, Medicaid, and the Children's Health Insurance Program.
Medicare Shared Savings Program Sec. 3022	A program that incentivizes groups of providers and suppliers to work together through accountable care organizations (ACOs) with the goal of promoting accountability, and thus better care coordination, for Medicare fee-for-service patient populations.
National Pilot Program on Payment Bundling Sec. 3023	A national pilot program encouraging hospitals, doctors, and postacute care providers to improve patient care and achieve savings for the Medicare program through bundled payment models.
Extension for Specialized Medicare Advantage Plans for Special Needs Individuals Sec. 3205	Extends the Medicare Advantage Special Needs Plan (SNP) program through 2013.
Establishing Community Health Teams to Support the Patient-Centered Medical Home Sec. 3502	Grants to states, state-designated entities, and Indian tribes to establish community health teams. The health teams will make it possible for local primary care providers to better address disease prevention and chronic illness management by facilitating collaboration between these providers and existing community-based health resources.
Medication Management Services in Treatment of Chronic Disease Sec. 3503	A grant program for medication management services provided through the Patient Safety Research Center (Section 3501) to aid pharmacists in implementing medication management services for the treatment of chronic illnesses.

ANNEX 3-1 Continued

Provision	Description
Patient Navigator System Sec. 3510	"Patient navigators" will coordinate health care services needed for the diagnosis and treatment of chronic illnesses. Patient navigators will also facilitate the involvement of community organizations in assisting individuals who are at risk for or who have chronic illnesses to receive better access to high-quality health care services.
Title IV	
National Prevention Council Sec. 4001	The National Prevention, Health Promotion and Public Health Council's main responsibilities will include coordination and leadership at the federal level and among all federal departments and agencies with respect to prevention, wellness, and health promotion practices, the public health system, and integrative health care in the United States; development of a national prevention strategy; and recommendations to the president and Congress concerning the nation's most pressing health issues.
Prevention and Public Health Fund Sec. 4002	Establishes a Prevention and Public Health Fund in HHS. The fund will provide for an expanded national investment in prevention and public health programs to improve health and help contain health care costs.
Medicare Personalized Prevention Plan Demonstration Project Concerning Individualized Wellness Plan Sec. 4103	Medicare must cover annual wellness visits and personalized prevention plan services with the creation of an individual plan that includes completion of a health risk assessment (HRA) and takes into account the results of the HRA.
Removal of Barriers to Preventive Services in Medicare Sec. 4104	Medicare will pay 100 percent (waiving beneficiary coinsurance and deductibles) for covered preventive services if the services are recommended with a grade of A or B by the U.S. Preventive Services Task Force.
Improving Access to Preventive Services for Eligible Adults in Medicaid Sec. 4106	Medicaid diagnostic, screening, preventive, and rehabilitation services are expanded to include approved clinical preventive services, recommended adult vaccinations, and any medical and remedial services recommended by a physician for the maximum reduction of physical or mental disability and restoration of an individual to the best possible functional level.

continued

ANNEX 3-1 Continued

Provision	Description
Incentives for Prevention of Chronic Disease in Medicaid Sec. 4108	A program to award grants to states to provide incentives for Medicaid beneficiaries who participate in programs and demonstrate changes in health risk and outcomes by meeting specific targets.
Community Transformation Grants Sec. 4201	Grants awarded to finance the policy, environmental, programmatic, and infrastructure changes needed to promote healthy living and reduce disparities in the community.
Healthy Aging, Living Well; Evaluation of Community-Based Prevention and Wellness Programs for Medicare Beneficiaries Sec. 4202	Grants awarded to state or local health departments for a 5-year pilot program to provide public health and community interventions, community preventive screenings, clinical referrals for individuals with chronic illness risk factors, and other preventive services to individuals who are between ages 55 and 64.
Employer wellness programs Sec. 4303	Programs to expand use of evidence-based prevention and health promotion approaches in the workplace.
Title V	
State Health Care Workforce Development Grants Sec. 5102	A competitive health care workforce development grant program to enable state partnerships to complete comprehensive planning and to carry out activities leading to coherent and comprehensive health care workforce development strategies at the state and local levels. First, for planning grants to help states plan for current and future health care workforce needs and, second, for implementation grants to help state partnerships implement activities that will result in a coherent and comprehensive plan for health care workforce development, addressing current and projected workforce demands in the state.
Training Opportunities for Direct Care Workers Sec. 5302	A grant program to fund eligible entities to provide new training opportunities for direct care workers who are employed in long-term care settings and agree to work in the field of geriatrics, disability services, long-term services and supports, or chronic care management for a minimum of 2 years following completion of the assistance period.
Grants to Promote the Community Health Workforce Sec. 5313	A grant program to support community health workers and to promote positive health behaviors and outcomes for populations in medically underserved communities.

ANNEX 3-1 Continued

Provision	Description
Co-Locating Primary and Specialty Care in Community-Based Mental Health Settings Sec. 5604	Grants for coordinated and integrated services through the colocation of primary and specialty care in community-based mental and behavioral health settings.
Title VI	
Patient Centered Outcomes Research Institute Sec. 6301(a)	A private, nonprofit institute to advance research on the comparative clinical effectiveness of health care services and procedures to prevent, diagnose, treat, monitor, and manage certain diseases, disorders, and health conditions. This research will assist patients, clinicians, purchasers, and policy makers in making informed health decisions.

REFERENCES

Ackermann, R.T. 2010. Description of an integrated framework for building linkages among primary care clinics and community organizations for the prevention of type 2 diabetes: Emerging themes from the CC-Link study. *Chronic Illness* 6(2):89–100.

Anderson, G. 2010. *Chronic Care: Making the Case for Ongoing Care.* Princeton, NJ: Robert Wood Johnson Foundation.

Bailit, M., K. Phillips, and A. Long. 2010. *Paying for the Medical Home: Payment Models to Support Patient-Centered Medical Home Transformation in the Safety Net.* Seattle, WA: Safety Net Medical Home Initiative.

Baker, B., and R. B. Doherty. 2009. *Reforming Physician Payments to Achieve Greater Value in Health Care Spending: A Position Paper of the American College of Physicians.* http:// acponline.org/advocacy/where_we_stand/policy/pay_reform.pdf (accessed November 3, 2011).

Bitton, A., C. Martin, and B. Landon. 2010. A nationwide survey of patient centered medical home demonstration projects. *Journal of General Internal Medicine* 25(6):584–592.

Burris, S., A.C. Wagenaar, J. Swanson, J.K. Ibrahim, J. Wood, and M.M. Mello. 2010. Making the case for laws that improve health: A framework for public health law research. *Milbank Quarterly* 88(2):169–210.

California Health in All Policies Task Force. 2010. *Report to the Strategic Growth Council.* http://sgc.ca.gov/HIAP/docs/publications/HIAP_Task_Force_Report.pdf (accessed November 3, 2011).

California Healthline. 2010. *GOP Launches Criticism of Berwick's Nomination as CMS Administrator.* http://www.californiahealthline.org/articles/2010/5/13/gop-launches-criticism-of-berwicks-nomination-as-cms-administrator.aspx (accessed September 22, 2011).

Campbell, J. 1994. Unintended consequences in public policy: Persons with psychiatric disabilities and the Americans with disabilities act. *Policy Studies Journal* 22(1):133–145.

CDC (Centers for Disease Control and Prevention) (a). *Designing and Building Healthy Places.* http://www.cdc.gov/healthyplaces/ (accessed January 16, 2012).

CDC (b). *Health Impact Assessment.* http://www.cdc.gov/healthyplaces/factsheets/Health_ Impact_Assessment_factsheet_Final.pdf (accessed January 16, 2012).

Chomik, T. 2007. *Lessons Learned From Canadian Experiences With Intersectoral Action to Address the Social Determinants of Health.* Ottawa, ON: The Public Health Agency of Canada. http://www.who.int/social_determinants/resources/isa_lessons_from_ experience_can.pdf (accessed December 15, 2011).

Choucair, B. 2011. *Feinberg PPH: Commencement Address Given by Bechara Choucair, May 4, 2011.* http://adonis49.wordpress.com/2011/05/22/feinberg-pph-commencement-address-given-by-bechara-choucair/ (accessed November 2, 2011).

Collins, J., and J. P. Koplan. 2009. Health impact assessment. *Journal of the American Medical Association* 302(3):315–317.

Council of Economic Advisors. 2009. The Economic Case for Health Care Reform. http:// www.whitehouse.gov/administration/eop/cea/TheEconomicCaseforHealthCareReform (accessed January 16, 2012).

Daly, M.C. 1997. Who is protected by the ADA? Evidence from the German experience. *Annals of the American Academy of Political and Social Science* 549(1):101–116.

Earle, A., and J. Heymann. 2011. Protecting the health of employees caring for family members with special health care needs. *Social Science and Medicine* 73(1):68–78.

Frieden, T. R. 2010. A framework for public health action: The health impact pyramid. *American Journal of Public Health* 100(4):590–595.

Goroll, A.H., R.A. Berenson, S.C. Schoenbaum, and L.B. Gardner. 2007. Fundamental reform of payment for adult primary care: Comprehensive payment for comprehensive care. *Journal of General Internal Medicine* 22(3):410–415.

Halpin, H.A., M.M. Morales-Suárez-Varela, and J.M. Martin-Moreno. 2010. Chronic disease prevention and the new public health. *Public Health Reviews* 32(1):120–154.

Hardcastle, L.E., K.L. Record, P.D. Jacobson, and L.O. Gostin. 2011. Improving the population's health: The affordable care act and the importance of integration. *Journal of Law, Medicine, and Ethics* 39(3):317–327.

Health Council of Canada. 2010. *Stepping It Up: Moving the Focus from Health Care in Canada to a Healthier Canada.* Toronto, ON: Health Council of Canada. http://www.healthcouncilcanada.ca/docs/rpts/2010/promo/HCCpromoDec2010.pdf (accessed December 15, 2011).

HHS (U.S. Department of Health and Human Services). 2000. *Reducing Tobacco Use: A Report of the Surgeon General.* Atlanta, GA: U.S. Department of Health and Human Services, Centers for Disease Control and Prevention, National Center for Chronic Disease Prevention and Health Promotion, Office on Smoking and Health.

Hinton, C.A. 2003. The perceptions of people with disabilities as to the effectiveness of the Americans with Disabilities Act. *Journal of Disability Policy Studies* 13(4):210.

IOM (Institute of Medicine). 2011. *For the Public's Health: Revitalizing Law and Policy to Meet New Challenges.* Washington, DC: The National Academies Press.

Koivusalo, M. 2010. The state of Health in All policies (HIAP) in the European Union: Potential and pitfalls. *Journal of Epidemiology and Community Health* 64(6):500–503.

Krech, R., and K. Buckett. 2010. The adelaide statement on Health in All Policies: Moving towards a shared governance for health and well-being. *Health Promotion International* 25(2):258–260.

Ku, L. 2010. Ready, set, plan, implement: Executing the expansion of Medicaid. *Health Affairs* 29(6):1173–1177.

Landon, B.E., J.M. Gill, R.C. Antonelli, and E.C. Rich. 2010. Prospects for rebuilding primary care using the patient-centered medical home. *Health Affairs* 29(5):827–834.

Longest, Jr., B.B., and G.A. Huber. 2010. Schools of public health and the health of the public: Enhancing the capabilities of faculty to be influential in policymaking. *American Journal of Public Health* 100(1):49–53.

Ministry of Social Affairs and Health and European Observatory on Health Systems and Policies. 2006. *Health in All Policies: Prospects and Potentials.* Finland: Ministry of Social Affairs and Health. http://ec.europa.eu/health/archive/ph_information/documents/health_in_all_policies.pdf (accessed December 15, 2011).

NAMI (National Alliance on Mental Illness). 2010. *Election 2010: The 60 to 140 Percent Bite; State-by-State Data on Disability Income, Housing Costs and People with Mental Illness; Are Candidates Addressing the Facts?* Arlington, VA: National Alliance on Mental Illness.

NCSL (National Conference of State Legislatures). 2011. *Providing Diabetes Coverage: State Laws and Programs.* http://www.ncsl.org/Default.aspx?TabId=14504 (accessed July 6, 2011).

Puska, P., and T. Ståhl. 2010. Health in all policies-the Finnish initiative: Background, principles, and current issues. *Annual Review of Public Health* 31:315–328.

Rajotte, B.R., C.L. Ross, C.O. Ekechi, and V.N. Cadet. 2011. Health in all policies: Addressing the legal and policy foundations of health impact assessment. *Journal of Law, Medicine, and Ethics* 39:27–29.

Robertson, C.T., R. Egelhof, and M. Hoke. 2008. Get sick, get out: The medical causes for home mortgage foreclosures. *Health Matrix* 18(1):65–104.

Shi, L., and D. A. Singh. 2010. *Essentials of the U.S. Health Care System.* 2nd ed. Burlington, MA: Jones and Bartlett.

Stapleton, D., G. Livermore, C. Thornton, B. O'Day, R. Weathers, K. Harrison, S. O'Neil, E.S. Martin, D. Wittenburg, and D. Wright. 2008. *Ticket to Work at the Crossroads: A Solid Foundation with an Uncertain Future.* Washington, DC: Mathematica Policy Research, Inc.

Starfield, B. 2010. Reinventing primary care: Lessons from Canada for the United States. *Health Affairs* 29(5):1030–1036.

Starfield, B., L. Shi, and J. Macinko. 2005. Contribution of primary care to health systems and health. *Milbank Quarterly* 83(3):457–502.

Starr, P. 1982. *The Social Transformation of American Medicine.* New York: Basic Books.

The Brookings Center on Children and Families and National Institute for Early Education Research. 2010. *Investing in Young Children: New Directions in Federal Preschool and Early Childhood Policy.* Edited by R. Haskins and W.S. Barnett. http://nieer.org/pdf/Investing_in_Young_Children.pdf (accessed November 30, 2011).

Tucker, B.P. 1997. The ADA and deaf culture: Contrasting precepts, conflicting results. *Annals of the American Academy of Political and Social Science* 549(1):24–36.

U.S. Census Bureau. 2010. *Facts for Features: 20th Anniversary of Americans with Disabilities Act: July 26.* http://www.census.gov/newsroom/releases/archives/facts_for_features_special_editions/cb10-ff13.html (accessed November 2, 2011).

U.S. Census Bureau. 2011. *Income, Poverty, and Health Insurance Coverage in the United States: 2010.* Washington, DC: U.S. Government Printing Office. http://www.census.gov/prod/2011pubs/p60-239.pdf (accessed December 28, 2011).

Wagner, E.H., B.T. Austin, and M. Von Korff. 1996. Organizing care for patients with chronic illness. *Milbank Quarterly* 74(4):511–544.

WHO (World Health Organization) (a). *Health Impact Assessment (HIA).* http://www.who.int/hia/en/ (accessed November 3, 2011).

4

Community-Based Intervention

INTRODUCTION

This chapter provides an overview of community-based interventions aimed at helping people live well with chronic illness. It starts with a discussion of the effects of preventive interventions, including healthy lifestyles, screening, and vaccination of persons living with chronic illness. The chapter then discusses other interventions, including self-management, disease management, treatment adherence management, complementary and alternative medicine, cognitive training, and efforts to increase access for and mobility among those with chronic illness. Finally, it makes the case for monitoring and evaluating implementation of these interventions and their effects and commenting on the need for dissemination and dissemination research.

PREVENTIVE INTERVENTIONS

Evidence-based preventive interventions recommended for the general population are relevant to living well with chronic illness. In some cases, such interventions can affect the disease process, progression, or complications of chronic disease. For example, the Look AHEAD trial for people with diabetes has shown than an intensive 1-year intervention focusing on diet, exercise, and weight loss improved weight, diabetes control, and cardiovascular risk factors, with effects persisting 4 years after the intervention (Look AHEAD Research Group and Wing, 2010; Look AHEAD Research Group et al., 2007). Even when a particular health behavior is not directly related to a person's chronic illness (e.g., smoking and arthritis), adoption of healthy lifestyles by individuals with chronic illnesses can serve to "strengthen the host," optimize overall health, and make them less vulnerable to further health threats and disability. Lifestyle behavior change cannot generally substitute for effective medical management of chronic illness, where it is available, but often supports "living well"—improving quality of life, ameliorating symptoms, and optimizing functional status. Below we summarize evidence related to benefits of preventive interventions for those with chronic illness as well as evidence-based strategies for optimizing adoption of the preventive intervention. For this overview we have relied primarily on systematic reviews and meta-analyses from such groups as the U.S. Preventive Services Task Force (USPSTF), Cochrane Database System Reviews, the Guide to Community Preventive Services of the Centers for Disease Control and Prevention (CDC), and the Advisory Committee on Immunization Practice (ACIP). In some cases, the research summarized in these reviews has emphasized the benefits of prevention for a particular chronic disease, but in general the body of research on living well with chronic disease is limited.

Lifestyle Behaviors

Physical Activity

Increasing physical activity has a number of benefits for those with chronic illnesses, including decreasing the risk of cardiovascular disease, some cancers, and diabetes, as well as improving physical functioning (Physical Activity Guidelines Advisory Committee, 2008). Physical activity interventions have been shown to benefit those with chronic illnesses as well as the general population. Whereas exercise can be expected to improve fitness in most individuals, for people with chronic illnesses, what is critical is determining the effects on quality of life, function, and progression of their illness. For example, a systematic review of physical activity trials in cancer survivors reports improvements related to fatigue, functional aspects of quality of life, anxiety, and self-esteem involving exercise (Speck et al., 2010). For type 2 diabetes patients, structured exercise programs, physical activity, and dietary advice from a physician potentially affect the disease course, reducing HbA1c levels (Umpierre et al., 2011). The American College of Sports Medicine and the American Diabetes Association have issued a joint position statement supporting participation in regular physical activity for individuals with type 2 diabetes (Colberg et al., 2010). Increasing physical activity through exercise also helps those with depression. A Cochrane review of 23 randomized controlled trials (RCT) showed that participants in exercise interventions showed greater reductions in depression both following treatment and at longer-term follow-up compared with a no-treatment control group (Mead et al., 2009), although, some methodological weaknesses were noted in the trials (e.g., inadequate blinding of outcome assessment). Evidence also exists that exercise may help relieve depressive symptoms of older adults who have osteoarthritis (OA) (Yohannes and Caton, 2010). The Arthritis Foundation and CDC, in their National Public Health Agenda for Osteoarthritis (2010), recommended promotion of low-impact aerobic and strength-building exercise for adults with OA in the hip and/or knee. OA research indicates that land-based exercise decreases pain, fatigue, and stiffness and improves performance on functional assessments (Callahan et al., 2008; Hughes et al., 2006). A Cochrane review of exercise for knee OA concluded that both land-based and aquatic exercise has short-term benefit in terms of reduced pain and improved physical functioning (Bartels et al., 2007; Fransen and McConnell, 2008).

Physical activity appears to be helpful to people with other chronic illnesses as well. For example, aerobic physical activity, alone or when included in multicomponent interventions, has also been shown to be beneficial to patients with fibromyalgia syndrome, having moderate-sized effects on pain, fatigue, depressed mood, and quality of life (Häuser et al., 2009, 2010). A Cochrane review on exercise for fibromyalgia indicated that moderate aerobic exercise may benefit overall well-being and physical function, whereas strength training appears more beneficial in terms of reducing pain, tender points, and depression (Busch et al., 2007). A limited number of studies have been conducted to test the effects of exercise on dementia. Results of the studies have been mixed, and the methodology has been of low to moderate quality, but some studies have indicated that participation in exercise is associated with such outcomes as better mobility and physical performance and improvement in activities of daily living (ADLs) (Blankevoort et al., 2010; Littbrand et al., 2011; Potter et al., 2011; Vreugdenhil et al., 2011); however, it is unclear whether exercise has an effect on cognitive functioning in this population (Littbrand et al., 2011).

Although substantial evidence has accrued for the benefits of physical activity for people with a range of chronic illnesses, there is limited evidence to indicate what type, duration, and intensity of exercise is most helpful for improving function, quality of life, and disease progression for most chronic illnesses, nor are there sufficient evidence-based programs to help individuals with chronic illnesses to successfully adopt and maintain exercise. A survey conducted of physical activity programs for the elderly in seven U.S. communities highlights the problems of both insufficient demands from this population as well as insufficient program capacity. The survey showed that the programs were serving only approximately 6 percent of the elderly population; however, less than 4 percent of the programs had waiting lists for their services (Hughes et al., 2005).

There are few evidence-based community programs specifically for individuals with chronic illnesses that have been shown to increase physical activity and improve outcomes, although programs developed for individuals with OA have been shown to be effective and successfully implemented. For example, a randomized trial of the 8-week Arthritis Foundation's Exercise Program intervention showed effects on pain, fatigue, and self-efficacy, with symptom improvements maintained at follow-up 6 months later. The prevalence of a particular chronic disease may limit the usefulness of having disease-specific physical activity programs for many chronic diseases. However, physical activity programs that are adaptable to individual needs may be appropriate for people with a range of chronic illnesses. An example is EnhanceFitness, an evidence-based physical activity program developed for older adults. EnhanceFitness is a 1-hour class that meets 3 times per week and includes moderate intensity aerobic exercise, strength training, flexibility, and balance-enhancing exercises. Benefits of the program include prevention of age-related decline in health status as measured via the SF-36 health survey (Wallace et al., 1998) and improved physical performance (Belza et al., 2006); participation in the program is also associated with reduced health care costs for individuals making heavy use of the program (Ackermann et al., 2008).

Several interventions are recommended by the CDC's Guide for Community Preventive Services to increase physical activity (Community Preventive Services Task Force, 2005a). Although these evidence-based interventions have not necessarily been tested in populations with chronic illnesses, several have been tested in older adults, who are more likely to suffer from chronic illnesses. Individually tailored health behavior programs also have sufficient evidence to be recommended by the task force. Such programs include evidence- and theory-based behavioral strategies to modify behavior, including goal setting and self-monitoring, rewarding positive changes in behavior, structured problem-solving skills, soliciting social support for the behavior changes, and preventing relapse. Interventions to increase social support for physical activity in community settings, such as exercise buddy systems or walking groups, are also recommended. Community-wide campaigns that involve sustained effort to promote high-visibility messages about increasing physical activity have been shown to be effective and may be combined with individual-level education/counseling efforts. Finally, recommended policy changes and environmental interventions include community-scale and street-scale urban design and land use policies, increased access to places for physical activity combined with informational outreach, and point of decision prompts to use stairs (Community Preventive Services Task Force, [d]). Urban design features that enhance activity include land use policies that influence the proximity of stores and other destinations to residential areas, aesthetics and safety, and connectivity/continuity of sidewalks and streets (Community Preventive Services Task Force, [b]).

Diet

Diet and physical activity are often linked when offering interventions for the prevention of chronic dieases. Although recommendations for healthy diets come from a variety of sources, they offer similar patterns of intake. Recommended Dietary Allowances (RDAs), Dietary Reference Intakes (DRIs), and the Dietary Guidelines for Americans are fairly consistent in recommending a diet that maintains a healthy weight, encouraging a rich intake of fresh fruits and vegetables (preferably those that are dark green, red, or orange), complex carbohydrates (whole grains), and low-fat dairy products and minimizing saturated fats (except for mono- or polyunsaturated fatty acids), lowering the consumption of salt, and taking in adequate fluids. These recommendations are also consistent with the *Healthy People 2010* and *Healthy People 2020* targets.

Individuals with chronic illnesses may encounter socioeconomic issues that contribute to food insecurity, a situation in which individuals have to make choices about how to spend limited income. Fresh fruits and vegetables may be expensive, whereas rice and potatoes are not. Food insecurity may also encompass challenges in procuring or preparing adequate food. Those with disabilities may have more problems with being able to independently shop or cook food and may rely on prepared or processed products, which are often high in salt and fat.

It is difficult for some older people to make healthy choices if they have not been educated in the basics of nutrition. Identifying nutritional deficiencies is often difficult, and both poor nutrition and obesity may have underlying etiologies that are not directly caused by poor choices about foods consumed. Eating can become a challenge for those who have to navigate making healthy food choices adhering to the multiple public health messages to consume less sodium, less fat, more unsaturated fats, less trans-fat, fewer triglycerides, more fruits and vegetables, as well as other dietary modifications associated with managing their chronic illness.

Tobacco

Smoking cessation is an important behavior-change target for people with chronic illnesses, particularly those whose illness is related to their tobacco use (HHS, 1990). Data from the National Health Interview Survey indicate that many individuals with smoking-related chronic illnesses continue to smoke; the prevalence of smoking among individuals with a smoking-related chronic illness is 36.9 percent, 23 percent among individuals with chronic illnesses that are not smoking related, and 19.3 percent in people with no chronic illness (Rock et al., 2007). Gritz et al. (2007) reviewed the literature with regard to benefits of smoking cessation and effectiveness of interventions for individuals with cardiovascular disease, chronic obstructive pulmonary disease, diabetes, asthma, cancer, and AIDS. For these diseases, continued smoking has been shown to increase the risk of disease exacerbation or complications. Smoking cessation interventions, delivered primarily in health care settings or in the context of self-management programs, have shown mixed results with regard to efficacy. More research is needed to determine optimal smoking cessation intervention approaches for individuals with chronic illnesses, as well as whether existing smoking cessation services are effective and accessible to individuals with chronic illness. A state of the science conference held by the National Institutes of Health (NIH) on smoking cessation in adults (including special populations) concluded that self-help strategies alone were not effective at increasing cessation rates, but combined counseling and pharmacotherapy were largely effective (Ranney et al., 2006). However, few studies focused on ways to reach special populations, such as those with chronic illness. One approach, intensive smoking cessation counseling delivered to hospitalized patients, has not been shown to be effective.

The 2008 nicotine dependence treatment guidelines (HHS and Public Health Service, 2008) conclude that cessation treatment, including both counseling and pharmacological treatment, is effective for smoking cessation in patients with cardiovascular disease, lung disease, and cancer, but that there were insufficient trials in HIV/AIDS populations. For individuals with psychiatric illnesses, who have high smoking rates compared with the general population, smoking cessation pharmacological (buproprion SR and nortriptyline for depressed individuals and nicotine replacement and buproprion SR for individuals with schizophrenia) and counseling interventions have also shown effectiveness. The guidelines concluded that there is insufficient evidence to indicate that individuals with psychiatric disorders benefit more from interventions tailored to the psychiatric disorder or symptoms than standard treatments. A more recent systematic review of smoking cessation interventions for individuals with severe mental illness confirmed that such individuals are able to quit smoking with pharmacological (buproprion and nicotine replacement therapy) and behavioral interventions (individual and group therapy) that are effective in the general population. Furthermore, those who are stable at the initiation of treatment do not suffer increases in psychiatric symptoms (Banham and Gilbody, 2010).

Individuals with chronic illnesses can also benefit from community efforts to encourage tobacco use cessation and reduce exposure to secondhand smoke. Tobacco policies in the community decrease exposure to secondhand smoke, and those in the workplace increase smoking cessation and decrease secondhand smoke exposure. In the workplace, incentives and competitions can be effective in increasing tobacco cessation when combined with other efforts. Recommended interventions for smoking cessation include mass media campaigns when combined with other interventions, an increase in the unit price of tobacco products, provider reminders with and without provider education, reduced out-of-pocket costs for tobacco cessation, and multicomponent interventions that include telephone counseling (Community Preventive Services Task Force, [a]).

Screening and Vaccination

USPSTF has developed recommendations for clinical preventive services based on systematic reviews of the literature. With few exceptions, recommendations of USPSTF apply as well to people with chronic illnesses as they do to people without chronic illness. The only exceptions to general prevention recommendations for people with chronic illnesses involve situations where the presence of the chronic illness changes the magnitude of benefit or harm from the specific preventive service. For example, if the chronic illness reduces life expectancy to a substantial degree, the potential benefit from the preventive service (e.g., screening mammography in women with metastatic lung cancer) may be reduced and the preventive service becomes inappropriate. Likewise, if the chronic illness increases the testing burden or the potential psychological or physical harm of the preventive service (e.g., colorectal cancer screening in people with advanced dementia), again the preventive service is inappropriate. As with individual preventive services for anyone, it is important for the health care system to assist people with chronic illnesses to consider the potential benefits and harms to make an informed decision about preventive services. Sometimes, people with chronic illnesses may decide that the burden of testing and possible work-up and treatment is not worth the potential benefit, or that the added burden of yet another medication (even if prophylactic) is more than they are willing to bear. Some people with chronic illnesses may decide that, given their situation, some preventive services are just not a high enough priority for them to spend the time and energy (both physical and emotional) to engage in them. In these situations, the health care systems should respect and support the person's decision (Sawaya et al., 2007).

Chronically ill individuals often suffer from multiple chronic conditions (MCCs) (HHS, 2010), and thus relevant outcomes for preventive interventions may be broader than those traditionally used to assess effectiveness of preventive services and include multiple domains. Some of these domains may be represented by a multiplicity of measures that create difficulties for clear, straightforward interpretation. The strategic framework on MCCs of the U.S. Department of Health and Human Services (HHS) identifies the definition of relevant health outcomes for individuals with MCCs as one of its priority objectives (HHS, 2010). Furthermore, the specific benefit of a preventive intervention for individuals with chronic illnesses may not be known. Randomized clinical trials of preventive services often exclude individuals with chronic illnesses or recruit them in insufficient numbers to allow subgroup analyses that could identify benefits and risks of the intervention. The risk of harm from the intervention might be higher for individuals with chronic illnesses. For example, in screening for cancer in those with heart failure or chronic obstructive pulmonary disease (COPD), consideration should be made of the risk of overtreatment and the individual's ability to tolerate treatment if a cancer is identified. As another example, people who are older and with chronic illnesses suffer more complications from screening colonoscopy than do younger people without chronic illnesses (Warren et al., 2009).

Influenza vaccines are one clinical preventive intervention for which there is evidence of benefit for individuals with chronic illness. The PRISMA study was a nested case-control study that evaluated the risk reduction of influenza vaccine among adults between the ages of 18 and 64 with chronic illness (Hak et al., 2005). In this age group, influenza vaccination prevented 78 percent of deaths, 87 percent of hospitalizations, and 26 percent of visits to a general practitioner. Influenza vaccine is recommended for all individuals age 6 months and older, but special emphasis is placed on immunizing individuals at higher risk of complications, including those with chronic illnesses, such as pulmonary and cardiovascular disease (except hypertension); renal, hepatic, and hematological diseases; neurological disorders; and metabolic disorders, such as diabetes. Individuals who are immunocompromised, because of either an illness or a treatment, are also a high priority for influenza vaccine outreach (CDC, 2011).

Because these clinical preventive services are for the most part delivered through health care settings, and individuals with chronic illnesses may have more contact with the health care system, they may have increased opportunities to receive preventive care. A study of preventive health care in individuals with lupus found that they had comparable levels of cancer screening to a general population sample and a sample of patients with other chronic illnesses (diabetes, asthma, and heart disease). The sample with lupus had higher rates of influenza vaccination and lower rates of pneumococcal vaccination than the general population had, and the patients with other chronic illnesses had lower rates of both types of vaccination (Yazdany et al., 2010). Having a primary care provider and a rheumatologist involved in care increased the likelihood that individuals with lupus received the influenza vaccine. Baldwin and colleagues (2011) studied preventive care in colorectal cancer survivors from the year prior to diagnosis to up to 8 years postdiagnosis using SEER (Surveillance, Epidemiology, and End Results)–Medicare data. Patients with stage 0 or 1 colorectal cancer had higher rates of mammography screening and having the influenza vaccine than did those with stage 2 or 3 cancer and controls. For individuals with stage 2 or 3 cancer, their use of mammography and influenza vaccine increased from prediagnosis through posttreatment and survivorship phases, indicating that perhaps either the "teachable moment" of the cancer diagnosis or their increased contact with the health care system facilitated their receipt of preventive services (Baldwin et al., 2011).

The Guide to Community Preventive Services recommends a number of measures to increase uptake of screening in the general population, which would be likely to impact those with chronic illnesses as well. Education efforts using one-to-one methods (breast and cervical cancer screening) or small-group education (breast cancer screening only) as well as small media (videos and print material to encourage people to obtain screening) have shown to increase screening uptake. Client reminder systems (breast and cervical cancer screening), a reduction in structural barriers (breast cancer screening only), and a reduction in out-of-pocket costs (breast cancer screening only) also increase screening rates (Community Preventive Services Task Force, [a]). Offering the influenza vaccination in the workplace to both health care and non–health care workers is recommended for increasing influenza vaccination rates and would be a useful adjunct to offering vaccinations in health care settings (Community Preventive Services Task Force, [c]).

Barriers to Lifestyle Behavior Change for Individuals with Chronic Illness

Efforts to increase adoption of healthy lifestyle behaviors among individuals affected by chronic illness should be undertaken with sensitivity to the additional barriers often faced by these populations. Individuals with low socioeconomic status, and African Americans and Hispanics, are more likely to experience chronic illnesses and impaired functional status (Kington and Smith, 1997), and therefore they may live in neighborhoods that have a high density of advertising of tobacco and alcohol products and outlets where such products may be purchased (Barbeau et al., 2005; Gentry et al., 2011), as well as poor access to fitness and recreation facilities, or supermarkets that sell fresh fruits and vegetables (Estabrooks et al., 2003; Larson et al., 2009). Furthermore, fitness and recreation facilities, as well as outdoor areas supporting physical activity, may not be accessible or welcoming to individuals with disabilities (Rimmer et al., 2004, 2005). Additionally, neighborhood safety is generally poorer in low socioeconomic status (SES) neighborhoods (Wilson et al., 2004) and may disproportionately affect people with chronic illnesses, particularly those with functional limitations who are more vulnerable to violence (Levin, 2011), falls, and physical barriers. Fear of violence in the community may suppress physical activity and also affects healthy eating patterns. Disparities such as these point to the need for environmental and policy approaches to supporting healthy lifestyle behavior among individuals with chronic illnesses (Brownson et al., 2006), including availability and accessibility of outlets for physical activity and healthy eating, and addressing violence in the community (Cohen et al., 2010); such approaches may be even more important for these populations than the general population.

Other Living Well Interventions

Self-Help Management

In 2005, 133 million people in America had at least one chronic illness (Partnership for Solutions National Program Office, 2004). About 25 percent of individuals with chronic illnesses have activity impairments (Partnership for Solutions National Program Office, 2004). The management of chronic illness often requires a multifactored approach among health care team members, informal caregivers, and the patient. One approach to minimizing the costs and instilling individual responsibility and confidence is the development of self-management programs. These programs offer information and behavioral strategies that provide tools for individuals to use in caring for their chronic illness. These programs need to be based on what the patients perceive as problematic, not on what health care providers think the focus of education should be (Lorig and Holman, 2003).

Self-management requires a set of skills that can be taught to individuals with chronic illness. These include problem solving, decision making, resource utilization, developing a patient-provider partnership, and taking action (Lorig and Holman, 2003). The development of self-management strategies is often done on an individual case basis. The dissemination of an evidence-based program for the self-management of chronic disease in the community is a recent phenomenon (Lorig et al., 2005). A 6-week program called the Chronic Disease Self-Management Program (CDSMP) was developed by a group of investigators at Stanford University in the 1990s. The program dissemination was implemented and evaluated at Kaiser Permanente, an integrated health care system that serves well over 8 million people (Lorig et al., 2005). In a 2-year follow-up, the investigators examined health status and health resource utilization (Lorig et al., 2001a). Health resource utilization, measured as the number of emergency room and outpatient visits, was reduced, and there was an improvement in self-efficacy or the confidence in one's ability to deal with health problems. In a smaller study that measured outcomes after one year, there were similar results: fewer emergency room and outpatient visits, although the results were not statistically significant (Lorig et al., 2001b).

Self-management of chronic diesases has since been evaluated in a variety of clinical trials. There are conflicting reports of their effectiveness and essential components (Chodosh et al., 2005). In a meta-analysis of the literature, 780 studies were reviewed and 53 were selected for analysis, including 26 diabetes programs, 14 osteoporosis studies, and 13 hypertension studies (Chodosh et al., 2005). The diabetes and hypertension studies reviewed showed clinical improvements in the participants' outcome measures (HbA1c and both systolic and diastolic blood pressure), but the osteoarthritis participants had only minimal impact on the outcome measures for pain and function. However, the investigators reported that the meta-analysis had limitations, in that the studies included were of variable quality. Self-management programs have been applied to different chronic disease interventions for osteoarthritis (Wu et al., 2011), depression (Zafar and Mojitabai, 2011), diabetes (Ismail et al., 2004; Moore et al., 2004), hypertension (Schroeder et al., 2004a, 2004b), and others (Chodosh et al., 2005; Gardetto, 2011).

There are other self-management programs, most notably Matter of Balance, a self-management program designed to decrease the risk of falls. The efficacy of a fall prevention program seems to be linked to a perception of need on the part of the individual (Calhoun et al., 2011). A recent meta-analysis concluded that fall prevention programs do reduce falls by 9–12 percent as reported in the literature (Choi and Hector, 2011).

Participation rates in patient self-management programs seem variable, depending on the program, the population, and the locale (Bruce et al., 2007). A recent study conducted in Canada that reviewed the implementation and success of a self-management program for individuals with chronic illnesses found a general lack of understanding about self-management, a minimum of evidence-based practices, and a tendency to focus on a single illness entity. The challenge was that most of the patients had multiple comorbidities and self-management programs did not account for this and proved to be a burden for patients and providers alike (Johnston et al., 2011).

Disease Management

Disease management programs are widely used by health plans and overlap with self-management programs. Disease management programs seek to detect patients with chronic illnesses and to increase their use of self-management and coordinated care with an eye toward improving outcomes and controlling costs (Bernstein et al., 2010). In 2010, 67 percent of large employers consisting of 200 or more workers included disease management in their most popular health plan (Kaiser Family Foundation and Health Research and Educational Trust, 2010). The effects of disease management programs have been well studied for a number of chronic diseases, including asthma, chronic obstructive pulmonary disease, congestive heart failure, coronary artery disease, depression, and diabetes but not for others, including Alzheimer's disease, cancer, dementia, and musculoskeletal disorders (Mattke et al., 2007).

Results are mixed for disease outcomes and costs. For fee-for-service Medicare beneficiaries, a recent analysis of 15 demonstration programs found little evidence of improved functioning or decreases in hospitalizations, and none of the programs produced net cost savings (Peikes et al., 2009). An earlier review of three large population-based programs and meta-analyses covering 317 studies concluded that disease management can improve quality of care and outcomes for congestive heart failure, coronary artery disease, diabetes, and depression, but effects on cost are inconclusive (Mattke et al., 2007). Characteristics of relatively effective programs include the use of individualized case management, personal contact (as opposed to phone-only contact), hospital discharge as a key disease management opportunity, and reduced or no cost sharing for effective medications and other treatments (Bernstein, 2011).

Management of Treatment Adherence

Individuals who live with chronic illness have interventions prescribed by their primary care providers in the form of medication regimens, dietary modification, or physical therapy and exercise. Success of any intervention requires that the patient comply with prescribed therapies to experience relief of symptoms associated with their chronic illness, but to also slow or stop progression of their illness. It has been reported, however, that only one-third of patients accurately follow their physicians' recommendations (Becker, 1985). In a review by Sackett (1976), it was reported that follow-up appointments were missed 20 to 50 percent of the time and 50 percent of patients did not take medications as prescribed. Behavior changes are even less successful, particularly when the outcome is smoking cessation, changes made in dietary habits, and self-management of physical therapy and exercise regimens (DiMatteo, 2004; Medina-Mirapeix et al., 2009; Rhodes and Fiala, 2009; Sackett, 1976). Noncompliance with health interventions is difficult to quantify and makes evaluation of the intervention's success invalid and unreliable (Becker, 1985). In a series of meta-analyses, patient adherence to prescribed therapies ranged from 4.6 to 100 percent, with a median of 76 percent and an overall average of 75.2 percent (DiMatteo, 2004).

Efforts by researchers to identify determinants of patient noncompliance have defined several categories of potential causes. One area explored is that of increasing patient knowledge, assuming that information about one's illness and its treatments will lead to greater compliance. Results of the studies revealed that individuals who were recently diagnosed (within 5 years) were more compliant with their medication regimen than were those who had lived with the illness for more than 20 years (Becker, 1985).

A second area of exploration is health-related decision making. The theory is that individuals are guided in their decision making by their attitudes and beliefs, which may be disconnected from the information provided by their care providers. The Health Belief Model (HBM), developed by compiling considerable empirical evidence, includes four factors: health motivation, susceptibility or sense of vulnerability, severity of their condition or perception of the seriousness of consequences of noncompliance, and the benefits and costs of the intervention (Becker, 1985). It has been pointed out that this is a psychosocial model that may not account for a lot of variability among patients.

Patients may find medical recommendations complicated, expensive, or inconvenient, particularly for chronic illnesses (Stephenson et al., 1993). Non-adherence is widespread and can occur for many reasons, including patients' misunderstanding physician recommendations, lack of social support, socioeconomic conditions, depression, and inadequate patient education, among others (Briesacher et al., 2007; DiMatteo, 2004). A significant factor that contributes to non-adherence is that medications for chronic illness management are often associated with unpleasant side effects (Barton, 2011). A consensus of many studies is that factors that are not subject to modification (i.e., age, gender, race, intelligence, and education) are not associated with level of compliance (Stephenson et al., 1993).

There is evidence that noncompliance with prescribed medication regimens among patients with chronic illness leads to potentially negative consequences, including hospital admissions (Bell et al., 2011). The more complex the drug therapy is, especially among older patients with MCCs, the more challenging the management. To best manage complex regimens, a multidisciplinary team is needed to address individual needs (Stegemann et al., 2010). Other approaches are being investigated to improve adherence to therapeutic regimens, including technology (Bosworth et al., 2011; Donkin et al., 2011; Reach, 2009) and other innovative approaches such as new packaging strategies (Mahtani et al., 2011) and behavioral motivations (Russell et al., 2011).

Complementary and Alternative Medicine

The National Institutes of Health has defined complementary and alternative medicine (CAM) as "a group of diverse medical and health care systems, practices, and products that are not generally considered part of conventional medicine" (NCCAM, [a]). It has been reported that nearly 40 percent of American adults and about 12 percent of children use some type of complementary and alternative medicine, including dietary supplements (Barnes et al., 2008). Data from the National Health Interview Study conducted in 1999 indicate that, of those who use complementary and alternative medicine, almost 31 percent were non-Hispanic whites, 20 percent were Hispanics, and 24 percent were non-Hispanic blacks (Ni et al., 2002).

The distinction between complementary medicine and alternative medicine is that complementary products are used in conjunction with conventional therapies, whereas alternative medicine practices are used in place of conventional medicine (Ventola, 2010a). In effect, the use of these interventions is a version of self-management in the prevention or treatment of chronic illness. The most commonly used complementary medicine products include herbal remedies, massage, megavitamins, self-help support groups, folk medicine, energy healing, and homeopathy (Ness et al., 1999). The most common ailments cited for selecting CAM therapies are back and neck pain, joint pain, and arthritis (Barnes et al., 2008; Ventola, 2010a). In a study conducted in the state of Washington, investigators found that participants who used CAM therapies exclusively were less likely to engage in preventive health behaviors than those who used conventional medicine or those who used conventional medicine in combination with CAM approaches (Downey et al., 2009). Physicians and pharmacists are often poorly informed about many CAM products, do not ask patients about their use, and are uncomfortable answering questions about the efficacy of these therapies due to the lack of evidence-based information in the literature (Ventola, 2010a).

The use of CAM approaches in the management of chronic illness raises some concerns among health care providers because of the lack of scientific evidence supporting the use of these products and the potential for ignoring traditional and effective therapies (but also in terms of safety and efficacy) (Ventola, 2010b). The Dietary Supplement Health and Education Act of 1994 did not mandate that manufacturers prove that their products are safe; rather, it put the burden on the U.S. Food and Drug Administration (FDA) to prove them unsafe (Ventola, 2010b).

Cognitive Training

The maintenance of cognitive abilities is a serious, chronic, and common issue for many older adults. Attempts to retain cognitive function are becoming an area of clinical research for geriatricians, psychologists, and others who work with older and disabled adults. Research has shown that declining cognitive ability is associated with increasing dependence and the potential for nursing home placement (Wolinsky et al., 2006a). A randomized control trial to evaluate cognitive training interventions (i.e., memory, reasoning, and speed of information processing) previously tried in laboratory settings or in small-scale groups under controlled conditions was conducted in a multisite RCT. The project, Advanced Cognitive Training for Independent and Vital Elderly (ACTIVE), began in 1998 and continued follow-up evaluations through early 2002 (Jobe et al., 2001). This study focused on primary outcomes that address the cognitive function skills needed to manage everyday functions, such as managing finances, food preparation, driving, and medication use. Secondary outcomes that were a part of this project included health service utilization and quality of life measures. These outcome measures should provide insight into the ability to maintain living independence and health care resource utilization. There were four groups in this study (memory training, reasoning, speed of processing, and a control); 25 percent of the study participants had an extensive health-related quality of life (HRQoL) decline. The speed-of-processing arm of the study showed the most promise with the least HRQoL decline, although the other arms of the study seemed to have equivalent outcomes (Wolinsky et al., 2006a). The same cohort was reevaluated at 2 and 5 years postintervention (Wolinsky et al., 2006b). Although the speed-of-processing intervention had stronger and longer effects on the retention of cognition, the two arms memory training and reasoning also had positive effects in decreasing age-related cognitive declines compared with a control group.

The ACTIVE study was a large RCT involving six research sites and potentially 4,970 participants. After initial screening, 2,802 subjects were randomly placed into one of the four arms of this study. Subsequent studies used different randomization groups to examine within-group variability of response to training. There were 703 subjects examined in the memory training arm. Results of data analysis demonstrated three distinct response patterns. Subjects tended to benefit most from learning specific mnemonic techniques (Langbaum et al., 2009). Despite the variability, the study results demonstrate that older adults do respond to memory training. Other investigators have confirmed that screening and cognitive training do have a positive impact on the retention of skills needed to maintain the ability to remain independent (Gross et al., 2011a, 2011b).

Another approach to improving cognitive function in older adults involves exercise. Physical training appears to be associated with a lower risk of cognitive impairment and dementia (Etgen et al., 2010; Geda et al., 2010; Laurin et al., 2001). A study conducted in Hong Kong compared two interventions for improving cognitive function in older adults. The methods compared were coordination exercises, including a set of simplified Tai Chi movements and exercises focused on upper body strength using a towel as a tool. Of the two, towel exercise is promoted as the more effective strength training method for persons with impaired locomotive abilities (Kwok et al., 2011); however, 40 individuals were recruited for this study, and after 8 weeks of intensive therapy, the coordination exercise groups both showed a significant improvement in the cognitive function scale used (Chinese Dementia Rating Scale).

Behavior, diet, and exercise programs have also been shown to improve both behavioral and cognitive symptoms in mild cognitive impairment (Hahn and Andel, 2011). Non-pharmacologic treatments are more cost-effective in a long-term intervention than are drugs to which there may be less adherence over time due to a variety of potential side effects.

Access and Mobility

Providing access opportunities for individuals with disabilities is a concept that has been important since the early 1960s, when disabled veterans of World War II and polio victims were excluded from social interactions, workplaces, and other communal spaces due to lack of access (Gossett et al., 2009). Spurring the development of an accessible built environment was the passage of the Americans with Disabilities Act of 1990.

The city of Chicago was among the first to institutionalize the concept of universal accessibility and conducted a citywide assessment of buildings; shared spaces, such as public bathrooms; and common areas, such as parks and playgrounds (Hanson, 2008). Chicago achieved the goal of accessibility by revising the building codes for new and renovated homes, office buildings, hospitals, clinics, and other built environments.

Although the original intent was to allow greater access for individuals with disabilities, the concept, also referred to as universal design, has broadened to other populations that might benefit from accessible environments (Canadian Human Rights Commission, 2006; Gossett et al., 2009). The concept of universal design is broader than access to physical structures, involving building ramps, automatic doors, and elevators. It includes the design of shampoo bottles, showers and baths, playgrounds and other communal areas, and devices for grooming, cooking, and other activities of daily living. In developing universal design facilities and products, investigators have found that the key themes include involving the stakeholders, considering aspects of "green" design, and addressing issues of diversity (Gossett et al., 2009).

Among the key concepts emerging from the development of universal design is that of Leadership in Energy and Environmental Design (LEED) certification. LEED is an internationally recognized green building certification system developed in March 2000 by the U.S. Green Building Council. Many of the aspects of LEED certification contribute to addressing the needs of individuals with pulmonary problems, disabilities that require flexibility in armrests or seat heights and require low physical effort to make adjustments, and lighting strategies that meet the needs of individuals with vision impairments, among others (Gossett et al., 2009).

A relatively recent trend in rehabilitation is the adoption of evidence-based guidelines. One approach is to use a "human factors perspective" (Fain, 2006). Accessibility evaluation can be performed using a direct measurement or a derived measurement. Direct measurement is accomplished by putting the patient or client in contact with the device or product and observing his or her ability to interact with the device (i.e., an assistive device, such as a walker or electric wheelchair or a computer, that can be used with nontraditional access), perform appropriate tasks, maintain safety, and achieve functionality. Derived measurement does not include a surrogate or patient but can be accomplished by a skilled evaluator who understands human performance as well as technical knowledge about how the product or device needs to perform (Fain, 2006).

Among the new approaches to enable disabled individuals to interact successfully with their environment is the use of assistive technology devices (Muncert et al., 2011; Zwijsen et al., 2011). An assistive technology device, as defined by the Assistive Technology Act of 1998 (Institute on Disabilities, Temple University, [a]), is "any item, piece of equipment, or product system, whether acquired commercially, modified, or customized, that is used to increase, maintain, or improve functional capabilities of individuals with disabilities." Disabled individuals may have a decreased quality of life due to social isolation, increased dependence, or reduced social interaction. Assistive technology, such as telehealth, may help to maintain a better quality of life and independent function. Individuals may be monitored or receive health care through technologies that allow telemedicine or telehealth assistance with sensory, cognitive, or physical disabilities. In one study, the devices that were valued highest were those that provided the most help to the individual user, saved time, were cost-effective, and were technologically advanced (Muncert et al., 2011).

Weight Control Programs

Being overweight or obese increases the risk of chronic illness, including heart disease, type 2 diabetes, stroke, and certain types of cancer (Kahn et al., 2009); therefore it is important to make weight control programs available to the public for health promotion. Participants in community-based weight management programs that implement national treatment guidelines can achieve significant weight loss, regardless of age or gender, which improves cardiovascular and other chronic illness risk factors (Graffagnino et al., 2006).

Lifestyle modification interventions are effective in reducing chronic

illness (Thorpe and Yang, 2011). The YMCA provides weight management programs, such as Diabetes Prevention Programs, at a community
level with proven success rates with significant improvement in weight loss
(Ackermann et al., 2011; Thorpe and Yang, 2011). More information about
the YMCA is provided in Chapter 6. Appel and colleagues (2011) found
that behavioral interventions, whether with in-person or remote support,
garner significant weight loss. In-person support consists of one-on-one and
group sessions with access to remote services. The remote intervention provides weight-loss support through a website, emails, and telephone support.

Weight Watchers International is an example of an effective
community-based program. It follows *Healthy People 2020*'s guideline
for a 10 percent improvement in healthy weight (HHS, 2011). Once the
short-term goal is met, participants focus on long-term goals. The program
educates participants in making healthy habits and food choices and ways
to be active, and it provides emotional support, which involves cognitive-
restructuring (Witherspoon and Rosenzweig, 2004). The program is widely
used across the United States, making it accessible to users, and is relatively
inexpensive compared with other corporate weight loss programs.

Respite Care

Respite care is "planned or emergency care to a child or adult with
special needs in order to provide temporary relief to the family caregiver"
(Virginia Department on Aging, 2011). Respite services are provided within
many settings, including home, adult day care centers, or residential care
facilities, and is the primary sector of family support and home- and
community-based care services. Respite care programs are essential for
maintaining strength within a family unit and act as an important resource
within a long-term care system. "Respite care protects the health and well-
being of both caregivers and care recipients" (Virginia Department on
Aging, 2011).

For those caregivers in need, respite services reduce a substantial amount
of stress. Based on an assessment of 23 appraisals of primary stressors (role
captivity [Pearlin], overload [Pearlin and new], worry and strain, depression
[CES-D], anger [Brief Symptom Inventory, and Pearlin], positive affect [posi-
tive and negative affect schedule]), one study found that those caregivers for
a loved one living with dementia using respite services had significantly lower
scores than did the control group on two of the three measures of primary
appraisals (overload and strain) and two of the three measures of well-being
(depression and anger). One year later, the treatment group still had significantly lower scores, most notably on overload and depression, than the
control group had (Zarit et al., 1998). In general, caregivers for loved ones
with dementia were found to experience far lower levels of stress when us-

ing respite services than when not (Zarit et al., 1998). Evidence consistently demonstrates an improvement in stress level and overall quality of life (Collins and Swartz, 2011; Empeño et al., 2011), but also an improvement in confidence and a feeling of empowerment (Gitlin et al., 2006).

Despite questions regarding actual service efficiency, caregivers tend to strongly report satisfaction for the services offered (Schoenmakers et al., 2010). In one study, in-person interviews held 3 months and a year after services started indicate high levels of satisfaction for service features such as staff friendliness, program activities or meals and benefits and drawbacks such as focusing on the behaviors of a care receiver before and after attending the day program (Jarrott et al., 1999).

As the evidence shows, although respite services provide proven benefits, most caregivers feel that what's out there is not enough (Paraponaris et al., 2011; Stirling et al., 2010). In addition, because a majority of those among lower socioeconomic status often experience difficulties in gaining access to these kinds of services, and because informal care consumes almost two-thirds of all care in a year, more services should be offered (Paraponaris et al., 2011).

Peer Support

The burden and demands of a chronic illness often reduce the patient's ability to self-manage their illness. Inadequate illness control and self-management reduces the patient's quality of life and increases poor psychological well-being (Bosworth et al., 2010). Peer support programs lend valuable firsthand experience knowledge to assist others with similar conditions in managing their own health (Ramirez and Turner, 2010). The focus of an illness is shifted from treatment to health promotion (Dennis, 2003). Evidence has consistently found that support groups are beneficial for addressing a variety of chronic illnesses—especially groups related to maintaining self-management regimens. These programs have been functioning since the 1970s and have been well documented (Boothroyd and Fisher, 2010). The Patient Protection and Affordable Care Act encourages peer support programs as part of community health initiatives.

Support ranges from remote assistance, including telephone, web- or email-based peer support, to face-to-face self-management programs (Ramirez and Turner, 2010). Such programs include assistance in learning and overcoming the challenges of diet, exercise and medication compliance, and self-monitoring illness control. Participants in diabetes peer support programs see success in decreased mean hemoglobin A_{1c} levels, and initiation of insulin therapy (Ramirez and Turner, 2010). Peers for Progress, which originated from the WHO, promotes peer support as, "a key part of health, health care, and prevention around the world" (Peers for Progress, [a]).

Social support has been demonstrated to be a protective factor of health, where social isolation—which the committee recognizes as a plausible consequence for person living with complex chronic illness—brings morbidity and mortality (Boothroyd and Fisher, 2010). Bosworth and colleagues (2010) discuss the important role of peer support in improving hypertension and cardiovascular disease, stating that patient self-management is "a crucial component of effective high-quality health care. . . . The patient must be a collaborator in this process, and methods of improving patients' ability and confidence for self-management are needed."

Caregiver Support

Caregivers of people living with chronic illnesses are greatly affected in numerous ways. Better than 65 million people in the United States are caregivers, or 29 percent of the total U.S. adult population (NAC, [a]). Family caregivers feel extreme stress, often leading to caregivers experiencing higher levels of depression, higher probability of chronic illnesses, premature aging, familial financial problems, and lower levels overall of well-being (NFCA, [a]). Additionally, caregivers experience higher rates of poverty, have lower income, and have higher out-of-pocket health care expenses. Six out of ten family caregivers are employed (NFCA, [a]).

Supporting caregivers is important for protecting their health and that of the person they are caring for. A sense of empowerment, acceptance of help from those around them, and prioritization of one's own health offers the best hope in maintaining caregivers' and dependents' mental and physical health (Carcone et al., 2011; Gitlin et al., 2006; Graff et al., 2007).

Supporting caregivers involves interventions with a multifaceted approach. A coach or mentor can provide training to build confidence and skills to be better advocates in activities of daily living with a chronic illness. Peer connections made among caregivers reduces feelings of isolation for caregivers (Amdur, 2011). Organizations such as the National Family Caregivers Association provide resources for caregivers to educate themselves as well as to connect with other caregivers and, ultimately, to empower those caring for others living with chronic illness.

MONITORING, EVALUATION, AND RESEARCH

As discussed earlier in this chapter, a number of community-based interventions have been developed and evaluated for their efficacy in serving individuals with chronic illness. These evidence-based programs include lifestyle interventions for physical activity, smoking cessation, and diet and nutrition, as well as other living-well interventions, such as disease self-management. Many of these programs have been rigorously evaluated in trials, but they have not been widely disseminated. As noted by Chambers and Kerner, "tested interventions are underutilized. Used interventions are under-tested" (Chambers and Kerner, 2007; Schillinger, 2010). Programs and interventions are not brought to scale for multiple, interacting reasons, including social, economic, cultural, and organizational factors (Glasgow and Emmons, 2007). In general, health promotion interventions that have been proven to be efficacious have tended to be intensive and demanding for both participants and program delivery staff (Glasgow and Emmons, 2007). The committee has included an article that discusses new models of health care and community-based programs to improve the functional autonomy and lives of those living with chronic illness (see Appendix B).

To ensure that more interventions designed to help individuals with chronic illness live well can be brought to the most people, more attention needs to be paid to the barriers to translating research into practice. Lack of dissemination and evaluation research and policy advocacy is one component that limits the impact of evidenced-based physical activity interventions on public health (Owen et al., 2006), particularly underserved groups. Evidence-based interventions recommended by government advisory bodies have proved to be less effective or ineffective in the aged, racial and ethnic minorities, and low-income groups, who experience a high burden of chronic illness and are among the most sedentary and understudied populations (Yancey et al., 2006). There are sociocultural, physical, economic, and environmental barriers to engaging certain evidenced-based interventions, like physical activity and exercise, with the elderly, racial and ethnic minorities, and low-income groups. Successful engagement of underserved populations in health-promoting evidenced-based interventions requires careful balance between embracing customs and values and recognizing the nonmonolithic nature of any sociodemographic group (Yancey et al., 2006).

To date, the focus on the efficacy of interventions rather than the effectiveness of interventions has resulted in sacrificing external validity in the hope of maximizing internal validity (Schillinger, 2010). Characteristics of the intervention, the target settings, the research or evaluation design, and the interactions of all three of these are areas that could potentially be addressed by public health researchers (Glasgow and Emmons, 2007). Interventions that are expensive, time- and staff-intensive, specific to a particular setting, not packaged for easy delivery or not customizable, difficult to learn, and not designed to be self-sustaining are difficult to bring to scale (Glasgow and Emmons, 2007). A theorem by Rose suggests that one solution to making sure interventions reach more individuals and diverse populations is to replace intensive interventions that engage fewer people with low-cost interventions (with frequent contact) that engage more people

(Schillinger, 2010). Although some level of intensity of intervention is desirable, the minimal intensity needed for change, rather than the maximum intensity, should be the focus of program designers (Schillinger, 2010).

Some of the issues related to program delivery that can result in huge barriers for scalability include competing demands for staff, financial or organizational instability, limited resources, time and organizational support, perverse incentives or regulations, and the specific needs of clients and the setting (Glasgow and Emmons, 2007; Glasgow et al., 2003). When program designers do not describe modifications of the intervention that are permissible, it can be difficult for practice settings that do not have the infrastructure or support of the trial settings to deliver the intervention with fidelity. It has been suggested that program designers should collect more process evaluation data to help make recommendations regarding program modifications (Schillinger, 2010).

Some of the other elements of the research design that can limit translation of programs include the failure to evaluate cost and reach or to assess adoption, implementation, maintenance, and sustainability. Recommendations have recently been made that interventions should be developed from the outset with dissemination and scalability in mind, with greater attention paid to replication and robustness (Kessler and Glasgow, 2011; Kleges et al., 2005).There are considerable challenges to assessing community and public health interventions, and the evidence is often far from complete (Community Preventive Services Task Force, 2005b; Leyland, 2010; Weatherly et al., 2009). Reasons for this include an insufficient number of studies on a given theme; the lack of truly experimental or even quasi-experimental designs; inclusion of inadequately representative study communities; inadequate statistical power for many study outcomes, including the primary one of interest; the short-term nature of many evaluations; the difficulty of replicating complex intervention protocols (Bell et al., 2007); and the uncertainty of outcomes outside those being directly addressed. In some deprived neighborhoods, often the target of public health interventions, it may not be logistically possible to conduct rigorous evaluations (Abbema et al., 2004). These challenges also apply to evaluation of cost-effectiveness, in which common problems include determining attribution of effects directly to the interventions, measuring and valuing the outcomes, calculating costs and consequences across many economic sectors—a particular problem for the Health in All Policy movement (Finland Ministry of Social and Health Affairs and European Observatory on Health Systems and Policies, 2006)—and taking equity into consideration (Weatherly et al., 2009). With respect to equity, it is possible for an intervention to have a net positive community effect and still perpetuate or even exacerbate disparities across various socioeconomic groups with respect to salient effects of the intervention. It must also be acknowledged that societal and individual perspectives may differ when it comes to what constitutes a life well lived with chronic illness. For example, although many physically inactive persons may wish to be active but are not for a variety of individual and societal reasons, others may be quite comfortable with their inactivity, and their wishes must be respected.

Another problem that occurs with assessing community interventions is the lack of attention or the inability to measure adverse effects of the intervention. Unlike studies of clinical interventions, in which all exposed can be routinely followed for a broad range of adverse health outcomes, evaluative studies of community respondents may involve many individuals who may have had adverse effects from the intervention but are never sampled or studied. Perhaps more importantly, it may not be possible to even anticipate potential adverse effects in community intervention programs; investigators may not even seek them, assuming that an educational or helping program could not encompass unwelcome effects. Some of this may result from inadequate formative evaluation of intervention programs (Whitehead, 2002) and the failure to do qualitative interviewing of groups and individuals exposed to the experimental intervention. Although CDC's Community Guide clearly notes the prospect of adverse effects (Community Preventive Services Task Force, 2005b), many of the "logic diagrams" of specific intervention do not even consider the possibility that they occur. Evaluation summaries that include such comments as "no adverse effects were found" often do not review the depth with which a search was conducted, over and above the possibility that the major effect was in the wrong direction.

Given this situation, it is difficult to know how many adverse effects were sought or evaluated, but examples exist. Pediatricians have anecdotally noted that some children were distraught after a school tobacco education program because they feared their parents who smoke would die. The whole issue of harm reduction, particularly aimed at substance abuse interventions, often generates substantial resistance in various community segments (Logan and Marlatt, 2010) such as for condom use or needle-sharing interventions, despite evidence of at least partial effectiveness.

The major message here is to acknowledge and anticipate that adverse effects of community interventions can occur. These adverse effects should be indentified to ensure that when the interventions become part of public health practice, they will not be impeded by such effects at a time of limited resources. As in clinical research, these adverse effects need not be a reason to avoid their incumbent programs, but they must be recognized and managed by the appropriate intervening organizations.

CONCLUSION

Like everyone, persons living with chronic illness need effective interventions aimed at prevention and early detection of additional illness. These interventions include healthy lifestyle behaviors (physical activity, healthy eating, maintenance of healthy weight, and tobacco avoidance), vaccination, screening, and chemoprevention. Issues in developing these interventions include their effectiveness in, their adaptation for, and their long-term maintenance among persons living with chronic illness. Although some interventions, such as physical activity, have been well studied and shown to improve the lives of persons living with many types of chronic illness, all interventions could benefit from further research on effectiveness, adaptation, and maintenance.

Persons living with chronic illness also need interventions aimed at controlling and limiting the effects of their illness. This chapter has explored the effectiveness of self-management, disease management, treatment adherence management, complementary and alternative medicine, cognitive training, and approaches to improving access and mobility. A large number of effective interventions have been developed, but important issues for further research include adaptation for specific illnesses and the relative cost-effectiveness of effective interventions.

Once interventions for both prevention of additional illness and control of existing illness are developed and shown to be effective, the hardest work begins. This is the work of scale-up, so that effective interventions reach all those in need, especially disadvantaged populations who are disproportionately affected by chronic illness. This work requires a different set of research that evaluates outcomes at both the individual level and the level of organizations seeking to disseminate and implement effective interventions. The public health community should join with health care systems and community organizations in giving much more attention to scale-up and the dissemination and implementation research required to achieve it.

The statement of task asks the committee to consider which population-based interventions can help achieve outcomes that maintain or improve quality of life, functioning, and disability?

- What is the evidence on effectiveness of interventions on these outcomes?
- To what extent do the interventions that address these outcomes also affect clinical outcomes?
- To what extent can policy, environmental, and systems change achieve these outcomes?

RECOMMENDATIONS 9–12

Recommendation 9

The committee recommends that CDC conduct rigorous evaluations of its funded chronic disease prevention programs to include the effects of those programs on health-related quality of life and functional status.

Recommendation 10

The committee recommends that all major CDC-funded research programs aimed at primary community-based chronic disease prevention or interventions be evaluated for their effect on persons with existing chronic illness to assess health- and social-related quality of life, management of existing illness, and efforts to prevent subsequent illnesses.

Recommendation 11

The committee recommends that public and private research funders increase support for research on and evaluation of the adoption and long-term maintenance of healthy lifestyles and effective preventive services (e.g., promoting physical activity, healthy eating patterns, appropriate weight, effective health care) in persons with chronic illness. Support should be provided for implementation research on how to disseminate effective long-term lifestyle interventions in community-based settings that improve living well with chronic illness.

Recommendation 12

The committee recommends that federally supported efforts to improve living with chronic illness have as an explicit goal the reduction of health disparities across affected populations.

- Barriers to obtaining complete assessments of community and public health interventions for populations experiencing health disparities should be identified and addressed.
- When interventions typically result in positive health outcomes for the general population of individuals living with chronic illness, they should be assessed and modified for adaptation and implementation in communities experiencing disparities in health outcomes.

REFERENCES

Abbema, E.A., P. Van Assema, G.J. Kok, E. De Leeuw, and N.K. De Vries. 2004. Effect evaluation of a comprehensive community intervention aimed at reducing socioeconomic health inequalities in The Netherlands. *Health Promotion International* 19(2):141–156.

Ackermann, R.T., B. Williams, H.Q. Nguyen, E.M. Berke, M.L. Maciejewski, and J.P. LoGerfo. 2008. Healthcare cost differences with participation in a community-based group physical activity benefit for Medicare managed care health plan members. *Journal of the American Geriatrics Society* 56(8):1459–1465.

Ackermann, R.T., E.A. Finch, H.M. Caffrey, E.R. Lipscomb, L.M. Hays, and C. Saha. 2011. Long-term effects of a community-based lifestyle intervention to prevent type 2 diabetes: The DEPLOY extension pilot study. *Chronic Illness* 7:279–290.

Amdur, D. 2011. *Assistance and Support Services for Family Caregivers.* PowerPoint presented at the National Training Summit on Women Veterans, Washington, DC. http://www.va.gov/WOMENVET/2011Summit/3B-Amdur7-15-11FINAL-1.pdf (accessed January 5, 2012).

Appel, L.J., J.M. Clark, H.C. Yeh, N.Y. Wang, J.W. Coughlin, G. Daumit, E.R. Miller, III, A. Dalcin, G.J. Jerome, S. Geller, G. Noronha, T. Pozefsky, J. Charleston, J.B. Reynolds, N. Durkin, R.R. Rubin, T.A Louis, and F.L. Brancati. 2011. Comparative effectiveness of weight-loss interventions in clinical practice. *New England Journal of Medicine* 365:1959–1968.

Arthritis Foundation and CDC. 2010. *A National Public Health Agenda for Osteoarthritis.* http://www.cdc.gov/arthritis/docs/oaagenda.pdf (accessed October 15, 2011).

Baldwin, L.M., S.A. Dobie, Y. Cai, B.G. Saver, P.K. Green, and C.Y. Wang. 2011. Receipt of general medical care by colorectal cancer patients: A longitudinal study. *Journal of the American Board of Family Medicine* 24(1):57–68.

Banham, L., and S. Gilbody. 2010. Smoking cessation in severe mental illness: What works? *Addiction* 105(7):1176–1189.

Barbeau, E.M., K.Y. Wolin, E.N. Naumova, and E. Balbach. 2005. Tobacco advertising in communities: Associations with race and class. *Preventive Medicine* 40(1):16–22.

Barnes, P.M., B. Bloom, and R.L. Nahin. 2008. Complementary and alternative medicine use among adults and children: United States, 2007. *National Health Statistics Reports* (12):1–23.

Bartels, E.M., H. Lund, K.B. Hagen, H. Dagfinrud, R. Christensen, and B. Danneskiold-Samsøe. 2007. Aquatic exercise for the treatment of knee and hip osteoarthritis. *Cochrane Database of Systematic Reviews* (4):CD005523.

Barton, D. 2011. Oral agents in cancer treatment: The context for adherence. *Seminars in Oncology Nursing* 27(2):104–115.

Becker, M.H. 1985. Patient adherence to prescribed therapies. *Medical Care* 23(5):539–555.

Bell, C.M., S.S. Brener, N. Gunraj, C. Huo, A.S. Bierman, D.C. Scales, J. Bajcar, M. Zwarenstein, and D.R. Urbach. 2011. Association of ICU or hospital admission with unintentional discontinuation of medications for chronic diseases. *Journal of the American Medical Association* 306(8):840–847.

Bell, S.G., S.F. Newcomer, C. Bachrach, E. Borawski, J.B. Jemmott, III, D. Morrison, B. Stanton, S. Tortolero, and R. Zimmerman. 2007. Challenges in replicating interventions. *Journal of Adolescent Health* 40(6):514–520.

Belza, B., A. Shumway-Cook, E.A. Phelan, B. Williams, S.J. Snyder, and J.P. LoGerfo. 2006. The effects of a community-based exercise program on function and health in older adults: The Enhance Fitness Program. *Journal of Applied Gerontology* 25(4):291–306.

Bernstein, J. 2011. The elusive benefits of chronic care management: Comment on "the effect of guided care teams on the use of health services." *Archives of Internal Medicine* 171(5):466–467.

Bernstein, J., D. Chollet, and G.G. Peterson. 2010. *Disease Management: Does It Work? Reforming Health Care Issue Brief #4*. Washington, DC: Mathematica Policy Research. http://www.mathematica-mpr.net/publications/PDFs/health/reformhealthcare_IB4.pdf (accessed November 3, 2011).

Blankevoort, C.G., M.J. van Heuvelen, F. Boersma, H. Luning, J. de Jong, and E.J. Scherder. 2010. Review of effects of physical activity on strength, balance, mobility and ADL performance in elderly subjects with dementia. *Dementia and Geriatric Cognitive Disorders* 30(5):392–402.

Boothroyd, R.I., and E.B. Fisher. 2010. Peers for progress: Promoting peer support for health around the world. *Family Practice* 27(Supplement 1):i62–i68.

Bosworth, H.B., B.J. Powers, and E.Z. Oddone. 2010. Patient self-management support: Novel strategies in hypertension and heart disease. *Cardiology Clinics* 28(4):655–663.

Bosworth, H.B., B.B. Granger, P. Mendys, R. Brindis, R. Burkholder, S.M. Czajkowski, J.G. Daniel, I. Ekman, M. Ho, M. Johnson, S.E. Kimmel, L.Z. Liu, J. Musaus, W.H. Shrank, E. Whalley Buono, K. Weiss, and C.B. Granger. 2011. Medication adherence: A call for action. *American Heart Journal* 162(3):412–424.

Briesacher, B.A., J.H. Gurwitz, and S.B. Soumerai. 2007. Patients at-risk for cost-related medication nonadherence: A review of the literature. *Journal of General Internal Medicine* 22(6):864–871.

Brownson, R.C., D. Haire-Joshu, and D.A. Luke. 2006. Shaping the context of health: A review of environmental and policy approaches in the prevention of chronic diseases. *Annual Review of Public Health* 27:341–370.

Bruce, B., K. Lorig, and D. Laurent. 2007. Participation in patient self-management programs. *Arthritis and Rheumatism* 57(5):851–854.

Busch, A.J., K.A. Barber, T.J. Overend, P.M. Peloso, and C.L. Schachter. 2007. Exercise for treating fibromyalgia syndrome. *Cochrane Database of Systematic Reviews* (4):CD003786.

Calhoun, R., H. Meischke, K. Hammerback, A. Bohl, P. Poe, B. Williams, and E.A. Phelan. 2011. Older adults' perceptions of clinical fall prevention programs: A qualitative study. *Journal of Aging Research* vol. 2011 (867341).

Callahan, L.F., T. Mielenz, J. Freburger, J. Shreffler, J. Hootman, T. Brady, K. Buysse, and T. Schwartz. 2008. A randomized controlled trial of the people with arthritis can exercise program: symptoms, function, physical activity, and psychosocial outcomes. *Arthritis and Rheumatism* 59(1):92–101.

Canadian Human Rights Commission. 2006. *International Best Practices in Universal Design. A Global Review*. Ottawa, ON: Human Rights Commission. http://www.chrc-ccdp.ca/pdf/bestpractices_en.pdf (accessed November 7, 2011).

Carcone, A.I., D.A. Ellis, A. Weisz, and S. Naar-King. 2011. Social support for diabetes illness management: Supporting adolescents and caregivers. *Journal of Developmental and Behavioral Pediatrics* 32(8):581–590.

CDC (Centers for Disease Control and Prevention). 2011. Chapter 11: Influenza. In *Epidemiology and Prevention of Vaccine-Preventable Diseases*, 12th ed. Edited by W. Atkinson, C. Wolfe, and J. Hamborsky. Washington, DC: Public Health Foundation. http://www.cdc.gov/vaccines/pubs/pinkbook/downloads/flu.pdf (accessed September 8, 2011).

Chambers, D.A., and J.F. Kerner. 2007. *Closing the Gap Between Discovery and Delivery*. Presented at the Dissemination and Implementation Research Workshop: Harnessing Science to Maximize Health. Rockville, MD. http://cancercontrol.cancer.gov/IS/pdfs/BackgroundDisseminationImplementationResearch.pdf (accessed September 20, 2011).

Chodosh, J., S.C. Morton, W. Mojica, M. Maglione, M.J. Suttorp, L. Hilton, S. Rhodes, and P. Shekelle. 2005. Meta-analysis: Chronic disease self-management programs for older adults. *Annals of Internal Medicine* 143(6):427–438.

Choi, M., and M. Hector. 2011. Effectiveness of intervention programs in preventing falls: A systematic review of recent 10 years and meta-analysis. *Journal of the American Medical Directors Association* Jun 14. [Epub ahead of print].

Cohen, L., R. Davis, V. Lee, and E. Valdovinos. 2010. *Addressing the Intersection: Preventing Violence and Promoting Healthy Eating and Active Living*. Oakland, CA: Prevention Institute. http://www.preventioninstitute.org/press/highlights/404-addressing-the-intersection.html (accessed December 7, 2011).

Colberg, S.R., R.J. Sigal, B. Fernhall, J.G. Regensteiner, B.J. Blissmer, R.R. Rubin, L. Chasan-Taber, A.L. Albright, B. Braun, American College of Sports Medicine, and American Diabetes Association. 2010. Exercise and type 2 diabetes: The American College of Sports Medicine and the American Diabetes Association: Joint position statement. *Diabetes Care* 33(12):e147–e167.

Collins, L.G., and K. Swartz. 2011. Caregiver care. *American Family Physician* 83(11): 1309–1317.

Community Preventive Services Task Force (a). *Cancer Prevention and Control: Client-Oriented Screening Interventions*. http://www.thecommunityguide.org/cancer/screening/client-oriented/index.html (accessed November 1, 2011).

Community Preventive Services Task Force (b). *Environmental and Policy Approaches to Increase Physical Activity: Community-Scale Urban Design Land Use Policies*. http://www.thecommunityguide.org/pa/environmental-policy/communitypolicies.html (accessed September 7, 2011).

Community Preventive Services Task Force (c). *Interventions to Promote Seasonal Influenza Vaccinations among Non-Healthcare Workers*. http://thecommunityguide.org/worksite/flunon-hcw.html (accessed November 2, 2011).

Community Preventive Services Task Force (d). *Promoting Physical Activity: Environmental and Policy Approaches*. http://www.thecommunityguide.org/pa/environmental-policy/index.html (accessed September 7, 2011).

Community Preventive Services Task Force. 2005a. Chapter 2. Physical activity. In *The Guide to Community Preventive Services: What Works to Promote Health?* Edited by S. Zaza, P.A. Briss, and K.W. Harris. Oxford University Press: New York. http://www.thecommunityguide.org/pa/Physical-Activity.pdf (accessed July 1, 2011).

Community Preventive Services Task Force. 2005b. *The Guide to Community Preventive Services: What Works to Promote Health?* Edited by S. Zaza, P.A. Briss, and K.W. Harris. Oxford University Press: New York. http://www.thecommunityguide.org/library/book/index.html (accessed November 28, 2011).

Dennis, C.L. 2003. Peer support within a health care context: A concept analysis. *International Journal of Nursing Studies* 40(3):321–332.

DiMatteo, M.R. 2004. Variations in patients' adherence to medical recommendations: A quantitative review of 50 years of research. *Medical Care* 42(3):200–209.

Donkin, L., H. Christensen, S.L. Naismith, B. Neal, I.B. Hickie, and N. Glozier. 2011. A systematic review of the impact of adherence on the effectiveness of e-therapies. *Journal of Medical Internet Research* 13(3):e52.

Downey, L., P.T. Tyree, and W.E. Lafferty. 2009. Preventive screening of women who use complementary and alternative medicine providers. *Journal of Women's Health* 18(8): 1133–1143.

Empeño, J., N.T. Raming, S.A. Irwin, R.A. Nelesen, and L.S. Lloyd. 2011. The hospice caregiver support project: Providing support to reduce caregiver stress. *Journal of Palliative Medicine* 14(5):593–597.

Estabrooks, P.A., R.E. Lee, and N.C. Gyurcsik. 2003. Resources for physical activity participation: Does availability and accessibility differ by neighborhood socioeconomic status? *Annals of Behavioral Medicine* 25(2):100–104.

Etgen, T., D. Sander, U. Huntgeburth, H. Poppert, H. Förstl, and H. Bickel. 2010. Physical activity and incident cognitive impairment in elderly persons: The INVADE study. *Archives of Internal Medicine* 170(2):186–193.

Fain, W.B. 2006. Assessment of workplace product accessibility: A human factors perspective. *Work* 27(4):371–379.

Finland Ministry of Social and Health Affairs and European Observatory on Health Systems and Policies. 2006. *Health in All Policies: Prospects and potentials.* Edited by T. Stahl, M. Wismar, E. Ollila, E. Lahtinen, and K. Leppo. Finland: Ministry of Social and Health Affairs. http://ec.europa.eu/health/archive/ph_information/documents/health_in_all_policies.pdf (accessed November 4, 2011).

Fransen, M., and S. McConnell. 2008. Exercise for osteoarthritis of the knee. *Cochrane Database of Systematic Reviews* (4):CD004376.

Gardetto, N.J. 2011. Self-management in heart failure: Where have we been and where should we go? *Journal of Multidisciplinary Healthcare* 4:39–51.

Geda, Y.E., R.O. Roberts, D.S. Knopman, T.J. Christianson, V.S. Pankratz, R.J. Ivnik, B.F. Boeve, E.G. Tangalos, R.C. Petersen, and W.A. Rocca. 2010. Physical exercise, aging, and mild cognitive impairment: A population-based study. *Archives of Neurology* 67(1):80–86.

Gentry, E., K. Poirier, T. Wilkinson, S. Nhean, J. Nyborn, and M. Siegel. 2011. Alcohol advertising at Boston subway stations: An assessment of exposure by race and socioeconomic status. *American Journal of Public Health* 101(10):1936–1941.

Gitlin, L., K. Reever, M. Dennis, E. Mathieu, and W. Hauck. 2006. Enhancing quality of life of families who use adult day services: Short-and long-term effects of the adult day services plus program. *The Gerontologist* 46(5):630–639.

Glasgow, R.E., and K.M. Emmons. 2007. How can we increase translation of research into practice? Types of evidence needed. *Annual Review of Public Health* 28:413–433.

Glasgow, R.E., E. Lichtenstein, and A.C. Marcus. 2003. Why don't we see more translation of health promotion research into practice? Rethinking the efficacy-to-effectiveness transition. *American Journal of Public Health* 93(8):1261–1267.

Gossett, A., M. Mirza, A.K. Barnds, and D. Feidt. 2009. Beyond access: A case study on the intersection between accessibility, sustainability, and universal design. *Disability and Rehabilitation. Assistive Technology* 4(6):439–450.

Graff, M.J., M.J. Vernooij-Dassen, M. Thijssen, J. Dekker, W.H. Hoefnagels, and M.G. Olderikkert. 2007. Effects of community occupational therapy on quality of life, mood, and health status in dementia patients and their caregivers: A randomized controlled trial. *Journals of Gerontology. Series A: Biological Sciences and Medical Sciences* 62(9): 1002–1009.

Graffagnino, C.L., J.M. Falko, M.L. Londe, J. Schaumburg, M.F. Hyek, L.E.T. Shaffer, R. Snow, and T. Caulin-Glaser. 2006. Effect of a community-based weight management program on weight loss and cardiovascular disease risk factors. *Obesity* 14:280–288.

Gritz, E.R., D.J. Vidrine, and M.C. Fingeret. 2007. Smoking cessation a critical component of medical management in chronic disease populations. *American Journal of Preventive Medicine* 33(6 Suppl):S414–S422.

Gross, A.L., G.W. Rebok, F.W. Unverzagt, S.L. Willis, and J. Brandt. 2011a. Cognitive predictors of everyday functioning in older adults: Results from the ACTIVE Intervention Trial. *Journals of Gerontology: Series B, Psychological Sciences and Social Sciences* 66(5):557–566.

Gross, A.L., G.W. Rebok, F.W. Unverzagt, S.L. Willis, and J. Brandt. 2011b. Word list memory predicts everyday function and problem-solving in the elderly: Results from the ACTIVE cognitive intervention trial. *Neuropsychology, Development, and Cognition: Section B, Aging, Neuropsychology and Cognition* 18(2):129–146.

Hahn, E.A., and R. Andel. 2011. Nonpharmacological therapies for behavioral and cognitive symptoms of mild cognitive impairment. *Journal of Aging and Health* 23(8):1223–1245.

Hak, E., E. Buskens, G.A. van Essen, D.H. de Bakker, D.E. Grobbee, M.A. Tacken, B.A. van Hout, and T.J. Verheij. 2005. Clinical effectiveness of influenza vaccination in persons younger than 65 years with high-risk medical conditions: The PRISMA study. *Archives of Internal Medicine* 165(3):274–280.

Hanson, D. 2008. The Chicago perspective on design for the disabled. *Topics in Stroke Rehabilitation* 15(2):75–79.

Häuser, W., K. Bernardy, B. Arnold, M. Offenbächer, and M. Schiltenwolf. 2009. Efficacy of multicomponent treatment in fibromyalgia syndrome: A meta-analysis of randomized controlled clinical trials. *Arthritis and Rheumatism* 61(2):216–224.

Häuser, W., P. Klose, J. Langhorst, B. Moradi, M. Steinbach, M. Schiltenwolf, and A. Busch. 2010. Efficacy of different types of aerobic exercise in fibromyalgia syndrome: A systematic review and meta-analysis of randomised controlled trials. *Arthritis Research and Therapy* 12(3):R79.

HHS (U.S. Department of Health and Human Services). 1990. *The Health Benefits of Smoking Cessation: A Report of the Surgeon General.* Rockville, MD: U.S. Department of Health and Human Services. http://profiles.nlm.nih.gov/NN/B/B/C/T/ (accessed November 2, 2011).

HHS. 2010. *Multiple Chronic Conditions: A Strategic Framework Optimum Health and Quality of Life for Individuals with Multiple Chronic Conditions.* http://www.hhs.gov/ash/initiatives/mcc/mcc_framework.pdf (accessed October 4, 2011).

HHS. 2011. *Nutrition and Weight Status.* http://healthypeople.gov/2020/topicsobjectives2020/objectiveslist.aspx?topicid=29 (accessed January 3, 2012).

HHS and Public Health Service. 2008. *Treating Tobacco Use and Dependence: 2008 Update. Clinical Practice Guideline.* Rockville, MD: U.S. Department of Health and Human Services and Public Health Service.

Hughes, S.L., B. Williams, L.C. Molina, C. Bayles, L.L. Bryant, J.R. Harris, R. Hunter, S. Ivey, and K. Watkins. 2005. Characteristics of physical activity programs for older adults: Results of a multisite survey. *The Gerontologist* 45(5):667–675.

Hughes, S.L., R.B. Seymour, R.T. Campbell, G. Huber, N. Pollak, L. Sharma, and P. Desai. 2006. Long-term impact of Fit and Strong! on older adults with osteoarthritis. *The Gerontologist* 46(6):801–814.

Institute on Disabilities, Temple University (a). *Pennsylvania's Initiative on Assistive Technology (PIAT).* http://disabilities.temple.edu/programs/assistive/piat/whatisAT.shtml (accessed September 20, 2011).

Ismail, K., K. Winkley, and S. Rabe-Hesketh. 2004. Systematic review and meta-analysis of randomized control trials of psychological interventions to improve glycaemic control in patients with type 2 diabetes. *Lancet* 363(9421):1589–1597.

Jarrott, S., S. Zarit, M.A. Paris-Stephens, A. Townsend, and R. Greene. 1999. Caregiver satisfaction with adult day service programs. *American Journal of Alzheimer's Disease* 14(4):233–244.

Jobe, J.B., D.M. Smith, K. Ball, S.L. Tennstedt, M. Marsiske, S.L. Willis, G.W. Rebok, J.N. Morris, K.F. Helmers, M.D. Leveck, and K. Kleinman. 2001. ACTIVE: A cognitive intervention trial to promote independence in older adults. *Controlled Clinical Trials* 22(4):453–479.

Johnston, S.E., C.E. Liddy, and S.M. Ives. 2011. Self-management support: A new approach still anchored in an old model of health care. *Canadian Journal of Public Health* 102(1): 68–72.

Kahn, L.K., K. Sobush, D. Keener, K. Goodman, A. Lowry, J. Kakietek, and S. Zaro. 2009. Recommended community strategies and measurements to prevent obesity in the United States. *Morbidity and Mortality Weekly* 58(RR07):1–26.

Kaiser Family Foundation and Health Research and Educational Trust. 2010. *Employer Health Benefits. 2010 Summary of Findings.* http://ehbs.kff.org/pdf/2010/8086.pdf (accessed September 19, 2011).

Kessler, R., and R.E. Glasgow. 2011. A proposal to speed translation of healthcare research into practice: Dramatic change is needed. *American Journal of Preventive Medicine* 40(6):637–644.

Kington, R.S., and J.P. Smith. 1997. Socioeconomic status and racial and ethnic differences in functional status associated with chronic disease. *American Journal of Public Health* 87(5):805–810.

Klesges, L.M., P.A. Estabrooks, D.A. Dzewaltowski, S.S. Bull, and R.E. Glasgow. 2005. Beginning with the application in mind: Designing and planning health behavior change interventions to enhance dissemination. *Annals of Behavioral Medicine* 29(2):66–75.

Kwok, T.C., K. Lam, P. Wong, W. Chau, K.S. Yuen, K. Ting, E.W. Chung, J.C. Li, and F.K. Ho. 2011. Effectiveness of coordination exercise in improving cognitive function in older adults: A prospective study. *Clinical Interventions in Aging* 6:261–267.

Langbaum, J.B., G.W. Rebok, K. Bendeen-Roche, and M.C. Carlson. 2009. Predicting memory training response patterns: Results from ACTIVE. *Journals of Gerontology: Series B, Psychological Sciences and Social Sciences* 64(1):14–23.

Larson, N.I., M.T. Story, and M.C. Nelson. 2009. Neighborhood environments: Disparities in access to healthy foods in the U.S. *American Journal of Preventive Medicine* 36(1):74–81.

Laurin, D., R. Verrcault, J. Lindsay, K. MacPherson, and K. Rockwood. 2001. Physical activity and risk of cognitive impairment and dementia in elderly persons. *Archives of Neurology* 58(3):498–504.

Levin, J. 2011. The invisible hate crime. *Miller-McCune*, March 1, 2011.

Leyland, A.H. 2010. Methodological challenges in the evaluation of community interventions. *European Journal of Public Health* 20(3):242–243.

Littbrand, H., M. Stenvall, and E. Rosendahl. 2011. Applicability and effects of physical exercise on physical and cognitive functions and activities of daily living among people with dementia: A systematic review. *American Journal of Physical Medicine and Rehabilitation* 90(6):495–518.

Logan, D.E., and G.A. Marlatt. 2010. Harm reduction therapy: A practice-friendly review of research. *Journal of Clinical Psychology* 66(2):201–214.

Look AHEAD Research Group and R.R. Wing. 2010. Long-term effects of a lifestyle intervention on weight and cardiovascular risk factors in individuals with type 2 diabetes mellitus: Four-year results of the Look AHEAD trial. *Archives of Internal Medicine* 170(17):1566–1575.

Look AHEAD Research Group, X. Pi-Sunyer, G. Blackburn, F.L. Brancati, G.A. Bray, R. Bright, J.M. Clark, J.M. Curtis, M.A. Espeland, J.P. Foreyt, K. Graves, S.M. Haffner, B. Harrison, J.O. Hill, E.S. Horton, J. Jakicic, R.W. Jeffery, K.C. Johnson, S. Kahn, D.E. Kelley, A.E. Kitabchi, W.C. Knowler, C.E. Lewis, B.J. Maschak-Carey, B. Montgomery, D.M. Nathan, J. Patricio, A. Peters, J.B. Redmon, R.S. Reeves, D.H. Ryan, M. Safford, B. Van Dorsten, T.A. Wadden, L. Wagenknecht, J. Wesche-Thobaben, R.R. Wing, and S.Z. Yanovski. 2007. Reduction in weight and cardiovascular disease risk factors in individuals with type 2 diabetes: One-year results of the look AHEAD trial. *Diabetes Care* 30(6):1374–1383.

Lorig, K.R., and H.R. Holman. 2003. Self-management education: History, definition, outcomes, and mechanisms. *Annals of Behavioral Medicine* 26(1):1–7.

Lorig, K.R., P. Ritter, A.L. Stewart, D.S. Sobel, B.W. Brown, Jr., A. Bandura, V.M. Gonzalez, D.D. Laurent, and H.R. Holman. 2001a. Chronic disease self-management program: 2-year health status and health care utilization outcomes. *Medical Care* 39(11):1217–1223.

Lorig, K.R., D.S. Sobel, P.L. Ritter, D. Laurent, and M. Hobbs. 2001b. Effects of a self-management program on patients with chronic disease. *Effective Clinical Practice* 4(6): 256–262.

Lorig, K.R., M.L. Hurwicz, D. Sobel, M. Hobbs, and P.L. Ritter. 2005. A national dissemination of an evidence-based self-management program: A process evaluation study. *Patient Education and Counseling* 59(1):69–79.

Mahtani, K.R., C.J. Heneghan, P.P. Glaziou, and R. Perera. 2011. Reminder packaging for improving adherence to self-administered long-term medications. *Cochrane Database of Systematic Reviews* 9:CDOO5025.

Mattke, S., M. Seid, and S. Ma. 2007. Evidence for the effect of disease management: Is $1 billion a year a good investment? *American Journal of Managed Care* 13(12):670–676.

Mead, G.E., W. Morley, P. Campbell, C.A. Greig, M. McMurdo, and D.A. Lawlor. 2009. Exercise for depression. *Cochrane Database Systematic Reviews* (3):CD004366.

Medina-Mirapeix, F., P. Escolar-Reina, J.J. Gascón-Cánovas, J. Montilla-Herrador, F.J. Jimeno-Serrano, and S.M. Collins. 2009. Predictive factors of adherence to frequency and duration components in home exercise programs for neck and low back pain: An observational study. *BMC Musculoskeletal Disorders* 10:155. http://www.biomedcentral. com/1471-2474/10/155. (accessed December 7, 2011).

Moore, H., C. Summerbell, L. Hooper, K. Cruickshank, A. Vyas, P. Johnstone, V. Ashton, and P. Kopelman. 2004. Dietary advice for treatment of type 2 diabetes mellitus in adults. *Cochrane Database of Systematic Reviews* (3):CD004097.

Muncert, E.S., S.A. Bickford, B.L. Guzic, B.R. Demuth, A.R. Bapat, and J.B. Roberts. 2011. Enhancing the quality of life and preserving independence for target needs populations through integration of assistive technology devices. *Telemedicine Journal and e-Health* 17(6):478–483.

NAC (National Alliance for Caregiving) (a). *Research.* http://www.caregiving.org/research (accessed on December 20, 2011).

NCCAM (National Center for Complementary and Alternative Medicine) (a). *Are You Considering Complementary and Alternative Medicine?* http://nccam.nih.gov/health/ decisions/consideringcam.htm (accessed September 19, 2011).

Ness, J., F.T. Sherman, and C.X. Pan. 1999. Alternative medicine: What the data say about common herbal therapies. *Geriatrics* 54(10):33–43.

NFCA (National Family Caregivers Association) (a). *Statistics on Family Caregivers and Family Caregiving.* http://www.thefamilycaregiver.org/who_are_family_caregivers/care_ giving_statstics.cfm (accessed on December 20, 2011).

Ni, H., C. Simile, and A.M. Hardy. 2002. Utilization of complementary and alternative medicine by United States adults: Results from the 1999 National Health Interview Survey. *Medical Care* 40(4):353–358.

Owen, N., K. Glanz, J.F. Sallis, and S.H. Kelder. 2006. Evidence-based approaches to dissemination and diffusion of physical activity interventions. *American Journal of Preventive Medicine* 31(4S):S35–S44.

Paraponaris, A., B. Davin, and P. Verger. 2011. Formal and informal care for disabled elderly living in the community: An appraisal of French care composition and costs. *European Journal of Health Economics.* http://www.springerlink.com/content/gn2006162584p756/. (accessed January 3, 2012).

Partnership for Solutions National Program Office. 2004. *Chronic Conditions: Making the Case for Ongoing Care: September 2004 Update.* Baltimore, MD: John Hopkins University. http://www.rwjf.org/pr/product.jsp?id=14685 (accessed September 9, 2011).

Peers for Progress (a). *About Us.* http://www.peersforprogress.org/about_us.php (accessed December 21, 2011).

Peikes, D., A. Chen, J. Schore, and R. Brown. 2009. Effects of care coordination on hospitalization, quality of care, and health care expenditures among Medicare beneficiaries: 15 randomized trials. *Journal of the American Medical Association* 301(6):603–618.

Physical Activity Guidelines Advisory Committee. 2008. *Physical Activity Guidelines Advisory Committee Report, 2008.* Washington, DC: U.S. Department of Health and Human Services. http://www.health.gov/paguidelines/report/ (accessed November 1, 2011).

Potter, R., D. Ellard, K. Rees, and M. Thorogood. 2011. A systematic review of the effects of physical activity on physical functioning, quality of life and depression in older people with dementia. *International Journal of Geriatric Psychiatry* 26(10):1000–1011.

Ramirez, A.G., and B.J. Turner, 2010. The role of peer patients in chronic disease management. *Annals of Internal Medicine* 153(8):544–545.

Ranney, L., C. Melvin, L. Lux, E. McClain, and K.N. Lohr. 2006. Systematic review: Smoking cessation intervention strategies for adults and adults in special populations. *Annals of Internal Medicine* 145(11):845–856.

Reach, G. 2009. Can technology improve adherence to long-term therapies? *Journal of Diabetes Science and Technology* 3(3):492–499.

Rhodes, R.E., and B. Fiala. 2009. Building motivation and sustainability into the prescription and recommendations for physical activity and exercise therapy: The evidence. *Physiotherapy Theory and Practice* 25(5-6):424–441.

Rimmer, J.H., B. Riley, E. Wang, A. Rauworth, and J. Jurkowski. 2004. Physical activity participation among persons with disabilities: Barriers and facilitators. *American Journal of Preventive Medicine* 26(5):419–425.

Rimmer, J.H., B. Riley, E. Wang, and A. Rauworth. 2005. Accessibility of health clubs for people with mobility disabilities and visual impairments. *American Journal of Public Health* 95(11):2022–2028.

Rock, V.J., A. Malarcher, J.W. Kahende, K. Asman, C. Husten, and R. Caraballo. 2007. Cigarette smoking among adults—United States, 2006. *MMWR* 56(44):1157–1161. http://www.cdc.gov/mmwr/preview/mmwrhtml/mm5644a2.htm (accessed November 2, 2011).

Russell, C.L., T.M. Ruppar, and M. Matteson. 2011. Improving medication adherence: Moving from intention and motivation to a personal systems approach. *Nursing Clinics of North America* 46(3):271–281.

Sackett, D.L. 1976. The magnitude of compliance and noncompliance. In *Compliance with Therapeutic Regimens,* edited by D.L. Sackett and R.B. Haynes. Baltimore, MD: Johns Hopkins University Press.

Sawaya, G.F., J. Guirguis-Blake, M. LeFevre, R. Harris, D. Petitti, and U.S. Preventive Services Task Force. 2007. Update on the methods of the U.S. Preventive Services Task Force: Estimating certainty and magnitude of net benefit. *Annals of Internal Medicine* 147(12):871–875.

Schillinger, D. 2010. *An Introduction to Effectiveness, Dissemination and Implementation Research. A Resource Manual for Community-Engaged Research.* Edited by P. Fleisher and E. Goldstein. San Francisco, CA: Clinical Translational Science Institute Community Engagement Program, University of California, San Francisco. http://ctsi.ucsf.edu/files/CE/edi_introguide.pdf (accessed November 7, 2011).

Schoenmakers, B., F. Buntinx, and J. DeLepeleire. 2010. Supporting the dementia family caregiver: The effect of home care intervention on general well-being. *Aging and Mental Health* 14(1):44–56.

Schroeder, K., T. Fahey, and S. Ebrahim. 2004a. Interventions for improving adherence to treatment in patients with high blood pressure in ambulatory settings. *Cochrane Database of Systematic Reviews* (2):CD004804.

Schroeder, K., T. Fahey, and S. Ebrahim. 2004b. How can we improve adherence to blood pressure-lowering medication in the ambulatory setting? Systematic review of randomized control trials. *Annals of Internal Medicine* 164(7):722–732.

Speck, R.M., K.S. Courneya, L.C. Mâsse, S. Duval, and K.H. Schmitz. 2010. An update of controlled physical activity trials in cancer survivors: A systematic review and meta-analysis. *Journal of Cancer Survivorship* 4(2):87–100.

Stegemann, S., F. Ecker, M. Maio, P. Kraahs, R. Wohlfart, J. Breitkreutz, A. Zimmer, D. Bar-Shalom, P. Hettrich, and B. Broegmann. 2010. Geriatric drug therapy: Neglecting the inevitable majority. *Ageing Research Reviews* 9(4):384–398.

Stephenson, B.J., B.H. Rowe, R.B. Haynes, W.M. Macharia, and G. Leon. 1993. The rational clinical examination. Is this patient taking the treatment as prescribed? *Journal of the American Medical Association* 269(21):2779–2781.

Stirling, C., S. Andrews, T. Croft, J. Vickers, P. Turner, and A. Robinson. 2010. Measuring dementia carers' unmet need for services—an exploratory mixed method study. *BMC Health Services Research* 10:22. http://www.biomedcentral.com/content/pdf/1472-6963-10-122.pdf (accessed January 3, 2012).

Thorpe, K.E., and Z. Yang. 2011. Enrolling people with prediabetes ages 60-64 in a proven weight loss program. *Health Affairs* 30(9):1673–1679.

Umpierre, D., P.A. Ribeiro, C.K. Kramer, C.B. Leitão, A.T. Zucatti, M.J. Azevedo, J.L. Gross, J.P. Ribeiro, and B.D. Schaan. 2011. Physical activity advice only or structured exercise training and association with HbA1c levels in type 2 diabetes: A systematic review and meta-analysis. *Journal of the American Medical Association* 305(17):1790–1799.

Ventola, C.L. 2010a. Current issues regarding complementary and alternative medicine (CAM) in the United States: Part 1: The widespread use of CAM and the need for better-informed health care professionals to provide patient counseling. *P&T* 35(8):461–468.

Ventola, C.L. 2010b. Current issues regarding complementary and alternative medicine (CAM) in the United States: Part II: Regulatory and safety concerns and proposed governmental policy changes with respect to dietary supplements. *P&T* 35(9):514–522.

Virginia Department on Aging. 2011. *Virginia Caregiver Coalition (VCC) Respite Care Message—October 2011.* http://www.vda.virginia.gov/respite.asp (accessed January 3, 2012).

Vreugdenhil, A., J. Cannell, A. Davies, and G. Razay. 2011. A community-based exercise programme to improve functional ability in people with Alzheimer's disease: A randomized controlled trial. *Scandinavian Journal of Caring Sciences*. May 12 [Epub ahead of print].

Wallace, J.I., D.M. Buchner, L. Grothaus, S. Leveille, L. Tyll, A.Z. LaCroix, and E.H. Wagner. 1998. Implementation and effectiveness of a community-based health promotion program for older adults. *Journals of Gerontology: Series A, Biological and Medical Sciences* 53(4):M301–M306.

Warren, J.L., C.N. Klabunde, A.B. Mariotto, A. Meekins, M. Topor, M.L. Brown, and D.F. Ransohoff. 2009. Adverse events after outpatient colonoscopy in the Medicare population. *Annals of Internal Medicine* 150(12):849–857.

Weatherly, H., M. Drummond, K. Claxton, R. Cookson, B. Ferguson, C. Godfrey, N. Rice, M. Sculpher, and A. Sowden. 2009. Methods for assessing the cost-effectiveness of public health interventions: Key challenges and recommendations. *Health Policy* 93(2-3):85–92.

Whitehead, T.L. 2002. *The Cultural Ecology of Health and Change (CEHC) Working Papers Series. Working Paper. Traditional Approaches to the Evaluation of Community Based Interventions: Strengths and Limitations.* College Park, MD: University of Maryland. http://www.cusag.umd.edu/documents/WorkingPapers/Traditional%20Apoproaches%20to%20Program%20Evaluation.pdf (accessed November 4, 2011).

Wilson, D.K., K.A. Kirtland, B.E. Ainsworth, and C.L. Addy. 2004. Socioeconomic status and perceptions of access and safety for physical activity. *Annals of Behavioral Medicine* 28(1):20–28.

Witherspoon, B., and M. Rosenzweig. 2004. Industry-sponsored weight loss programs: Description, cost and effectiveness. *Journal of the American Academy of Nurse Practitioners* 16(5):198–205.

Wolinsky, F.D., F.W. Unverzagt, D.M. Smith, R. Jones, E. Wright, and S.L. Tennstedt. 2006a. The effects of the ACTIVE cognitive training trial on clinically relevant declines in health-related quality of life. *Journals of Gerontology: Series B, Psychological Sciences and Social Sciences* 61(5):S281–S287.

Wolinsky, F.D., F.W. Unverzagt, D.M. Smith, R. Jones, A. Stoddard, and S.L. Tennstedt. 2006b. The ACTIVE cognitive training trial and health-related quality of life: Protection that lasts 5 years. *Journals of Gerontology: Series A, Biological Sciences and Medical Sciences* 61(12):1324–1329.

Wu, S.F., M.J. Kao, M.P. Wu, M.W. Tsai, and W.W. Chang. 2011. Effects of osteoarthritis self-management programme. *Journal of Advanced Nursing* 67(7):1491–1501.

Yancey, A.K., M.G. Ory, and S.M. Davis. 2006. Dissemination of physical activity promotion interventions in underserved populations. *American Journal of Preventive Medicine* 31(4 Suppl):S82–S91.

Yazdany, J., C. Tonner, L. Trupin, P. Panopalis, J.Z. Gillis, A.O. Hersh, L.J. Julian, P.P. Katz, L.A. Criswell, and E.H. Yelin. 2010. Provision of preventive health care in systemic lupus erythematosus: Data from a large observational cohort study. *Arthritis Research and Therapy* 12(3):R84.

Yohannes, A.M., and S. Caton. 2010. Management of depression in older people with osteoarthritis: A systematic review. *Aging and Mental Health* 14(6):637–651.

Zafar, W., and R. Mojtabai. 2011. Chronic disease management for depression in US medical practices: Results from the Health Tracking Physician Survey. *Medical Care* 49(7): 634–640.

Zarit, S., M. Stephens, A. Townsend, and R. Greene. 1998. Stress reduction for family caregivers: Effects of adult day care use. *Journal of Gerontology: Social Sciences* 53B(5): S267–S277.

Zwijsen, S.A., A.R. Niemeijer, and C.M. Hertogh. 2011. Ethics of using assistive technology in the care for community-dwelling elderly people: An overview of the literature. *Aging and Mental Health* 15(4):419–427.

5

Surveillance and Assessment

INTRODUCTION

Surveillance, one of the three core functions of public health, is defined as the ongoing, systematic collection, analysis, interpretation, and dissemination of data regarding a health-related event for use in public health action to reduce morbidity and mortality and to improve health (German et al., 2001; IOM, 1988). During the latter half of the 20th century, much of the focus of surveillance activities in the United States was on describing variations in the major causes of death and associated risk factors for fatal diseases. The results of these surveillance activities have been used to guide research investments and subsequent public health and health care interventions to address the major causes of mortality, including cardiovascular diseases and cancer; the associated chronic diseases, including obesity, hypertension, and hyperlipidemia; and behavioral risk factors, including poor diet, physical inactivity, and smoking.

Life expectancy has improved over the past century, primarily as a result of public health interventions, such as tobacco control efforts, that have reduced the risk of the leading chronic diseases, such as heart disease, stroke, and cancer (Remington and Brownson, 2011). More recent evidence suggests that the increases in life expectancy during the past 20 years have come from improvements in disease management rather than in disease prevention (McGovern et al., 1996). However, mortality data from 2000 to 2007 demonstrate wide variation in life expectancy across counties in the United States and an overall relative decline in life expectancy for most communities compared with other nations (Kulkarni et al., 2011).

In addition to life expectancy, available evidence suggests that self-reported health status has not improved among retirees (Hung et al., 2011) or has declined in the general population (Jia and Lubetkin, 2009; Zack et al., 2004) and persons with certain chronic illnesses (Pan et al., 2006). However, these findings are not consistent (Salomon et al., 2009), as some data suggest that the prevalence of disability is decreasing (Manton, 2008), and in some surveys health status is improving (Salomon et al., 2009), over time. These disparate findings likely result from lack of standardized methods of measurement of the complex components and determinants of health status and disability (NRC, 2009), and they suggest that the current surveillance systems are insufficient for tracking progress in efforts to monitor trends in quality of life in the United States overall or within communities.

Despite uncertainty about trends in quality of life in the United States, the evidence is clear that *more* people are living with chronic illnesses as a result of increasing prevalence of some illnesses (e.g., obesity) and longer survival among patients diagnosed with chronic illness. Moreover, the rising costs of health care, along with evidence from research focused on patterns of health care utilization and costs, have focused attention on the societal burden of chronic diseases, particularly multiple chronic conditions (MCCs) (Tinetti and Studenski, 2011). Together, the aging of the population, the decline in relative life expectancy and possibly the quality of life, and unsustainable increases in health care costs combine to create a rapidly growing burden of chronic illness that demands more comprehensive surveillance beyond mortality and risk factors to address these problems.

The goal of living well with chronic illness and efforts to control the growing societal burden of chronic illness start with enhanced surveillance to provide data necessary to plan, implement, and evaluate effectiveness of interventions at the individual and population levels. This chapter has several objectives:

1. To describe a conceptual framework for chronic disease surveillance.
2. To describe how public health surveillance may be used to inform public policy decisions to improve the quality of life of patients living with chronic illnesses.
3. To examine current data sources and methods for surveillance of certain chronic diseases and identify gaps.
4. To describe potential for surveillance system integration.
5. To describe future data sources, methods, and research directions for surveillance to enhance living well with chronic illness.

CONCEPTUAL FRAMEWORK FOR CHRONIC
DISEASE SURVEILLANCE

The ultimate goal of public health is to promote health and prevent disease occurrence or to limit progression from preclinical to symptomatic disease through primary and secondary prevention, respectively. Health promotion is the process of enabling people to gain increasing control over and improve their health. Primary prevention is usually addressed through interventions targeting lifestyle risk factors or environmental exposures among illness-free persons, including smoking, physical inactivity, and over-weight/obesity. Secondary prevention among asymptomatic persons with preclinical illness may include a range of interventions comprised of early detection, immunizations, and chemoprevention.

Because of the public health emphasis on health promotion and disease prevention (especially primary and secondary prevention), chronic disease surveillance has traditionally focused on major risk factors for disease and the occurrence of chronic diseases. However, although primary and secondary prevention may have relevance for persons with chronic illnesses to prevent the development of other comorbid illnesses, a more immediate concern for individuals is how to live well, which involves a balance between their experience living with chronic illness(es) and associated costs (i.e., value).

Moreover, from a societal perspective, interventions to improve the patient experience need to be cost-effective and contribute to improving the health of the population. Thus, there is a strong rationale for expanded surveillance of chronic diseases to measure not only the factors that increase the "upstream" risk of chronic diseases but also the relevant health "downstream" outcomes associated with living well with chronic illness (Porter, 2010).

Table 2-1 provides an excellent framework for establishing a comprehensive chronic disease surveillance system. Such a surveillance system should collect data along the entire chronic disease continuum—from upstream risk factors to end of life care and for the purposes of promoting living well among persons with chronic illness. Such systems should collect information on symptoms, functional impairment, self-management burden, and burden to others.

Integrating the multiple potential measures of health status and determinants of health, including risk factors and interventions and costs, will be necessary for the ideal surveillance system to assess the status of patients living well with chronic illness and the societal impacts. The need to integrate these multiple measures has been emphasized in a recent Institute of Medicine (IOM) report on a framework for surveillance of cardiovascular and chronic respiratory diseases (IOM, 2011) and in reviews by others

(Fielding and Teutsch, 2011; Porter, 2010). Briefly, the conceptual framework for an ideal surveillance system to enhance living well with chronic illness incorporates the life course model that describes health status on a spectrum from illness-free to death and the ecological model of multiple determinants of health, including individual characteristics (i.e., biological makeup, health literacy and beliefs, health-related behaviors), family and community environments (i.e., social, economic, cultural, physical), and health-related interventions (i.e., public health, policy, clinical care). Measuring variations and disparities among subpopulations—for example, by age, race, gender, residence, and other factors—is a critical part of any public health surveillance system.

Surveillance of chronic diseases may also be used to monitor progress in achieving the triple aim of health care improvement: that is, to improve the patient experience, to control costs, and to improve the health of the population (Institute for Healthcare Improvement, [a]). These three aims provide further dimensions for defining relevant metrics and data sources of an enhanced surveillance system to monitor the multiple determinants and outcomes of living well with chronic illness, including the individual, the health system, and the population/community levels (Table 5-1). Moreover, these metrics and data sources reflect the multi-pronged interventions necessary for optimizing management and outcomes for patients with chronic illness, as described in the enhanced Chronic Care Model (Barr et al., 2003).

Although there is abundant evidence that the health status of patients with chronic illnesses and the quality of health care and associated costs (i.e., value) is not optimal in the United States (IOM, 2001; Porter, 2010), limited data are available on what it means at the individual level to live well (Porter, 2010; Thacker et al., 2006). Ideally, living well is defined by patients' values and goals regarding their physical, emotional, and social functioning. However, wide variation in patients' perspectives presents a major challenge for conducting surveillance of living well with chronic illness; the definition of living well was discussed in detail in Chapter 1. Moreover, because of barriers to access and the low value of health care in the United States, the current policy focus is largely on enhancing access and increasing value by improving quality, reducing costs by decreasing use of ineffective and/or high-cost interventions, and improving the processes of care. However, the determinants of living well with chronic illness are more complex, and these efforts alone will not adequately support patients in these circumstances.

Porter (2010) has described a health outcome hierarchy focused on health care delivery, which can be applied to provide a framework for designing a comprehensive measurement system to enhance living well with chronic illness. The principles described in this framework are as follows:

- Outcomes have multiple dimensions, which ideally include one dimension at each tier and level
  — Tier 1: health status achieved or retained
    o Survival
    o Degree of health/recovery (e.g., quality of life, functional status)
  — Tier 2: Process of recovery
    o Time to recovery and return to normal activities (e.g., time to achieve functional status)
    o Disutility of care process (e.g., acute complications)
  — Tier 3: Sustainability of health
    o Sustainability of health/recovery and nature of recurrences (e.g., frequency of exacerbations)
    o Long-term consequences of therapy (e.g., care-induced illnesses)
- Outcomes must be relevant to patients and their specific illness(es) (i.e., valid)
- Multiple determinants of outcomes (e.g., disease-related, psychological, social, lifestyle) must be measured
- Measurement instruments must be standardized to provide reliability and comparability
- Measurement instruments must be sensitive to change
- Measurements must be ongoing and sustained

In addition to the measurement of health status or outcomes at the individual level, comprehensive surveillance must incorporate measures of characteristics, exposures, and processes that affect health outcomes comprising the multiple determinants of living well and their interactions at the levels of the individual, the family, and the community; health care–related interventions; and public policy. Individual health-related behaviors, including lifestyle (e.g., smoking, physical activity, diet) and self-management (e.g., medication adherence, action plans), are all influenced by patient characteristics, such as education level, health literacy, beliefs, activation, and self-efficacy. In turn, these characteristics and other exposures are partly influenced by an individual's larger cultural, socioeconomic, and physical environments, comprised of family, work, and community. Finally, measurement of access to and utilization of health care and public health resources/interventions (e.g., structural interventions; see Katz, 2009) and coordination of care are needed to complete the assessment of factors that may contribute to patients living well with chronic illness.

Given the complexity of measuring the multiple determinants and dimensions of living well (i.e., quality of life, functional status), there is no single-best measure of living well for patients with chronic illness (Thacker

TABLE 5-1 Matrix for Surveillance for Living Well with Chronic Illness

Health Factors and Outcomes	Examples	Patient-Reported, Individual-Level Information	Health Care Administrative Data and Illness Registries	Population-Based Surveys and Assessments
Environmental, Social, and Personal Determinants of Health				
Physical and built environment	Air/water quality, walking paths, food deserts	Self-report	Geo-coded addresses	County health rankings, EPA, census
Social and economic factors	Education, income, employment, social support	Self-report (personal health record), social support, caregiver burden		County health rankings, Dept of Education, Dept of Justice, census
Policy, law, and regulation	Workplace policies on smoking, immunization; taxes on tobacco, sugar-sweetened beverages	Self-report on awareness, enforcement of policies and laws (BRFSS)	JCAHO data (e.g., hospital smoking bans, health worker flu vaccination levels)	State- and county-level databases of public health laws and taxes
Health care access, coordination, quality, and costs	Insurance coverage, immunizations, cancer screening	Self-report (e.g., ACOVE RAND)	Claims data, hospital discharge data, RHIOs	MEPS, HCAHPS

Health literacy, beliefs, motivations	Health literacy, self-efficacy, activation	Health risk appraisal (HRA)		BRFSS, NHIS, NHANES
Health behaviors	Smoking, diet, physical activity, unsafe sex	HRA		
Health Outcomes				
Social health outcomes	Relationships and function	Self-report (personal health record)		National surveys
Mental health outcomes	Affect, behavior, cognition, PHQ-9	Self-report (personal health record)		BRFSS (limited), NHIS
Physical health outcomes	ADLs, symptoms, functioning	Self-report (personal health record)		BRFSS (limited), NHIS
Illness-specific outcomes	Diabetes, arthritis, cancer, dementia	Electronic medical record (EMR)	Vital stats, SEER, claims data (e.g., costs)	NHIS, NHANES, BRFSS, disability from CPS
Primary uses of data		Improve quality and health outcomes (living well)	Improve quality, manage costs, find "hot spots"	Assess trends, burden, disparities (by person and place), research

NOTE: ACOVE RAND = Assessing Care of Vulnerable Elders—A RAND Health Project; ADLs = activities of daily living; BRFSS = Behavioral Risk Factor Surveillance System; CPS = Current Population Survey; EPA = Environmental Protection Agency; HCAHPS = Hospital Consumer Assessment of Healthcare Providers and Systems; JCAHO = Joint Commission on Accreditation of Healthcare Organizations; MEPS = Medical Expenditure Panel Survey; NHANES = National Health and Nutrition Examination Survey; NHIS = National Health Interview Survey; PHQ-9 = Patient Health Questionnaire-9; RHIO = Regional Health Information Organization; SEER = Surveillance, Epidemiology, and End Results.

et al., 2006), and illness-specific measures may not detect the entire patient experience (Monninkhof et al., 2004; Yeh et al., 2004). Therefore,
an aggregate index of living well will consist of multiple measures from
the individual, health care system, community, and policies to characterize
the population (Table 5-1). However, a further challenge for surveillance
of living well with chronic illness is that the majority of patients may have
MCCs, which further supports the need for generic measures of health
outcomes in contrast to illness-specific measures.

In summary, the best way to meet the goal of living well with chronic
illness is to prevent chronic illness in the first place and, if that fails, to
manage the illness to improve quality of life and prevent the development
of additional chronic illness. Doing so requires a comprehensive surveillance system that includes incentives for individuals and organizations to
participate in surveillance activities. The characteristics of a surveillance
system to enhance living well with chronic illness are complex and integrate
a number of measures of the multiple determinants and multiple dimensions
of outcome most relevant to patients. Individual patient-level measures are
discussed in the section below on Current Data Sources and Surveillance
Methods.

USE OF SURVEILLANCE TO INFORM PUBLIC POLICY DECISIONS

Public health surveillance systems may be used to inform public policy
decisions to improve the prevention and control of chronic illnesses at the
individual or population level. In this section, we review how surveillance
(i.e., data collection and reporting) at various levels (e.g., individual, community, health system, state, national) may be used to promote living well
with chronic illness. In broad terms, these systems may be used to

- promote dissemination of evidence-based programs and policies,
  especially when a gap exists between research and practice;
- target interventions to areas or populations of greatest need (e.g.,
  where health disparities are greatest); and
- evaluate the effectiveness of new or emerging interventions.

When the evidence is strong for interventions that could effectively
address a gap, the surveillance effort should be focused on closing this gap
by promoting the implementation of an evidence-based intervention. For
example, surveillance systems have been used to demonstrate continued
exposure to cigarette smoke in the workplace, the lack of advice given
by physicians to quit smoking, or the slow uptake of breast, cervical, or
colorectal cancer screening. Because of the complexity of the determinants
of living well, effective dissemination of interventions will most often re-

quire system-level changes at the local, state, or national level (i.e., policy, rules, regulation, culture), which are discussed in greater detail in Chapters 3 and 4.

Public health surveillance systems can also be used to identify disparities in all aspects of chronic disease prevention and control. Monitoring and reducing health disparities has been a central focus of the U.S. Department of Health and Human Services (HHS) *Healthy People* efforts over the past 30 years. In *Healthy People 2000*, the focus was to reduce health disparities among Americans. *Healthy People 2010* emphasized eliminating, not just reducing, health disparities. In *Healthy People 2020*, that goal was expanded even further to achieve health equity, to eliminate disparities, and to improve the health of all groups.

Surveillance efforts in chronic disease should build on the *Healthy People 2020* effort by carefully monitoring health disparities, defined as "a particular type of health difference that is closely linked with social, economic, and/or environmental disadvantage. Health disparities adversely affect groups of people who have systematically experienced greater obstacles to health based on their racial or ethnic group; religion; socioeconomic status; gender; age; mental health; cognitive, sensory, or physical disability; sexual orientation or gender identity; geographic location; or other characteristics historically linked to discrimination or exclusion."

Finally, when evidence of effective interventions is not strong, surveillance systems can provide information about the effect of programs or policies in actual populations and guide future improvement efforts. Ideally, the evidence base for effective chronic disease prevention programs and policies would be developed through an explicit public health research agenda. However, evidence often evolves during the implementation of programs and policies in actual practice, using data collected in well-designed surveillance systems or population-based surveys. As more programs and policies are directed toward helping people live well with chronic illness, comprehensive surveillance systems will help evaluate their impact on populations throughout the United States.

CURRENT DATA SOURCES AND SURVEILLANCE METHODS

As described in previous sections, surveillance of living well with chronic illness is a complex phenomenon requiring multiple methods and data sources to adequately characterize and track. Overall, there are three levels of data, including patient, health system, and population. A detailed review of current population-based and health system data sources was recently conducted by IOM on the surveillance of cardiovascular and chronic respiratory diseases (IOM, 2011). In this section we provide an overview of available data sources (Table 5-2) and methods specific to the surveil-

TABLE 5-2 Selected Chronic Disease Data Sources and Surveillance Systems

Data System	Example	Strengths	Limitations
Notifiable diseases[a,b,c]	State-based lead poisoning reporting systems	• Data are available at the local level. • Usually coupled with a public health response (e.g., lead paint removal). • Detailed information can be collected to aid in designing control programs. • Laboratory-based systems are inexpensive and effective.	• Requires participation by community-based clinicians. • Clinician-based systems have low reporting rates. • Active reporting systems are time-consuming and expensive.
Vital statistics[a,b,c]	Death certificates	• Data are widely available at the local, state, and national levels. • Population-based. • Can monitor trends in age-adjusted disease rates. • Can target areas with increased mortality rates.	• Cause of death information may be inaccurate (e.g., lack of autopsy information). • No information about risk factors.
Sentinel surveillance[b,c]	Sentinel Event Notification System for Occupational Risks (SENSOR)	• Low-cost system to monitor selected diseases. • Usually coupled with a public health response (e.g., asbestos removal following report of mesothelioma). • Provides information on risk factors and disease severity.	• Requires motivated reporting providers. • May not be representative.
Disease registries[b,c]	Cancer registries	• Data are increasingly available throughout the United States. • Includes accurate tissue-based diagnoses. • Provides stage-of-diagnosis data available.	• Systems are expensive. • Data are affected by patient out-migration from one geographic unit to another. • Risk factor information is seldom available.

Data source	Example	Advantages	Limitations
Health surveys[b,c]	Behavioral risk factor surveillance telephone surveys	• Monitors trends in risk factor prevalence. • Can be used for program design and evaluation.	• Information is based on self-reports. • May be too expensive to conduct at the local level. • May not be representative due to nonresponse (e.g., telephone surveys).
Administrative data collection systems[b,c]	Hospital discharge systems	• Reflects regional differences on disease hospitalization rates. • Can capture cost information. • Data are readily available. • One of few sources of morbidity data.	• Often lacks personal identifiers. • Rates may be affected by changing patterns of diagnosis based on reimbursement mechanisms. • Difficult to separate initial from recurrent hospitalizations.
U.S. census[a,b,c]	Poverty rates by county	• Required to calculate rates. • Important predictors of health status. • Available to all communities and readily available online.	• Collected infrequently (every 10 years). • May undercount certain populations (e.g., the poor, homeless persons).

[a]Data are available from most local public health agencies.
[b]Data are available from most state departments of health.
[c]Data are available from many U.S. federal health agencies (e.g., Centers for Disease Control and Prevention, National Cancer Institute, Health Care Financing Administration).

SOURCE: Remington, P.L., M.V. Wegner, and A.M. Rohan. 2010. Chronic disease surveillance. In *Chronic Disease Epidemiology and Control*, 3rd ed., edited by P.L. Remington, R.C. Brownson, and M.V. Wegner. Pp. 98–99. Washington, DC: America Public Health Association.

lance of living well with chronic illness and consider their strengths and limitations.

Patient-Level Data and Methods

Direct reports from the patient, including patient-reported outcomes (PROs) or measures of functional and cognitive performance, are the most direct measure of whether a patient is living well or not. PROs may consist of generic or illness-specific measures of health-related quality of life (HRQoL), the ability to perform activities of daily living (ADLs), symptoms of one's chronic illness (Table 5-3), and measures of psychological distress. Although the Behavioral Risk Factor Surveillance System (BRFSS) includes a brief PRO instrument, patient-level measures are most commonly used for specific research purposes and are not routinely used for public

TABLE 5-3 Symptoms That Interfere with Living Well

Symptom	Examples of Illnesses
Fatigue	• Congestive heart failure • Chronic respiratory diseases (e.g., chronic obstructive pulmonary disease) • Arthritis • Depression • Sleep disorders • Posttraumatic injury/critical illness
Dyspnea	• Chronic respiratory diseases (e.g., chronic obstructive pulmonary disease) • Congestive heart failure • Cardiovascular diseases • Deconditioning
Pain	• Arthritis • Cardiovascular diseases
Distress	• Depression • Anxiety • Anger • Suffering
Cognitive impairment	• Dementia • Posttraumatic injury/critical illness • Vision/hearing impairment • Cataracts • Macular degeneration • Noise-induced hearing loss

TABLE 5-4 Generic Patient Reported Outcome Measures

Measure	Description
EuroQol (EQ-5D)[a]	Five single item measures of mobility, self-care, usual activities, pain/discomfort, and anxiety/depression.
Nottingham Health Profile[b]	Two part survey to measure subjective physical, emotional, and social aspects of health. Part I measures six dimensions of health: physical mobility, pain, social isolation, emotional reactions, energy, and sleep. Part II measures seven areas of life most affected by health status.
Short Form-36 Health Survey (SF-36)[c]	36 questions with eight different sub-scores that measure physical functioning, physical role limitations, bodily pain, general health perceptions, vitality, social functioning, emotional role limitations, mental health, and two composite scores: physical component and mental component score.
SF-12 Health Survey[d]	Shorter version of SF-36, measuring functional health being and well-being from patient's point of view, using 12 questions.
SF-8 Health Survey[e]	Condensed version of SF-36 that relies on a single item to measure each of the eight domains of health as defined in the SF-36 Health Survey.

[a]The EuroQol Group. 1990. EuroQol-a new facility for the measurement of health-related quality of life. *Health Policy* 16(3):199–208.

[b]Hunt, S.M., S.P. McKenna, J. McEwen, J. Williams, and E. Papp. 1981. The Nottingham Health Profile: Subjective health status and medical consultations. *Social Science and Medicine, Part A, Medical Sociology* 15(3 Part 1):221–229.

[c]Ware, J.E., Jr., and C.D. Sherbourne. 1992. The MOS 36-Item Short-Form Health Survey (SF-36): I. Conceptual framework and item selection. *Medical Care* 30(6):473–483.

[d]Ware, J.E., Jr., M. Kosinski, and S.D. Keller. 1996. A 12-Item Short-Form Health Survey: Construction of scales and preliminary tests of reliability and validity. *Medical Care* 34(3):220–233.

[e]Ware, J.E., Jr., M. Kosinski, J.E. Dewey, and B. Gandek. 2001. *How to Score and Interpret Single-Item Health Measures: A Manual for Users of the SF-8 Health Survey.* Lincoln, RI: QualityMetric Incorporated.

health surveillance. Moreover, functional performance may be assessed with observer-assessed physical measurements (e.g., short physical performance battery, 6-minute walk), and cognitive performance may be assessed with standardized instruments (e.g., Mini-Mental State Exam).

Generic and disease-specific PRO measures of HRQoL (Tables 5-4 and 5-5) and other outcomes related to chronic disease were developed and began to be used in the research environment in the 1980s (Fries et al., 1980; Meenan et al., 1980; Stewart et al., 1988). PROs, such as the Health Assessment Questionnaire (HAQ) used in arthritis, have been shown to predict morbidity and mortality in some chronic diseases as effectively as labora-

TABLE 5-5 Illness-Specific Patient-Reported Outcome Measures

Measure	Description
Adult Asthma Quality of Life Questionnaire (AQLQ)[a]	32 items that produce 4 dimension scores relating to activity limitations, symptoms, emotional function, and environmental exposure.
Arthritis Impact Measurement Scales (AIMS)[b]	9 scales that measure physical, psychological, and social health status outcomes in rheumatoid arthritis patients.
Arthritis Self-efficacy Scale (ASES)[c]	20-item scale across 3 domains, including coping with pain, function and other symptoms to measure self-efficacy in patients with rheumatoid arthritis.
Chronic Respiratory Questionnaire (CRQ)[d]	20 items that produce 4 dimension scores relating to dyspnea, fatigue, emotional functioning, and mastery to measure health-related quality of life in patients with difficulty breathing.
EXAcerbations of Chronic Pulmonary Disease Tool (EXACT)[e]	14-item daily diary to evaluate frequency, severity and duration of acute exacerbation of chronic obstructive pulmonary disease and chronic bronchitis.
Stanford Health Assessment Questionnaire (HAQ)[f]	Five-dimension comprehensive outcome measure that assesses patient outcomes in four domains: disability, discomfort and pain, drug side-effects (toxicity), and dollar costs, developed for those with arthritis but now used more generically.
Seattle Angina Questionnaire (SAQ)[g]	19 items across 5 dimensions of coronary artery disease: anginal stability and frequency, physical limitation, treatment satisfaction, quality of life.
St. George Respiratory Questionnaire (SGRQ)[h]	50-item, 76 weighted responses divided into 3 components: symptoms, activity, and impacts to quantify health-related health status in patients with chronic airflow limitation.
Western Ontario McMasters University Osteoarthritis Index (WOMAC)[i]	24 items across 3 subscales that assess pain, stiffness and physical function in patients with hip and/or knee osteoarthritis (OA).

[a]Juniper, E.F., G.H. Guyatt, P.J. Ferrie, and L.E. Griffith. 1993. Measuring quality of life in asthma. *American Review of Respiratory Disease* 147(4):832–838.

[b]Meenan, R.F., P.M. Gertman, and J.H. Mason. 1980. Measuring health status in arthritis. *Arthritis and Rheumatism* 23(2):146–152.

[c]Lorig, K., R.L. Chastain, E. Ung, S. Shoor, and H.R. Holman. 1989. Development and evaluation of a scale to measure perceived self efficacy in people with arthritis. *Arthritis and Rheumatism* 32(1):37–44.

[d]Guyatt, G.H., L.B. Berman, M. Townsend, S.O. Pugsley, and L.W. Chambers. 1987. A measure of quality of life for clinical trials in chronic lung disease. *Thorax* 42(10):773–778.

[e]Leidy, N.K., T.K. Wilcox, P.W. Jones, L. Murray, R. Winnette, K. Howard, J. Petrillo, J. Powers, S. Sethi, and EXACT-PRO Study Group. 2010. Development of the EXACerbations of Chronic Obstructive Pulmonary Disease Tool (EXACT): A Patient-Reported Outcome (PRO) measure. *Value Health* 13(8):965–975.

[f]Fries, J.F., P. Spitz, R.G. Kraines, and H.R. Holman. 1980. Measurement of patient outcomes in arthritis. *Arthritis and Rheumatism* 23(2):137–145.

[g]Spertus, J.A., J.A. Winder, T.A. Dewhurst, R.A. Deyo, J. Prodzinski, M. McDonell, and S.D. Fihn. 1995. Development and evaluation of the Seattle Angina Questionnaire: A new functional status measure for coronary artery disease. *Journal of the American College of Cardiology* 25(2):333–341.

[h]Jones, P.W., F.H. Quirk, C.M. Baveystock, and P. Littlejohns. 1992. A self-complete measure of health status for chronic airflow limitation. The St. George's Respiratory Questionnaire. *The American Review of Respiratory Disease* 145(6):1321–1327.

[i]Bellamy, N., W.W. Buchanan, C.H. Goldsmith, J. Campbell, and L.W. Stitt. 1988. Validation study of WOMAC: A health status instrument for measuring clinically important patient relevant outcomes to antirheumatic drug therapy in patients with osteoarthritis of the hip or knee. *Journal of Rheumatology* 15(12):1833–1840.

tory, radiographic, and performance-based measures of physical function in longitudinal observational studies (Pincus and Sokka, 2003; Wolfe and Pincus, 1999). In clinical trials, PROs have been demonstrated to have a higher relative efficiency when analyzing differences between active versus placebo treatments in patients with chronic illness (Strand et al., 1999, 2005; Tugwell et al., 2000). The SF-36v2, SF-12v2, and SF-8 health surveys are the most widely used generic PRO measures for assessing eight health domains (Ware et al., 1994, 1997, 2001). Psychometrically based physical component summary (PCS) scores and mental component summary (MCS) scores can be derived from each survey. In addition to the generic PRO measures, there are many disease-specific PRO measures. These commonly used generic and disease-specific PROs have been demonstrated to be reliable, valid, and sensitive to change—properties that are essential for all patient-level measures, whether they are self-reported or performance-based.

The common measures discussed above were developed using classical test theory. The Patient Reported Outcomes Measurement Information System (PROMIS), a National Institutes of Health (NIH) Roadmap network project, is intended to improve the reliability, validity, and precision of PROs using modern measurement techniques, including item-response theory and computerized adaptive testing. The measures being developed from the initiative may be very useful for surveillance of patient-level outcomes (see the section "The Use of Patient-Reported Outcomes in Surveillance Systems"). Much of the research focus has been on illness-specific instruments because of enhanced responsiveness, but for MCCs and public health, more generic instruments that are cross-cutting and characterize living well are needed. PROMIS measures are designed to be cross-cutting for individuals with any illness (or none).

Although self-reported measures of functional performance may be most feasible for surveillance, the validity of these measures for assessing physical performance is limited (Reuben et al., 1995). Performance-based measures of physical function are often measured for research purposes and in clinical settings; however, their use in population-based surveillance has been largely limited to cross-sectional surveys, such as the National Health and Nutrition Examination Survey (NHANES), a cross-sectional, population-based survey (Kuo et al., 2006). Two measures of physical performance that have been used in NHANES are peak leg power and usual gait speed (Kuo et al., 2006), which are associated with late-life disability. The short physical performance battery (SPPB) and the composite of standing balance, walking speed, and ability to rise from a chair are predictors of future disability among the elderly (Guralnik et al., 1995). The Senior Fitness Test has been developed to assess physical performance in older adults across a wide range of age groups and abilities (Rikli and Jones, 2001). The items in the test reflect a cross-section of the major fitness components associated with independent functioning in later years. The Senior Fitness Test includes measures of upper and lower body strength, aerobic endurance, upper and lower body flexibility, gait speed, and agility/dynamic balance.

Surveillance of cognitive performance is uncommon, but it has been included in the NHANES using the Mini-Mental State Examination (Obisesan et al., 2008). This instrument consists of six orientation, six recall, and five attention items. For NHANES respondents over age 70, these items have been associated with hypertension and uncontrolled hypertension (Obisesan et al., 2008).

In addition to PROs and measures of functional and cognitive performance, other patient-level measures with potential relevance to living well may include patient reports of quality of care and employee surveys. RAND health researchers developed a set of quality indicators that reflect the most comprehensive examination of the quality of medical care provided to vulnerable older Americans, the Assessing Care of Vulnerable Elders (ACOVE) indicators (Chodosh et al., 2004). In it, 22 illnesses that account for the majority of health care received by older adults were identified; these included illnesses, syndromes, physiological impairments, and clinical situations. After review by expert panels and the American College of Physicians Task Force on Aging, 236 quality indicators were accepted. These indicators factor in four stages of the health care process: prevention, diagnosis, treatment, and follow-up. ACOVE researchers found that patients who receive better care are more likely to be alive 3 years later than those who received poor care. Patients with MCCs were the least likely to receive adequate care.

Surveillance of both employee workplace attendance and productivity may provide an indicator of functional impact among workers with chronic illnesses. For example, "presenteeism is defined as 'lost productivity that occurs when employees come to work but perform below par due to any kind of illness.' While costs associated with absenteeism of employees have been studied for some time, only recently have costs of presenteeism been studied" (Levin-Epstein, 2005).

Health-System Data and Methods

Although not direct measures of living well, access to and quality of health care services partly influence health outcomes among patients with chronic illnesses and are frequently used as process measures to evaluate how well health systems address patient care needs. Health insurance status and health care utilization claims data are often used as measures to infer access to and quality of health care services. For example, examination of variations in hospitalization rates for selected chronic diseases, termed ambulatory care sensitive conditions (e.g., congestive heart failure, chronic obstructive pulmonary disease [COPD], diabetes), has demonstrated that loss of Medicaid coverage is associated with higher hospitalization rates for these conditions, suggesting suboptimal disease control because of inadequate access to primary care services (Bindman et al., 2008). Disparities in access to health care associated with poor health outcomes has also been suggested by higher hospitalization rates (Jackson et al., 2011) and mortality rates (Abrams et al., 2011) among rural residents with COPD using state and Department of Veterans Affairs (VA) data on hospitalizations, respectively.

On a national level, measurement of performance in health care is relatively new and started with U.S. hospitals in 1998 as a condition of accreditation (Chassin et al., 2010). It has expanded to include measures of outpatient performance in 2007, termed the Physician Quality Reporting Initiative (Metersky, 2009). These measurements and reporting initiatives, termed pay-for-performance or value-based purchasing, are part of the evolving transformation of the health care system in the United States with a growing emphasis on quality of care at lower costs (Berwick, 2011; Conway and Clancy, 2009; Lindenauer et al., 2007). Moreover, the electronic health record (EHR), discussed in greater detail in the next section, will provide the foundation for enhanced data collection and reporting with the goal of "meaningful use" to improve quality of care and health outcomes (Classen and Bates, 2011; Maxson et al., 2010). A limitation of these data sources and measures is that performance on process measures does not reliably predict health outcomes that are relevant to living well with chronic illness (Chassin et al., 2010; Porter, 2010).

Administrative health care claims data from a number of sources, including Medicare and Medicaid (Schneider et al., 2009; The Dartmouth Atlas of Health Care, [a]), the VA (Abrams et al., 2011), and hospital consortia (Lindenauer et al., 2006), are frequently used to assess the quality and cost of health care services. Moreover, with the growing recognition of the need for data to evaluate health system performance and public health policy, a number of states are developing all-payer claims databases (Love et al., 2010).

In addition to health care claims data, patient registries provide a method for directly measuring whether patients are living well. The Agency for Healthcare Research and Quality (AHRQ) has defined a patient registry as "an organized system that uses observational study methods to collect uniform data (clinical and other) to evaluate specified outcomes for a population defined by a particular illness, condition, or exposure and that serves predetermined scientific, clinical or policy purpose(s)." There are a number of different types of patient registries, such as illness, treatment, device, and after-care registries. The use of registries and health care services claims data for chronic disease surveillance was reviewed in greater detail in a recent IOM report (2011).

Population-Based Data and Methods

Population-based data and information about chronic diseases, including measures of living well, are available from a number of sources (Table 5-2). The methods used to support these systems vary, depending on the type of data system and the population it covers. In addition, data from these systems, such as illness occurrence and health-related quality of life, may be used to derive estimates of illness burden and construct cost-effectiveness analyses—for example, disability-adjusted life-years (DALYs) and quality-adjusted life-years (QALYs).

The most robust surveillance systems are census-based, collecting information from the entire population and including vital statistics (birth, death) records similar to those of the U.S. Census Bureau. These systems could provide precise estimates of occurrence of chronic illnesses or other health determinants since they include the entire population, but they would be expensive to support.

Population-based samples are used to conduct surveys to measure self-reported factors related to living well with chronic illness (e.g., quality of life) at the national level and, since 1984, at the state level as part of the BRFSS (Mokdad and Remington, 2010). Methods also exist to survey people in person, in order to measure chronic illness occurrence and its impacts on functional and cognitive performance at the national level (e.g., NHANES) and in some states (e.g., Survey of Health of Wisconsin). Examples of these systems include population-based surveys (e.g., the BRFSS, the National Health Interview Survey, NHANES, state and local surveys) to estimate the prevalence of disability (Brault et al., 2009) or quality of life (Centers for Disease Control and Prevention [CDC]: BRFSS healthy days core module HRQoL-4) (four questions), activity limitations module (five questions), and healthy days symptoms module (five questions) (http://www.cdc.gov/hrqol/ hrqol14_measure.htm). A number of systems use administrative data:

- Hospital Consumer Assessment of Healthcare Providers and Systems (HCAHPS): patient survey of hospital care experience
- Prevention Quality Indicators: www.qualityindicators.ahrq.gov/pqi_overview.htm
- Healthcare Cost and Utilization Project: http://hcupnet.ahrq.gov/

A number of organizations have developed web-based systems to access population-based data either to conduct primary data analysis (Friedman and Parish, 2006) or to retrieve summary reports. Examples of such systems include

- Community Health Status Indicators: www.communityhealth.hhs. gov
- County Health Rankings: www.countyhealthrankings.org
- The Community Health Data Initiative: www.hhs.gov/open/data sets/communityhealthdata.html
- The Health Indicators Warehouse: http://www.healthindicators. gov/
- The American Community Survey of the U.S. Census Bureau

Population-based data on illness occurrence and health-related quality of life may be used for estimating DALYs (Grosse et al., 2009) for use in cost-effectiveness analyses. However, because DALYs are not estimated using direct measures of disability, the validity of this estimate is suspect (Grosse et al., 2009).

Limitations/Data Gaps

Current surveillance of chronic diseases emphasizes risk factors and disease occurrence, and few longitudinal data are obtained on PROs or functional and cognitive performance at the level of health care systems or local, state, and national populations. Despite advances in public health surveillance and health information systems (e.g., electronic health records), few communities have comprehensive surveillance systems to measure chronic diseases and related health risk factors and quality of life. Few health care systems routinely collect information on health-related quality of life as part of the electronic medical record. And, because available process measures do not reliably predict health outcomes, they have limited usefulness for measuring and rewarding performance relevant to living well at the health system or community level.

Data collection is further complicated because of the many potential confounding variables (e.g., age, gender, geography, race/ethnicity, number of comorbid illnesses, health literacy, social support) that may influence living well and are needed to appropriately analyze and interpret results. Moreover, although many people have MCCs, this factor has received limited attention. Finally, rare diseases cannot be accurately measured in population-based surveys. Overcoming these limitations for conducting surveillance for living well with chronic illness is further complicated by the dramatically increasing costs of collecting this information at the population level, as fewer homes have landline telephones and telephone surveys response rates continue to fall. Future systems should be able to capture this information within the health care system and build up to provide information on community, state, and national health risk behavior, chronic disease, and quality of life.

PUBLIC HEALTH SURVEILLANCE SYSTEM INTEGRATION

One of the biggest weaknesses of the current surveillance systems for chronic illness is the lack of integration between information collected at the patient, health system, and population levels. Detailed information may be collected from patients about chronic diseases, risk factors, and quality of life, but it is rarely captured in comprehensive health system databases. Health system information, primarily derived from administrative billing systems, is rarely used to assess chronic disease control at population levels. Finally, information collected at the population level, ranging from detailed census information to characteristics of the built environment, is rarely included in health system information systems.

Another limitation is the lack of information about health outcomes of individual patients over time so that transitions in health status can be monitored. Most available data are on process outcomes rather than health outcomes, and longitudinal data are rarely available. In addition, despite advances in health information technology, these information systems are not well integrated, and the number and variety of systems are likely to increase with advances in electronic data interchange and integration. These changes will also heighten the importance of patient privacy, data confidentiality, and system security. Finally, the value of health care and other interventions to improve health outcomes can be determined only by examining costs and health outcomes, but few data sources include costs (Rosen and Cutler, 2009).

It is technically feasible to integrate existing surveillance systems along the entire continuum of prevention, starting with patient-reported information, to improving the performance of health care systems, to monitoring risk factor and outcome trends over time at the community, state, or national level (i.e., population level). This integration at the level of health care system, with examples, has been extensively reviewed in a series of Institute of Medicine workshops on "The Learning Healthcare System" (IOM, 2007). Figure 5-1 shows how health information can be collected and potentially integrated at three different levels. This section describes these three levels of information systems, provides examples of existing systems, and describes barriers and opportunities for improving systems in the future.

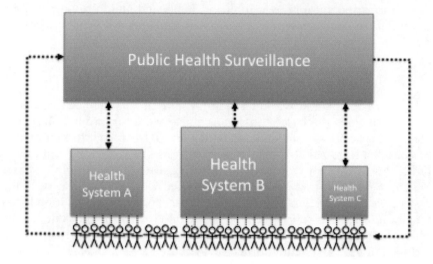

FIGURE 5-1 Integration of health system and public health surveillance systems.
SOURCE: Committee on Living Well with Chronic Disease: Public Health Action
to Reduce Disability and Improve Functioning and Quality of Life.

Patient-Level Surveillance Systems

Surveillance systems of chronic illnesses may be used to evaluate the
effectiveness of patient care and public health interventions and should
include outcome information relevant to living well collected directly from
patients. However, although the patient-reported perspective of living well is
the "gold standard" (e.g., living well or patient-reported health outcomes),
this remains a major gap in surveillance for chronic illnesses (Porter, 2010).
This is a rapidly growing area of research and, with the growing use of
electronic medical records (EMRs), an emerging opportunity for chronic
disease surveillance.

An example of the relevance and feasibility of self-reported ratings of
living well was provided by Strine and colleagues (2008), who analyzed
data from a national sample in excess of 340,000 noninstitutionalized
adults using the BRFSS and found that even a single question rating life satisfaction, a surrogate for living well, was strongly associated with unhealthy
lifestyles, decreased health status, disability, and chronic illness. However,
this measure has not been used to assess interventions among patients with
chronic illnesses. Moreover, although measures of self-reported health-
related quality of life are the major outcomes in research trials of clinical

and public health interventions, they are not often used in routine clinical care or related surveillance systems. However, widespread implementation of electronic medical records (discussed below) may provide the opportunity to conduct widespread surveillance of patient-reported outcomes.

Finally, recent advances in the application of the genetics and molecular biology to patient illnesses are likely to change the nature and interpretation of surveillance over the next few years. This has sometimes been called "personalized medicine" (Offit, 2011), leading to changes in illness risk, classification, clinical behavior, and outcomes. Some implications include

- Altered classification of diseases and conditions according to molecular or genetic characteristics, such as subgroups of breast cancer with the HER-2-neu marker.
- Differential treatment approaches based on molecular markers, such as levels of P450 enzymes, leading to varied medication applications.
- Altered risk of incident diseases based on molecular markers. A large number of genetic variants have now been related to disease risk and occurrence. Although these altered risks for chronic diseases have not been large, such risks may be large enough to change screening practices.

Health Care System–Level Surveillance Systems

Information about chronic illness care and outcomes is collected by health systems as part of routine patient care. These data systems include descriptive information about patient demographics, residence, and insurance status. Using patient addresses, area-level information can be appended to patient records, such as median household income, census tract rates of poverty or crime, and characteristics of the built environment. Billing information is available on most patients (e.g., fee-for-service) on procedures, diagnoses, and hospitalization.

Health care organizations have used health information systems to improve processes of care and to reduce costs. Most of these systems have focused on measuring quality of health care using process measures, but relatively few routinely incorporate measures of health outcomes. These systems hold promise for improving health outcomes, as long as there is a strong link between the process measure and the expected health outcome. Berwick and others have described how improving the U.S. health care system requires simultaneous pursuit of three aims: improving the experience of care, improving the health of populations, and reducing per capita costs of health care (Berwick et al., 2008).

However, those working on the Triple Aim projects may focus on the two more concrete goals of improving the experience of health care and reducing per capita costs of health care and less on the aim of improving population health (Kindig, 2011). Kindig states that "the reality is that even major progress in these two areas over the next decade will not help us achieve our goals related to healthy life expectancy and disparity reduction."

Since the late 1990s—and partly as a result of two IOM reports, which describe the frequency of errors and mortality associated with hospitalization (*To Err Is Human*) and gaps in quality of care in the U.S. health care system (*Crossing the Quality Chasm*)—there has been increasing attention on measuring health care safety and quality, which is linked to hospital accreditation and reimbursement (Chassin et al., 2010) (see below). Moreover, these surveillance activities have resulted in nationwide initiatives to enhance the capacity of health systems to use the data and drive performance improvement (Institute for Healthcare Improvement, [a]). However, these activities have largely focused on improving safety and outcomes associated with acute care rather than improving longer-term outcomes for patients with chronic illnesses.

According to Porter, outcome measurement is perhaps the single most powerful tool that could be used to improve the quality of care among persons with chronic illness. As the true measures of quality in chronic illness care, it is necessary to measure, report, and compare specific and multidimensional outcomes. Understanding the outcomes achieved is also critical to ensuring that cost reduction is value enhancing (Porter, 2010). In his review, Porter suggests that although outcome measurement in the health care system is uncommon, there are examples that have proven practical and economically feasible. Moreover, accepted risk adjustment has been developed and implemented and although measurement initially revealed major variation in outcomes in each case over time, striking outcome improvement and narrowing of variation across providers were the result (Porter, 2010).

Despite consensus of the importance of measuring health outcomes in efforts to help patients live better with chronic illness, there is little consensus about what constitutes an optimal outcome and the distinctions among care processes, biological indicators, and outcomes remain unclear in practice (Porter, 2010). Currently used outcome measures tend to focus on the immediate results of particular interventions rather than the overall success of the full care cycle longitudinally for medical diseases or primary and preventive care. In addition, measured outcomes often fail to capture dimensions that are highly important to living well with chronic illness (Porter, 2010).

According to Porter, generalized outcomes, such as overall hospital infection rates, mortality rates, medication errors, or surgical complications, are too broad to permit proper evaluation of a provider's care in a way that is relevant to patients. Porter states that these generalized outcomes also obscure the causal connections between specific care processes and outcomes, since results are heavily influenced by many different processes (Porter, 2010). However, these system-level measures may be valuable for guiding organizational or public health interventions and future research (Conway and Clancy, 2009; Dougherty and Conway, 2008).

In addition to measuring health outcomes to drive performance improvement, analyzing health care costs has demonstrated wide geographic variations in risk-adjusted costs, which are not consistently associated with health outcomes (The Dartmouth Atlas of Health Care, [a]). These observations have partly contributed to recent health reform policies and regulations at the national and state levels to minimize variation in costs in an attempt to control rising health care costs.

Population-Based Surveillance Systems

Public health surveillance systems are an essential complement to patient- and health system–based information systems. These population-based health information systems have evolved over the past 50 years, broadening the scope from infectious to chronic diseases. Traditional surveillance systems that focused on infectious diseases have been expanded to include chronic diseases and chronic disease risk factors. CDC's National Program of Cancer Registries now supports central cancer registries in 45 states, the District of Columbia, Puerto Rico, and the U.S. Pacific Island jurisdictions, representing 96 percent of the U.S. population. Together with the National Cancer Institute's (NCI's) Surveillance, Epidemiology, and End Results (SEER) Program, cancer incidence data are available for the entire U.S. population.

During the 1980s, CDC established surveillance systems to monitor trends in risk factors for chronic diseases among adults (Behavioral Risk Factor Surveillance System) and children (Youth Risk Behavior Surveillance System, or YRBSS). These state-based systems for the first time provided information for state and selected local health departments for program planning and evaluation. The colored maps showing the increasing rates of obesity in every state during the past several decades have been seen by countless professionals, students, and members of the public.

In addition, there has been a growing awareness of the impact the built environment has on people's physical and mental health. Therefore, several interesting new surveillance methodologies have been developed that aim to monitor the health of individuals in the context of the communities in which they live, involving a complex interaction of health determinants, health outcomes, physical measurements, biological samples, policies, and the built environment (Nieto et al., 2010).

Public health surveillance systems are used to assess the causes and consequences of chronic illnesses, including measuring the burden, monitoring changes over time, and evaluating the effectiveness of broad-based interventions. These systems are generally developed and operated by governmental public health agencies at the local, state, or national level and vary from a simple system collecting data from a single source, to electronic systems that receive data from many sources in multiple formats, to complex population-based surveys. Accordingly, these systems address a range of public health needs:

a.   "guide immediate action for cases of public health importance;
b.   measure the burden of a disease (or other health-related event), including changes in related factors, the identification of populations at high risk, and the identification of new or emerging health concerns;
c.   monitor trends in the burden of a disease (or other health-related event), including the detection of epidemics (outbreaks) and pandemics;
d.   guide the planning, implementation, and evaluation of programs to prevent and control disease, injury, or adverse exposure;
e.   monitor adverse effects of interventions (e.g., the U.S. Food and Drug Administration and drugs);
f.   evaluate public policy;
g.   detect changes in health practices and the effects of these changes;
h.   prioritize the allocation of health resources;
i.   describe the clinical course of disease; and
j.   provide a basis for epidemiological research" (German et al., 2001).

Summary

Multidimensional surveillance of risk factors and health outcomes data at the patient, health organization, and population levels is essential for informing decisions on priorities and interventions to enhance living well with chronic illness at the level of patients, health organizations, and communities. However, many barriers continue to exist that prevent optimal integration and use of these data for program planning and evaluation.

Future chronic disease surveillance systems should integrate information from patient-, health system–, and population-based surveillance systems. The County Health Rankings (www.countyhealthrankings.org) is an example of an integrated system for surveillance of the overall health of a community that could be adapted for measuring living well with chronic illness. For example, rather than relying on estimates of quality of life from telephone surveys, health outcomes for communities could integrate information about quality of life from patient and health system databases.

FUTURE DATA SOURCES, METHODS, AND RESEARCH DIRECTIONS

The need for improved chronic disease surveillance systems is great, given the increasing demands for better patient experiences, lower costs, and improved population health outcomes. Future decisions about these systems will be driven by multiple factors, including the burden of illnesses and effectiveness, adoption, implementation, and maintenance of interventions, along with cost-benefit considerations (Glasgow et al., 1999). This section describes methods, data sources, and research needed to meet this increasing demand in the future.

Although many environmental, social, and health care factors contribute to health outcomes for persons with chronic illnesses, the current health care reform initiatives at the federal level are largely targeting health care access and quality. In addition, these initiatives include a number of policies and programs intended to enhance surveillance for chronic disease and enhance coordination of care. However, given the many determinants of health, the focus on enhancing access to care and transforming delivery of health care alone will be insufficient for helping persons with chronic illness to live well.

Measurement and incentives will drive health system change to improve chronic illness care. The Health Information Technology for Economic and Clinical Health (HITECH) Act (Blumenthal, 2010) provides incentives to facilitate the adoption of health information technology/electronic medical records, which will provide the foundation for surveillance data of health care and decision support. There are several provisions in the Affordable Care Act (ACA) to promote chronic disease surveillance. A provision of the ACA states that "any federally conducted or supported health care or public health program, activity or survey collects and reports, to the extent practicable data on ... disability status" and data collection standards have been developed to address this mandate (http://minorityhealth.hhs. gov/templates/browse.aspx?lvl=2&lvlid=208). Group health plans will be required to report annually to the HHS on their benefits and reimbursement structures that improve quality of care and health outcomes for individuals with chronic health illnesses (http://www.scribd.com/doc/57950324/ Health-Care-Shalls-in-the-Affordable-Care-Act). Tax-exempt hospitals will be required to conduct community health needs assessments every 3 years. Although this provision acknowledges the relevance of integrating data from the health care system and the community to drive performance improvement, no details are provided about what should be measured.

Recent developments in health information technology provide numerous avenues for the collection of individual-level health information that is relevant to living well with chronic illness. However, in using such data, consideration is needed to determine the extent to which the data are using measures that are reliable, valid (i.e., internally and externally), and responsive to change. In subsequent sections, we review potential methods and data sources for future surveillance to enhance living well, and research needs to address current gaps in knowledge relevant to surveillance for chronic illnesses.

The Use of Patient-Reported Outcomes in Surveillance Systems

PRO measures are considered essential for monitoring outcomes and quality of life in individuals with chronic illness. Recent years have seen a number of advances in the science of PROs, particularly by the PROMIS group, which funded the development of item banks as well as short forms and computer-adaptive tests to measure a range of PROS. Health domains for PROMIS were built on the World Health Organization framework of physical, mental, and social health (Cella et al., 2007). Domain definitions were created for physical function, fatigue, pain, emotional distress (including anxiety, depression, and anger), social health (including social function and social support), and global health. PROMIS instruments available as of June 2011 are listed in Table 5-6.

PROMIS instruments were validated and calibrated in samples from the U.S. general population and multiple illness populations, including individuals with arthritis, congestive heart failure, COPD, cancer, and other illnesses. The instruments are designed to measure feelings, functions, and perceptions applicable to a range of chronic illnesses, enabling efficient and interpretable clinical research and clinical practice application of patient-reported outcomes. The instruments have been validated against legacy illness-specific instruments.

New Modes of Data Collection

There is an increasing number of modes for the collection of health information, including patient-reported outcomes, that may be used for surveillance efforts in the future. For example, many employers use health risk appraisals (HRAs) as feedback tools for their employees to improve their health. Although these assessments are meant to be tools to help individuals improve their health status and thus tend to focus on health behavior and preventive health care utilization, it could be particularly

TABLE 5-6 Available PROMIS Instruments

Domain	Bank	Short Forms
Emotional distress—anger	29	8
Emotional distress—anxiety	29	4, 6, 7, 8
Emotional distress—depression	28	4, 6, 8a, 8b
Applied cognition—abilities	33	4, 6, 8
Applied cognition—general concerns	34	4, 6, 8
Psychosocial illness impact—positive	39	4, 8
Psychosocial illness impact—negative	32	4, 8
Fatigue	95	4, 6, 7, 8
Pain—behavior	39	7
Pain—interference	41	4, 6a, 6b, 8
Pain intensity	3	
Physical function	124	4, 6, 8, 10, 20
Mobility		
Upper extremity		
Physical function for samples with mobility aid users	114	12
Sleep disturbance	27	4, 6, 8a, 8b
Sleep-related impairment	16	8
Sexual function: global satisfaction with sex life and 10 other subscales	7	
Satisfaction with participation in discretionary social activities	12	7
Satisfaction with participation in social roles	14	4, 6, 7, 8
Satisfaction with social roles and activities	44	4, 6, 8
Ability to participate in social roles and activities	35	4, 6, 8
Companionship	6	4, 6
Informational support	10	4, 6, 8
Emotional support	16	4, 6, 8
Instrumental support	11	4, 6, 8
Social isolation	14	4, 6, 8
Peer relationships		
Asthma impact		
Global health	10	

SOURCE: PROMIS Assessment Center. Instruments Available for Use. http://assessmentcenter.net/documents/InstrumentLibrary.pdf.

useful for individuals with chronic illness to track health outcomes, such as PROs, over time.

Online personal health records (PHRs), like the Health Vault by Microsoft, may also eventually provide data for surveillance of living well with chronic illness. Such tools allow individuals to record and track their own health information online. Some systems have the ability to link with a health care system's electronic health record, and so adoption of EHRs by health care systems is important to the usefulness of such tools, as is the interoperability between the PHR and health care system EHR (Archer et al., 2011). A further limitation is that not all PHRs include the type of outcomes that are relevant to living well with chronic illness. In particular, valid and reliable PRO measures are not widely available in these systems, although there may be value to a person living with a chronic illness in tracking an outcome like pain or fatigue. Incorporation of such measures into PHRs could help increase their usefulness to surveillance efforts as well. However, the use of PHRs requires long-term use and considerable effort on the part of the health consumer. More research is needed to identify ways to optimize the usefulness of PHRs for individuals and identify methods to motivate and increase their use (Archer et al., 2011).

Registries have long been used as a method for studying diseases. Traditional registries (e.g., cancer registries) usually involve information submitted by the health care provider. Although such registries are used for surveillance (the SEER registry being a prime example), they rarely assess the patient-reported outcomes that are relevant to living well with chronic illness. Often, the patient has not consented to follow-up contact; conducting surveillance that involves recontacting patients therefore often requires several costly steps, such as requesting permission from the health care provider. However, a number of registries are emerging in which individuals themselves volunteer for the registry, expressing their willingness to participate in health research. Examples include two state-based registries—the Illinois Women's Health Registry and the Kentucky Women's Health Registry—and a disease-specific registry, the Susan Love Foundation's Army of Women, a registry of breast cancer survivors and women without breast cancer who are willing to participate in research related to breast cancer. Also, for some registries, information is submitted by health care providers rather than the participants themselves (e.g., cancer registries). Registries could be used for surveillance efforts related to living well with chronic illness, but attention needs to be paid to assessing selection bias in who enrolls in registries.

Online networks for individuals with chronic illness may also provide opportunities for surveillance. For example, networks, such as Patients Like Me and Cure Together, have as part of their goal information gathering and sharing that can help patients understand their illness course and effective treatments. Patients Like Me has a membership of 114,953 patients. They routinely collect patient-reported outcomes on their website, although participation in this data collection is voluntary. It is a for-profit organization whose business model includes selling the patient information to clients like pharmaceutical companies. The network started by serving primarily the ALS community. It conducted an observational study with matched controls on the use of lithium among their members with ALS. The study found the same result as subsequent trials, that lithium was of no benefit in slowing the progression of this illness (Wicks et al., 2011). Cure Together has approximately 25,000 members. It asks members to provide data on symptoms, treatments they have tried, and effectiveness of treatments and then share the results online with other members. Another example is registries of patients with chronic lung diseases (http://www.alpha1registry.org/index.html). Such networks could be tapped for surveillance efforts in the future, but consideration of selection bias is still necessary. Furthermore, it is unclear to what extent these networks use validated assessment tools that are reliable and sensitive to change in their data gathering, which would be important for surveillance measures (Thacker et al., 2006).

With the increasing adoption as well as incentives and support for adoption of electronic medical records, future surveillance methods may be able to utilize this information to monitor whether patients are living well. One of the components of meaningful use is submitting clinical quality and other measures, but this does not currently include measures of living well (Classen and Bates, 2011). Although it is common to use medical care records to monitor quality of care, the potential exists to use these data to track outcomes as well. However, available research evidence does not include patient-level outcomes for assessing the effectiveness of EMRs, and only recently has cross-sectional evidence suggested that the use of EMRs is associated with improvements in standards of care processes and intermediate outcomes compared with paper records for patients with diabetes (Cebul et al., 2011). If brief patient-reported outcome measures are incorporated into the EMR for patients with chronic illnesses, these data could be used to provide longitudinal information on quality of life indicators of importance to this population, extending current systems that primarily monitor statistics related to illness mortality. While the entire nation does not have access to electronic medical records at this time, there is still widespread availability of EMR covering large segments of the population. The use and availability of EMR will continue to expand, which supports the incremental approach to enhanced chronic disease surveillance. The PROMIS measures are ideal for such a system because they are reliable and validated, brief, and applicable across a range of chronic diseases.

Syndromic surveillance refers to the detection of outbreaks or disease trends using automated surveillance of pre-diagnostic data, including, for example, sales of over-the-counter medications or emergency room visits. Movement toward electronic medical records may make such surveillance feasible with medical records, but innovative applications of more population-based data have also been explored. Data mining of information collected by search engines or in either general or disease-specific online social networks may be more sensitive to such detection methods. However, one limitation of this approach is that such methods are more sensitive to short-term changes (e.g., influenza epidemics; see Signorini et al., 2011). In addition, people with chronic illness are less likely to have Internet access than others, raising the possibility of selection bias in who provides information. However, people with chronic illnesses who go online are more likely to seek out others with similar health concerns than are those without chronic illness (Fox, 2011), indicating that this may be a fruitful area for surveillance, as more people with chronic illness obtain access to the Internet.

Research on Measurement of Chronic Disease

Although the need for surveillance is a well-established function of public health, surveillance of chronic illness to enhance living well is complex and presents a number of challenges that will require further investigation at the individual, health organization, and population levels. Moreover, the effectiveness of potential future methods and data sources for surveillance to drive improvement will need to be determined.

Individual Level

The measurement of patient-reported outcomes continues to be an active area of investigation (as previously described for PROMIS), and much of the research focus has been on reliability, validity, and responsiveness to change. For example, there is limited evidence on sources of variation of HRQoL, including gender (Cherepanov et al., 2010), season (Jia and Lubetkin, 2009), and MCCs (Chen et al., 2011). Further research is needed to determine other sources of variation (e.g., health literacy, socioeconomic factors). Moreover, the reliability of surveillance of HRQoL remains controversial, in need of further research (Avendano et al., 2009; Salomon et al., 2009). For specific illnesses, further qualitative research to obtain the patient's perspective (e.g., illness intrusiveness, regrets about treatment decisions) may be needed to strengthen the validity of measures of patient-reported outcomes for measuring living well. In addition to patient-reported outcomes, little is known about the feasibility and potential usefulness of objective, longitudinal measures of functional and cognitive capacity for surveillance. Finally, in the context of health care reform and concern about costs, the burden and costs versus benefits of surveillance of patient-reported outcomes and other individual-level measures will need to be determined.

Health Organization Level

A major component of the transformation process currently under way in the U.S. health care system is comparative effectiveness research (Conway and Clancy, 2009; Dougherty and Conway, 2008); although this research agenda is focused on health care interventions, chronic disease surveillance is the first step in the intervention process. Ongoing health services research is needed to assess the effectiveness of surveillance methods using the EMR (Kmetik et al., 2011) and of methods for public reporting of health care organization performance (Mukamel et al., 2010). Chassin and colleagues (2010) recently reviewed the current status of surveillance measurement of hospital performance and outline four criteria for accountability measures, which provide a framework for future research focused on surveillance of health care organizations: (1) there is a strong evidence base showing that the care process leads to improved outcomes; (2) the measure accurately captures whether the evidence-based care process has, in fact, been provided; (3) the measure addresses a process that has few intervening care processes that must occur before the improved outcome is realized; and (4) implementing the measure has little or no chance of inducing unintended adverse consequences. The rising costs of health care and wide geographic variation in health care costs has increasingly focused attention on determining the value of health care. However, there are a number of challenges in estimating the cost of disease (Rosen and Cutler, 2009), which will require ongoing research.

The rapid growth in new technology and research evidence, combined with gaps between evidence and practice, along with unsustainable growth in health care costs has focused nationwide attention on innovative, collaborative efforts to "learn about the best uses of new technologies at the same rate that it produces new technologies"—termed the rapid learning health system (IOM, 2007, p. 210). The foundation for the learning health care system is large EMR research databases (IOM, 2007), and current examples of where these research databases are being used for health care improvement include the Veterans Administration and Kaiser Permanente.

Population Level

The general surveillance-related research needs at the population level are similar to the needs described for the individual and health organization level, including the reliability, validity, and responsiveness to change of surveillance measures. At the population level, these measurement characteristics will apply to the social and environmental determinants of living well, including policies and regulations.

Summary

Because of the complex determinants of living well, including factors at the patient, health care system, and population levels, surveillance to drive and monitor the effectiveness of public health action to reduce disability and improve function and quality of life requires multidimensional longitudinal measurement. In addition to fundamental research on measurement reliability, validity, and responsiveness to change, overarching questions remain on what measurements are minimally needed for effective surveillance and how frequently data collection should be performed. At the patient level, recent population-based studies suggest that relatively simple individual-level measures of life satisfaction (Strine et al., 2008) and well-being (Gerstorf et al., 2010) are associated with a number of health outcomes; when measured longitudinally, a rapid slope of decline is predictive of mortality 3 to 5 years before death (Gerstorf et al., 2010). Further research is needed, but these results suggest that surveillance using a composite of relatively simple measures of life satisfaction and well-being, combined with measures at the health care system (e.g., access) and population (e.g., policies) levels, may be useful for monitoring the effectiveness of health care and public health interventions to promote living well among patients with chronic illness.

CONCLUSION

The committee's statement of task asks "How can public health surveillance be used to inform public policy decisions to minimize adverse life impacts?" This question can be answered first by considering the types of public policy decisions that can affect the quality of life among persons living with chronic illness. Surveillance is the first step in the change process to drive interventions to address gaps for patients with chronic illnesses to live well and to improve the nation's health and economic well-being by reducing disability and improving quality of life and functioning. This shift in focus from only extending life to living well has the potential to facilitate decision making at the individual, health care system, and population levels that optimizes outcomes not only for patients and families but also for society.

For example, advanced care planning using evidence from surveillance on prognosis and options enables patients and families to make more informed decisions that improve satisfaction and quality of life and reduce suffering (Curtis, 2011). Although this evidence may be obtained from clinical trials, longitudinal population-based surveillance of patients with chronic illnesses provides the strongest external validity. Moreover, this enhanced decision making is associated with lower health care costs (Morrison et al., 2011).

For the second question—What consequences of chronic diseases are most important to the nation's health and economic well-being?—the response is more complex and cannot be limited only to consequences, because of the multiple determinants of chronic disease. Therefore, measures used for surveillance of living well must be multidimensional and include measures of determinants of health at the individual, health system, and population levels as well as health-related outcomes (e.g., patient-reported outcomes, functioning) that are relevant to patients living well. Moreover, these individual-level consequences should be associated with lower societal costs. Finally, it must be feasible to collect these data elements longitudinally.

If providers and communities are going to be rewarded for preventing and controlling chronic disease, better data systems are needed. These data systems should draw on individual-level data (e.g., from the electronic health record) and include three types of information:

- Risk of chronic illness (e.g., through a health risk appraisal)
- Presence of chronic illnesses
- Measures of quality of life and functioning

Risk factor information is needed in order to reward chronic disease prevention efforts. Providers who invest in clinical or community-based prevention programs are unlikely to see the outcomes in lower rates of chronic diseases given the low incidence and lag between interventions and outcomes. However, these interventions can produce short-term changes in behaviors and other risk factors.

Information about chronic diseases should be collected on all persons. Some of this information can be obtained from electronic health records. However, signs and symptoms of chronic illnesses are often lacking in health care systems and should be collected as part of a health assessment.

Finally, information on disability and quality of life should be collected at the individual level. A variety of methods exist, but standard definitions are needed (similar to the risk factor definitions developed for the BRFSS) to permit comparison between communities and over time (NRC, 2009).

The technology exists today to collect comprehensive health information on everyone living in a community. However, there are a number of barriers to be overcome, such as budget constraints, organizational inertia for prioritizing/replacing existing methods, lack of sharing agreements, lack of incentives, lack of standard definitions, and limitations of workforce capacity. Decision-making processes are needed to optimize surveillance activities despite limited resources. Research and demonstration projects will be needed to address the many barriers to enhancing surveillance systems to promote "living well." Grants could be provided to first demonstrate the feasibility of collecting this information in large health systems, and eventually in entire communities. Ultimately, priorities for surveillance need to be driven by a number of factors, including the burden of illness (e.g., frequency, disability, costs) for individuals and society, and availability of cost-effective interventions.

RECOMMENDATIONS 16–17

The committee provides two recommendations to address the question how can public health surveillance be used to inform public policy decisions to minimize adverse life impacts.

Recommendation 16

The committee recommends that the secretary of HHS encourage and support pilot tests by health care systems to collect patient-level information, share deidentified data across systems, and make them available at the local, state, and national levels in order to monitor and improve chronic illness outcomes. These data should include patient self-reported outcomes of health-related quality of life and functional status in persons with chronic illness.

Recommendation 17

The committee recommends that the secretary of HHS establish and support a standing national work group to oversee and coordinate multidimensional chronic diseases surveillance activity, including obtaining patient-level data on health-related quality of life and functional status from electronic medical records and data on the implementation and dissemination of effective chronic disease interventions at the health care system and the community level, including longitudinal health outcomes.

REFERENCES

Abrams, T.E., M. Vaughan-Sarrazin, V.S. Fan, and P.J. Kaboli. 2011. Geographic isolation and the risk for chronic obstructive pulmonary disease–related mortality. *Annals of Internal Medicine* 155(2):80–86.

Archer, N., U. Fevrier-Thomas, C. Lokker, K. McKibbon, and S. Straus. 2011. Personal health records: A scoping review. *Journal of the American Medical Informatics Association* 18(4):515.

Avendano, M., T. Huijts, and S. Subramanian. 2009. Re: "Are Americans feeling less healthy? The puzzle of trends in self-rated health." *American Journal of Epidemiology* 170(12):1581.

Barr, V., S. Robinson, B. Marin-Link, L. Underhill, A. Dotts, D. Ravensdale, and S. Salivaras. 2003. The expanded chronic care model. *Hospital Quarterly* 7(1):73–82.

Berwick, D. M. 2011. Launching accountable care organizations—the proposed rule for the Medicare shared savings program. *New England Journal of Medicine* 364(16):e32.

Berwick, D.M., T.W. Nolan, and J. Whittington. 2008. The triple aim: Care, health, and cost. *Health Affairs* 27(3):759–769.

Bindman, A. B., A. Chattopadhyay, and G. M. Auerback. 2008. Interruptions in Medicaid coverage and risk for hospitalization for ambulatory care–sensitive conditions. *Annals of Internal Medicine* 149(12):854–860.

Blumenthal, D. 2010. Launching HITECH. *The New England Journal of Medicine* 362(5): 382–385.

Brault, M., J. Hootman, C. Helmick, K. Theis, and B. Armour. 2009. Prevalence and most common causes of disability among adults—United States, 2005. *Morbidity and Mortality Weekly Report* 58(16):421–426.

Cebul, R.D., T.E. Love, A.K. Jain, and C.J. Hebert. 2011. Electronic health records and quality of diabetes care. *New England Journal of Medicine* 365(9):825–833.

Cella, D., S. Yount, N. Rothrock, R. Gershon, K. Cook, B. Reeve, D. Ader, J.F. Fries, B. Bruce, and M. Rose. 2007. The patient-reported outcomes measurement information system (PROMIS): Progress of an NIH roadmap cooperative group during its first two years. *Medical Care* 45(5 Suppl 1):S3–S11.

Chassin, M.R., J.M. Loeb, S.P. Schmaltz, and R.M. Wachter. 2010. Accountability measures—using measurement to promote quality improvement. *New England Journal of Medicine* 363(7):683–688.

Chen, H.Y., D.J. Baumgardner, and J.P. Rice. 2011. Health-related quality of life among adults with multiple chronic conditions in the United States, Behavioral Risk Factor Surveillance System, 2007. *Preventing Chronic Disease* 8(1):A09.

Cherepanov, D., M. Palta, D.G. Fryback, and S.A. Robert. 2010. Gender differences in health-related quality-of-life are partly explained by sociodemographic and socioeconomic variation between adult men and women in the US: Evidence from four us nationally representative data sets. *Quality of life research* 19(8):1115–1124.

Chodosh, J., D.H. Solomon, C.P. Roth, J.T. Chang, C.H. MacLean, B.A. Ferrell, P.G. Shekelle, and N.S. Wenger. 2004. The quality of medical care provided to vulnerable older patients with chronic pain. *Journal of the American Geriatrics Society* 52(5):756–761.

Classen, D.C., and D.W. Bates. 2011. Finding the meaning in meaningful use. *New England Journal of Medicine* 365(9):855–858.

Conway, P.H., and C. Clancy. 2009. Transformation of health care at the front line. *Journal of the American Medical Association* 301(7):763.

Curtis, J.R. 2011. Reimbursement for advance care planning: Why should intensivists care? *American Journal of Respiratory and Critical Care Medicine* 184(4):387.

Dougherty, D., and P.H. Conway. 2008. The "3t's" road map to transform US health care. *Journal of the American Medical Association* 299(19):2319.

Fielding, J.E., and S.M. Teutsch. 2011. An opportunity map for societal investment in health. *Journal of the American Medical Association* 305(20):2110–2111.

Fox, S. 2011. *The social life of health information.* http://pewinternet.org/Reports/2011/Social-Life-of-Health-Info.aspx (accessed September 21, 2011).

Friedman, D.J., and R. Parrish. 2006. Characteristics, desired functionalities, and datasets of state web-based data query systems. *Journal of Public Health Management and Practice* 12(2):119.

Fries, J.F., P. Spitz, R.G. Kraines, and H.R. Holman. 1980. Measurement of patient outcome in arthritis. *Arthritis & Rheumatism* 23(2):137–145.

German, R.R., L.M. Lee, J.M. Horan, R.L. Milstein, C.A. Pertowski, and M.N. Waller; Guidelines Working Group Centers for Disease Control and Prevention. 2001. Updated guidelines for evaluating public health surveillance systems: Recommendations from the Guidelines Working Group. *Morbidity and Mortality Weekly Report* 50(RR-13):1–35.

Gerstorf, D., N. Ram, G. Mayraz, M. Hidajat, U. Lindenberger, G.G. Wagner, and J. Schupp. 2010. Late-life decline in well-being across adulthood in Germany, the United Kingdom, and the United States: Something is seriously wrong at the end of life. *Psychology and Aging* 25(2):477.

Glasgow, R.E., T.M. Vogt, and S.M. Boles. 1999. Evaluating the public health impact of health promotion interventions: The re-aim framework. *American Journal of Public Health* 89(9):1322.

Grosse, S.D., D.J. Lollar, V.A. Campbell, and M. Chamie. 2009. Disability and disability-adjusted life years: Not the same. *Public Health Reports* 124(2):197.

Guralnik, J.M., L. Ferrucci, E.M. Simonsick, M.E. Salive, and R.B. Wallace. 1995. Lower-extremity function in persons over the age of 70 years as a predictor of subsequent disability. *New England Journal of Medicine* 332(9):556–561.

Hung, W., J. Ross, K. Boockvar, and A. Siu. 2011. Recent trends in chronic disease, impairment and disability among older adults in the United States. *BMC geriatrics* 11(1):47.

Institute for Healthcare Improvement (a). *The IHI Triple Aim.* http://www.ihi.org/offerings/Initiatives/TripleAim/Pages/default.aspx (accessed December 19, 2011).

IOM (Institute of Medicine). 1988. *The Future of Public Health.* Washington, DC: National Academy Press.

IOM. 2001. *Crossing the Quality Chasm: A New Health System for the 21st Century.* Washington, DC: National Academy Press.

IOM. 2007. *The Learning Healthcare System: Workshop Summary.* Washington, DC: The National Academies Press.

IOM. 2011. *A National Surveillance System for Cardiovascular and Select Chronic Diseases.* Washington, DC: The National Academies Press.

Jackson, B.E., S. Suzuki, K. Lo, F. Su, K.P. Singh, D. Coultas, A. Bartolucci, and S. Bae. 2011. Geographic disparity in COPD hospitalization rates among the Texas population. *Respiratory Medicine* 105(5):734–739.

Jia, H., and E.I. Lubetkin. 2009. Time trends and seasonal patterns of health-related quality of life among U.S. adults. *Public Health Reports* 124(5):692.

Katz, M.H. 2009. Structural interventions for addressing chronic health problems. *Journal of the American Medical Association* 302(6):683–685.

Kindig, D.L. 2011. *Unpacking the Triple Aim Model.* http://www.improvingpopulationhealth.org/blog/2011/01/unpacking_triple_aim.html (accessed November 2, 2011).

Kmetik, K.S., M.F. O' Toole, H. Bossley, C.A. Brutico, G. Fischer, S.L. Grund, B.M. Gulotta, M. Hennessey, S. Kahn, K.M. Murphy, T. Pacheco, L.G. Pawlson, J. Schaeffer, P.A. Schwamberger, S.H. Scholle, and G. Wozniak. 2011. Exceptions to outpatient quality measures for coronary artery disease in electronic health records. *Annals of Internal Medicine* 154(4):227–234.

Kulkarni, S.C., A. Levin-Rector, M. Ezzati, and C.J.L. Murray. 2011. Falling behind: Life expectancy in US counties from 2000 to 2007 in an international context. *Population Health Metrics* 9(1):16.

Kuo, H.K., S.G. Leveille, C.J. Yen, H.M. Chai, C.H. Chang, Y.C. Yeh, Y.H. Yu, and J.F. Bean. 2006. Exploring how peak leg power and usual gait speed are linked to late-life disability: Data from the National Health and Nutrition Examination Survey (NHANES), 1999-2002. *American Journal of Physical Medicine and Rehabilitation* 85(8):650–658.

Levin-Epstein, J. 2005. *Presenteeism and Paid Sick Days.* http://www.clasp.org/admin/site/publications/files/0212.pdf (accessed November 2, 2011).

Lindenauer, P.K., P. Pekow, S. Gao, A.S. Crawford, B. Gutierrez, and E.M. Benjamin. 2006. Quality of care for patients hospitalized for acute exacerbations of chronic obstructive pulmonary disease. *Annals of Internal Medicine* 144(12):894.

Lindenauer, P.K., D. Remus, S. Roman, M.B. Rothberg, E.M. Benjamin, A. Ma, and D.W. Bratzler. 2007. Public reporting and pay for performance in hospital quality improvement. *New England Journal of Medicine* 356(5):486–496.

Love, D., W. Custer, and P. Miller. 2010. All-payer claims databases: State initiatives to improve health care transparency. *Issue Brief (Commonwealth Fund)* 99:1–14.

Manton, K.G. 2008. Recent declines in chronic disability in the elderly US population: Risk factors and future dynamics. *Annual Review of Public Health* 29:91–113.

Maxson, E., S. Jain, M. Kendall, F. Mostashari, and D. Blumenthal. 2010. The regional extension center program: Helping physicians meaningfully use health information technology. *Annals of Internal Medicine* 153(10):666.

McGovern, P.G., J.S. Pankow, E. Shahar, K.M. Doliszny, A.R. Folsom, H. Blackburn, and R.V. Luepker. 1996. Recent trends in acute coronary heart disease—mortality, morbidity, medical care, and risk factors. *New England Journal of Medicine* 334(14):884–890.

Meenan, R.F., P.M. Gertman, and J.H. Mason. 1980. Measuring health status in arthritis. *Arthritis & Rheumatism* 23(2):146–152.

Metersky, M.L. 2009. The Medicare physician quality reporting initiative. *Chest* 136(6):1644.

Mokdad, A.H., and P.L. Remington. 2010. Measuring health behaviors in populations. *Preventing Chronic Disease* 7(4):A75.

Monninkhof, E., M. van der Aa, P. van der Valk, J. van der Palen, G. Zielhuis, K. Koning, and M. Pieterse. 2004. A qualitative evaluation of a comprehensive self-management programme for COPD patients: Effectiveness from the patients' perspective. *Patient Education and Counseling* 55(2):177–184.

Morrison, R.S., J. Dietrich, S. Ladwig, T. Quill, J. Sacco, J. Tangeman, and D. E. Meier. 2011. Palliative care consultation teams cut hospital costs for Medicaid beneficiaries. *Health Affairs* 30(3):454.

Mukamel, D.B., L.G. Glance, A.W. Dick, and T.M. Olser. 2010. Measuring quality for public reporting: Making it meaningful to patients. *American Journal of Public Health* 100(2):264–269.

Nieto, F.J., P.E. Peppard, C.D. Engelman, J.A. McElroy, L.W. Galvao, E.M. Friedman, A.J. Bersch, and K.C. Malecki. 2010. The Survey of the Health of Wisconsin (SHOW), a novel infrastructure for population health research: Rationale and methods. *BMC Public Health* 10:785.

NRC (National Research Council). 2009. *Improving the Measurement of Late-Life Disability in Population Surveys: Beyond ADLs and IADLs: Summary of a Workshop.* Washington, DC: The National Academies Press.

Obisesan, T.O., O.A. Obisesan, S. Martins, L. Alamgir, V. Bond, C. Maxwell, and R.F. Gillum. 2008. High blood pressure, hypertension, and high pulse pressure are associated with poorer cognitive function in persons aged 60 and older: The third national health and nutrition examination survey. *Journal of the American Geriatrics Society* 56(3):501–509.

Offit, K. 2011. Personalized medicine: New genomics, old lessons. *Human Genetics* 130(1):3–14.

Pan, L., Q. Mukhtar, S. Geiss, M. Rivera, A. Alfaro-Correa, and R. Sniegowski. 2006. Self-rated fair or poor health among adults with diabetes—United States, 1996-2005. *Journal of the American Medical Association* 296:2919-2920.

Pincus, T., and T. Sokka. 2003. Quantitative measures for assessing rheumatoid arthritis in clinical trials and clinical care. *Best Practice & Research Clinical Rheumatology* 17(5):753-781.

Porter, M.E. 2010. What is value in health care? *New England Journal of Medicine* 363(26): 2477-2481.

Remington, P.L., and R.C. Brownson. 2011. Fifty years of progress in chronic disease epidemiology and control. MMWR. Surveillance summaries: Morbidity and mortality weekly report. *Surveillance summaries/CDC* 60(4):70.

Remington, P.L., M.V. Wegner, and A.M. Rohan. 2010. Chronic disease surveillance. *Chronic Disease Epidemiology and Control, 3rd ed.*, edited by P.L. Remington, R.C. Brownson, and M.V. Wegner. Washington, DC: American Public Health Association.

Reuben, D.B., L.A. Valle, R.D. Hays, and A.L. Siu. 1995. Measuring physical function in community-dwelling older persons: A comparison of self-administered, interviewer-administered, and performance-based measures. *Journal of the American Geriatrics Society* 43(1):17-23.

Rikli, R.E., and C.J. Jones. 2001. *Senior Fitness Test Manual.* Champaign, IL: Human Kinetics.

Rosen, A., and D. Cutler. 2009. Reconciling national health expenditure accounts and cost-of-illness studies. *Medical Care* 47:S7-S13.

Salomon, J.A., S. Nordhagen, S. Oza, and C.J.L. Murray. 2009. Are Americans feeling less healthy? The puzzle of trends in self-rated health. *American Journal of Epidemiology* 170(3):343.

Schneider, K.M., B.E. O' Donnell, and D. Dean. 2009. Prevalence of multiple chronic conditions in the United States' Medicare population. *Health and Quality of Life Outcomes* 7(1):1-11.

Signorini, A., A.M. Segre, and P.M. Polgreen. 2011. The use of twitter to track levels of disease activity and public concern in the US during the influenza A H1N1 pandemic. *PloS One* 6(5):e19467.

Stewart, A.L., R.D. Hays, and J.E. Ware, Jr. 1988. The MOS short-form general health survey. Reliability and validity in a patient population. *Medical Care* 26(7):724.

Strand, V., P. Tugwell, C. Bombardier, A. Maetzel, B. Crawford, C. Dorrier, A. Thompson, and G. Wells. 1999. Function and health-related quality of life: Results from a randomized controlled trial of leflunomide versus methotrexate or placebo in patients with active rheumatoid arthritis. Leflunomide rheumatoid arthritis investigators group. *Arthritis & Rheumatism* 42(9):1870-1878.

Strand, V., D.L. Scott, P. Emery, J.R. Kalden, J.S. Smolen, G.W. Cannon, P. Tugwell, and B. Crawford. 2005. Physical function and health related quality of life: Analysis of 2-year data from randomized, controlled studies of leflunomide, sulfasalazine, or methotrexate in patients with active rheumatoid arthritis. *The Journal of Rheumatology* 32(4):590.

Strine, T.W., D.P. Chapman, L.S. Balluz, D.G. Moriarty, and A.H. Mokdad. 2008. The associations between life satisfaction and health-related quality of life, chronic illness, and health behaviors among U.S. Community-dwelling adults. *Journal of Community Health* 33(1):40-50.

Thacker, S.B., D.F. Stroup, V. Carande-Kulis, J.S. Marks, K. Roy, and J.L. Gerberding. 2006. Measuring the public's health. *Public Health Reports* 121(1):14-22.

The Dartmouth Atlas of Health Care (a). http://www.dartmouthatlas.org/ (accessed November 2, 2011).

Tinetti, M.E., and S.A., Studenski. 2011. Comparative effectiveness research and patients with multiple chronic conditions. *New England Journal of Medicine* 364(26):2478-2481.

Tugwell, P., G. Wells, V. Strand, A. Maetzel, C. Bombardier, B. Crawford, C. Dorrier, and A. Thompson. 2000. Clinical improvement as reflected in measures of function and health-related quality of life following treatment with leflunomide compared with methotrexate in patients with rheumatoid arthritis: Sensitivity and relative efficiency to detect a treatment effect in a twelve-month, placebo-controlled trial. *Arthritis & Rheumatism* 43(3):506–514.

Ware, J.E., M. Kosinski, and S.D. Keller. 1994. *SF-36 Physical and Mental Health Summary Scales: A Users' Manual.* Boston, MA: The Health Institute, New England Medical Center.

Ware, J., K. Snow, M. Kosinski, and B. Gandek. 1997. *SF-36 Health Survey: Manual and Interpretation Guide.* Boston, MA: The Health Institute, New England Medical Center.

Ware, J.E., Jr., M. Kosinski, J.E. Dewey, and B. Gandek. 2001. *How to Score and Interpret Single-Item Health Measures: A Manual for Users of the SF-8 Health Survey.* Lincoln, RI: QualityMetric Incorporated.

Wicks, P., T. E. Vaughan, M. P. Massagli, and J. Heywood. 2011. Accelerated clinical discovery using self-reported patient data collected online and a patient-matching algorithm. *Nature biotechnology* 29:411–414.

Wolfe, F., and T. Pincus. 1999. Listening to the patient: A practical guide to self-report questionnaires in clinical care. *Arthritis & Rheumatism* 42(9):1797–1808.

Yeh, M.L., H.H. Chen, Y.C. Liao, and W.Y. Liao. 2004. Testing the functional status model in patients with chronic obstructive pulmonary disease. *Journal of Advanced Nursing* 48(4):342–350.

Zack, M. M., D. G. Moriarty, D. F. Stroup, E. S. Ford, and A. H. Mokdad. 2004. Worsening trends in adult health-related quality of life and self-rated health—United States, 1993-2001. *Public Health Reports* 119(5):493.

6

Interface of the Public Health System, the Health Care System, and the Non–Health Care Sector

INTRODUCTION

An aligned system with a strong interface among public health, health care, and the community and non–health care sectors could produce better prevention and treatment outcomes for populations living with chronic illness. In part, these systems are natural allies, as they often serve the same populations and see themselves as contributing to the public's health, and they often share the burden of poor chronic disease outcomes. They could serve as powerful partners because only together can they achieve the goal of living well across populations and across chronic illnesses.

Imagining how public health, health care, and community-based organizations could align to improve outcomes in chronic disease led the committee to develop a conceptual model that frames the interaction among the factors and systems associated with chronic disease and its management. We examined how these various factors and systems produce better health for individuals and populations living with chronic illness. Many of these factors in the model impact health outside traditional health care settings and are understood at the population level rather than through an individual focus. Interventions at the population level can be implemented to prevent disease and promote health, and the committee was interested in the roles and effectiveness of organizations that do now or could in the future contribute to living well with chronic illness. This chapter reviews how public health, health care, and community and non–health care organizations approach the prevention and management of chronic disease and opportunities for improvement.

PUBLIC HEALTH SYSTEM STRUCTURES AND APPROACHES

Perhaps the programs that impact chronic disease that are least well understood lie within the constellation of agencies that serve the public's health, working primarily across populations. Governmental public health agencies (GPHAs) are the primary providers of these programs. In many cases, community-based organizations (CBOs) also provide care. Governmental public health agencies have been and likely will be important in helping people live well with chronic disabling conditions and other chronic illnesses particularly in their shared role with clinical services to education and support the transition of care. Over the past 25 years, these agencies have moved from a focus on clinical care for the underserved to improving population health, and they have changed their role from doing to leading.

The Institute of Medicine (IOM) helped to encourage this redirection of focus through two reports on the future of public health. The first report (IOM, 1988) focused almost exclusively on GPHAs. It documented their disarray and attributed it to their being torn between trying to improve population health and serving as care providers, of last resort, of clinical care to the underserved, including the uninsured, all with inadequate resources. The report emphasized both population health and leadership as it described three roles for GPHAs: (1) assessment—to "systematically collect, assemble, analyze, and make available information on the health of the community"; (2) policy development—to "serve the public interest in the development of comprehensive public health policies by promoting use of the scientific knowledge base in decision-making about public health and by leading in developing public health policy"; and (3) assurance—to "assure their constituents that services necessary to achieve agreed upon goals are provided, either by encouraging actions by other entities (private or public sector), by requiring such action through regulation, or by providing services directly" (IOM, 1988).

The second report (IOM, 2002) was much less focused on government and placed the role of GPHAs in a broader context as one of many public health partners with an important role in improving population health. These partners include communities, the health care delivery system, employers and businesses, the media, and the academic community. Specific recommendations to GPHAs again emphasized leadership and included "1) adopting a population health approach that considers the multiple determinants of health; 2) strengthening the governmental public health infrastructure, which forms the backbone of the public health system; 3) building a new generation of intersectoral partnerships that also draw on the perspectives and resources of diverse communities and actively engaging them in health action; 4) developing systems of accountability to assure the quality and availability of public health services; 5) making evidence the foundation of decision making and the measure of success; and 6) enhancing and facilitating communication within the public health system (e.g., among all levels of the governmental public health infrastructure and between public health professionals and community members" (IOM, 2002).

This redirection of GPHAs over the past 25 years—in content, from clinical care to population health, and in role, from doing to leading—has been echoed in the development of programs for chronic disease prevention. The Centers for Disease Control and Prevention (CDC) has led the development of these programs through its National Center for Chronic Disease Prevention and Health Promotion, initiated in 1989 (Collins et al., 2009). CDC's initial focus was on state-level programs aimed at preventing and controlling often-fatal chronic diseases. One of the first, and still largest, programs was a clinical prevention program, the National Breast and Cervical Cancer Early Detection Program, which promoted and paid for clinical screening for breast and cervical cancer for uninsured women (CDC, [e]). As of 2009, other fatal disease–oriented programs existing in all 50 states focused on diabetes and comprehensive cancer control (Collins et al., 2009). Less widespread programs focus on heart disease and stroke (Collins et al., 2009).

From the beginning, CDC has also focused on state-level programs to measure and reduce leading chronic disease risk behaviors, in particular tobacco use, physical inactivity, unhealthy eating, and obesity (Collins et al., 2009; McGinnis and Foege, 1993). As of 2009, CDC-funded programs existing in all 50 states included the Behavioral Risk Factor Surveillance System and tobacco control (Collins et al., 2009). More recently, CDC has also initiated state-level programs focused on chronic disabling diseases, and one of the largest of these, begun in 1999, focuses on arthritis. CDC initially funded smaller arthritis programs in many states, ultimately 36; however, in 2008, after an external review, CDC began funding fewer states, now 12, with a minimum of $500,000 per year (CDC, [b]). These state arthritis programs "work to increase awareness that something can be done for arthritis and promote self-management education and physical activity" (CDC, [b]).

An additional theme of the CDC programs in recent years has been a transition from state-level categorical programs aimed largely at communication and service provision to community-level integrated programs aimed more at policies and environments. This transition has accelerated with the recognition that many local GPHAs have had difficulty mounting chronic disease prevention (Frieden, 2004). The first such CDC program, Racial and Ethnic Approaches to Community Health (REACH), began in 1999 and has focused on community-level approaches to eliminating racial and ethnic disparities in chronic illnesses (CDC, [f]; Collins et al., 2009). Others that have followed include Steps, begun in 2003 and later transitioned to Healthy Communities, funding states and large and small communities to reduce fatal chronic diseases and related risk behaviors (CDC, [c]); ACHIEVE (Action Communities for Health, Innovation, and Environmental Change), begun in 2008 and focused broadly on reducing chronic diseases and risk behaviors in smaller communities (CDC, [c]); and Communities Putting Prevention to Work, begun in 2010 and focused on policy and environmental approaches to reducing obesity and tobacco use, through MAPPS (Media, Access, Point of decision information, Price, and Social support services) strategies (CDC, [a], [c]). These programs have had little or no explicit focus on arthritis or other chronic disabling diseases. An interesting new model from CDC is support for the development of workforce capacity for translating the CDC Division of Diabetes Translation (DDT) lifestyle intervention to be delivered by community organizations. This is a primary prevention initiative with CDC positioned in the role as a convener of commercial, CBO (e.g., the YMCA and others), and public health partners (diabetes prevention and control programs in 50 states) to scale the Diabetes Prevention Program (DPP) nationally. CDC funding through Emory University to run a national recognition center to publish standards for DDT delivery, data management of outcomes, and public reporting of results could motivate health payers and other third parties to offer payment to CBOs that offer the program (CDC, [d]; Diabetes Training and Technical Assistance Center, [a]).

Going forward, the Affordable Care Act (ACA) promises to further redirect the focus of GPHAs and their work on chronic diseases. The availability of near-universal health insurance may mean that GPHAs will need to focus even less on direct provision of care to the underserved. ACA-mandated coverage of clinical preventive services in health insurance should also decrease the need for GPHAs to deliver cancer screening and other preventive care. The ACA's Prevention and Public Health Fund (PPHF) is slated to provide $2 billion a year that is heavily focused on chronic disease prevention. CDC is already using the PPHF to fund its Community Transformation Grants, a new set of integrated community-level programs with a focus on policy and environmental approaches to reducing risk behaviors. Even $2 billion a year in PPHF support to GPHAs, however, is grossly inadequate for tackling fatal chronic diseases and their risk behaviors. As a comparison, the tobacco industry spends $10.5 billion a year on marketing its tobacco products (Campaign for Tobacco Free Kids, 2011).

What is known about the effectiveness of many population-focused efforts to improve outcomes for individuals with chronic illness is somewhat limited. This has been a particular barrier to galvanizing changes in the financing and alignment of public health, health care, and community efforts.

Structures that Support Population Health

The structure and function of state and local public health agencies has been documented over time by public health–related associations, such as the Association of State and Territorial Health Officials, the National Association of County and City Health Officials, the National Association of Local Boards of Health, and the American Public Health Association. The data from these various surveys enumerate the workforce, financing, activities, and general structure of public health agencies. Data related to the structure and function of state-level public health agencies in 2001 and 2007 were compared to evaluate changes in program responsibilities. New areas of practice included bioterrorism preparedness, perinatal epidemiology, toxicology, tobacco control and prevention, violence prevention, cancer and chronic disease epidemiology, and environmental epidemiology. At the same time that programs and services were increasing, funding for state public health agencies programs remained flat, with median state spending at approximately $29 per capita (Madamala et al., 2011).

The extent to which these structures effectively impact outcomes of chronic disease is less well known. Much of what public health does to impact or prevent disease is structural in nature. Interventions, such as zoning regulations, building codes, infrastructure improvements, and policies, have been designed to address such factors as physical activity, exposure to tobacco, nutrition, and environmental hazards. These types of interventions have either not been widely implemented or evaluated because of lack of understanding or interest on the part of policy makers, lack of concern on the part of the business sector, and limited collaboration between public health agencies and organizations that develop structural interventions (Katz, 2009).

Structures that are designed to assist in the evaluation of programs and interventions aimed at populations are essential to understanding which programs are of value in terms of outcomes and cost. Dilley, Bekemeier, and Harris (unpublished) completed a systematic review of the quality improvement literature related to interventions in public health. The types of quality initiatives included organization-wide efforts, program or service-related interventions, and administrative or management practice improvements. The authors concluded that the evidence for public health quality initiatives directed at improving public health practice and health-related outcomes is weak and the studies related to quality initiatives in public health contained a number of limitations, including the lack of a link to health outcomes. With the promise of a public health accreditation process (Public Health Accreditation Board) capable of reporting on a set of performance standards (National Public Health Performance Standards, [a]), the field may begin to move closer to outcome-level data at the public health organization level.

Approaches That Support Population Health

Setting priorities for population health requires a methodology for defining and measuring health status and a framework for intervention. One of the challenges for public health agencies in directing and focusing efforts has been the multiple and varied methods derived over time to create interest on the part of the public and policy makers in the economic, environmental, social, and ethical impacts of disease. An example of priority setting that could influence the focus of public health on chronic disease prevention in selected areas and the alignment of public health and health care is the CDC report *Winnable Battles* (CDC, [g]). These priority areas with associated strategies could result in large-scale impact on improving health throughout the nation. Another example of a methodology to set health priorities emerged from Wisconsin's Division of Public Health (2010). The Division of Public Health developed a four-step process to identify major health conditions, prioritize those health conditions, identify risk factors, and prioritize the risk factors. The process aligned the magnitude and severity of major health conditions with their associated risk factors. The resulting report, *Healthiest Wisconsin 2010: A Partnership Plan to Improve the Health of the Public* (2010), contains focus areas for health, including policy initiatives, collaborative partnerships, necessary public health resources and infrastructure, needed research, and the data required to track progress.

Indicators and Measurement of Population Health

Measurement of population health status has traditionally been the role of public health agencies as part of their assessment and assurance functions. The infrastructure to measure population health and the tools and methods used to gather and analyze data are well described in the literature. Surveillance in most public health agencies is a high-priority practice, as it often drives decisions about the allocation of resources and programming. However, some activities in public health are important to the health of the public but remain difficult to measure. These include the quality of services and the performance of public health agencies. Thacker and colleagues (2006) determined that beyond the current measures of mortality, morbidity, cost, and functional status are activities that, while difficult to measure, are essential to public health. The authors note when the burden of a disease or event on the population's health is substantial but the methods to measure the impact are difficult.

A recent review of the U.S. Department of Health and Human Services (HHS) national agenda for *Healthy People 2020* resulted in the renewal of a set of topics, indicators, and objectives for the nation's health. The list of leading indicators includes chronic disease, with specific objectives for reducing coronary heart disease deaths, reducing the proportion of persons in the population with hypertension, and reducing the overall cancer death rate (IOM, 2011). This determination of a set of indicators for the nation can help set a course for public health agencies focused on the prevalence and mortality of specific chronic diseases and serve to provide opportunities for public health and health care to collaborate.

Responses to Emerging Population Health Threats

The response of public health to chronic disease has been varied across the nation depending on the infrastructure, workforce, and partners available to the agency and whether they have the resources to pursue interventions at all levels of risk. Although work continues on the development of the evidence base for interventions aimed at risk factors associated with chronic disease, public health efforts to pursue the prevention of disease are complicated by the fact that they must respond at the policy and societal levels, where interventions to modify environments and laws are most effective; at the community level, where public awareness, community campaigns, and school-based and workforce interventions are most effective; and at the individual and family levels, where clinical preventive services are delivered (Halpin et al., 2010). Rare is the public health system that has the resources to address each of these levels effectively all of the time.

As policy makers have focused on the implementation of various features of the Affordable Care Act, the public health community may see this as an opportunity to refocus efforts on interventions at the population level essential to the prevention of chronic disease and reducing their role in interventions aimed at the management of chronic disease. The Affordable Care Act has some provisions for the development of programs related to healthier nutrition choices, reduction of risky behaviors, and increasing healthy behaviors (Compilation of Patient Protection and Affordable Care Act, 2010). Orza (2010) argues that health reform efforts have not focused primarily on health care but rather on those dimensions of health—personal behavior, genetics, education, economic resources, neighborhood conditions, and the global and local environment—that are dominant contributors to health status. Faced with the need to define, measure, and report to policy makers outcomes related to cost-effectiveness, public health has had a limited voice in the development of framing reform. Orza (2010) described the role of public health in the prevention of chronic disease and other diseases as "community population-based" and focused primarily on the alteration of community and environment to promote healthy lifestyles; development opportunities for screening; and, when needed, promoting self-care and disease management at home, work, and school. The author clearly distinguished between the roles of clinical prevention and community-level prevention.

Alignment Among Structures and Approaches

Aligning public health with potential and current partners, including community-based agencies, health care systems, voluntary health-related organizations, and policy-making bodies, has policy and political dimensions. To be a fully participating partner in the debate around health reform, it will take political and collective action to realize cost-effective strategies for reducing chronic disease; the transition of safety net services to the health care sector; and the strengthening of public health infrastructure to respond to the heightened needs for measurement, surveillance, and population strategies to reduce the impact and development of chronic disease. Gostin and others (2004) discussed strategies for improving the public's health from the perspective of past and current IOM reports on public health. They cite the report *The Future of the Public's Health in the 21st Century*, which describes the need to strengthen the governmental public health infrastructure, engage nongovernmental actors in partnerships for public health, and improve multiple conditions for the public's health (IOM, 2002). The authors stress that this agenda may be seen as an overreach on the part of a public health agenda that strives to link causal pathways between determinants of health and disease. These links are not well understood or researched. At the same time, waiting until definitive evidence exists before public health is assured that poor health outcomes will respond to societal changes would result in undue delay in implementing health policies directed at socioeconomic conditions.

The literature reporting efforts to structurally align public health and health care to achieve a balance among population and individually based interventions to impact chronic illness has primarily come from work in Canada. These reports described the literature on collaboration between primary care and public health, a framework for the prevention and management of chronic disease, and the structural integration of public health and primary care. Although not developed as a set of evidence-based interventions at the system level, they nevertheless point to an important direction. A report to the Canadian Health Services Research Foundation (Martin-Misener and Valaitis, 2008) reviewed existing literature on structures and processes for successful collaboration among public health and primary care, outcomes from collaboration among these two systems, and factors related to successful collaboration. Results of this review showed that collaboration between public health and primary care has grown since the 1990s, especially in Canada and the United Kingdom. The majority of the collaboration occurred in urban settings, and its purpose was primarily to improve quality and cost-effectiveness; identify community health problems through clinical practices; and improve health care through collaboration focused on policy, training, and research. *The Cochrane Database of Systematic Reviews* (Hayes et al., 2011) reported a limited number of studies with results on the impact of local partnerships on health. Almost all of the 11 comparative studies reviewed had methodological problems, and none showed evidence of improvement in health outcomes due to collaboration among governmental and health agencies.

The Canadian Ministry of Health and Long-Term Care's Ontario Framework (2007) is based on the Chronic Care Model and the Expanded Chronic Care Model described earlier in this chapter. The framework brings together efforts around developing individual skills necessary for health, the reorientation of health services to a stronger focus on prevention and health promotion, the development of public policy that promotes health and prevents disease, the creation of environments that support health, and extra strength to community action. These are common themes in the majority of the literature that call for a stronger focus on prevention and management of chronic disease.

Rowan et al. (2007) report some evidence suggesting that models that integrate primary care and public health have successfully addressed individual and community-based approaches to influence population health. The prominent link among these systems is through data and surveillance systems poised to detect health events and changes in a variety of determinants of health and to rapidly communicate health information across sectors. The models ranged in development and focus from planning to integrate to fully integrating and evaluating basic chronic disease prevention into primary care settings. The models reviewed in the report were primarily outside the United States except for the Community-Oriented Primary Care (COPC) model. Iliffe and Lenihan (2003) reviewed COPC efforts to combine a primary care and a public health perspective in delivering care to communities. Much of the experience of COPC has been with an underserved population through targeting high-priority services to a select population. The results of this review revealed that participation on the part of community organizations has not been highly active or influential in developing the COPC targeted programs. The efforts have largely been through action in the health care sector. This is particularly true in examples in studies of COPC programs in North America. The major criticism related to efforts in the United States to align public health and primary care is that they were focused on balancing responsibilities between medical care and public health rather than true alignment (Iliffe and Lenihan, 2003).

Although the literature supports new models and approaches to the prevention and management of chronic disease, much of it is not specific to chronic disease, and few of the models have been tested. A few emerging community-based models of care for people with multiple chronic conditions (MCCs) is described in this report (see Appendix B).

HEALTH CARE SYSTEM APPROACHES

The health care system has not benefited from or pursued in a comprehensive way incentives to align with public health and community-based organizations in developing approaches and structures for the prevention and management of chronic disease. Given what is known about the contribution of nondisease determinants to health and disease, one would expect a comprehensive system of primary and tertiary care interacting continually with the community, social, and physical environments and the public policy structure in seeking improved access, quality, and cost-effectiveness in the care and prevention of chronic disease. Instead, the current approach is often fragmented, costly, inefficient, difficult to access, and, at times, of poor quality. This has been documented extensively in the IOM Quality Chasm series (2000–2007), an 11-report series that includes *Crossing the Quality Chasm: A New Health System for the 21st Century* (IOM, 2001) and such workshops as *The Healthcare Imperative: Lowering Costs and Improving Outcomes: Workshop Series Summary* (IOM, 2010). One of the messages in *Crossing the Quality Chasm* is that "the goals of any payment method should be to reward high-quality care and to permit the development of more effective ways of delivering care to improve the value obtained for the resources expended" (IOM, 2001).

System Design

The design of health care systems can have tremendous impact on the costs and quality of care of persons living with chronic illness. The current health care system in the United States was designed to address acute disease rather than chronic disease. Health care systems are currently organized to respond to patients' acute illnesses by relying primarily on patients to contact the health care system when they have a health problem or concern and on physicians to provide curative treatment with little or no patient participation in the process. Clearly these features are not supportive of the type of care needed for most chronic diseases.

The quality of care of chronic diseases could be improved if health systems were designed on the basis of the characteristics and needs of patients with chronic illnesses (Canadian Ministry of Health and Long-Term Care,

2007). The Ontario Framework emphasizes that "a more responsive approach to chronic disease would recognize that chronic disease:

- Is ongoing, and therefore warrants pro-active, planned, integrated care within a system that clients can easily navigate;
- Involves clients living indefinitely with the [illness] and symptoms, requiring those persons be active partners in managing their condition, rather than passive recipients of care;
- Requires multi-faceted care which calls for clinicians and nonclinicians from multiple disciplines to work closely together, to meet the wide range of needs of the chronically ill; and
- Can be prevented and therefore warrants health promotion and disease prevention strategies targeted to the whole population, especially those at high risk for chronic [illness]."

It should also be noted that individuals with chronic illness may have complications that can be prevented, and they are therefore able to live well with the support of health care, public health, community engagement, and self-management strategies. Considerable evidence already exists about ways to prevent chronic illnesses and to manage the care of those who already have them. As described earlier in this chapter, most of these programs and policies are based on components of the Chronic Care Model, which summarizes the basic elements for improving care in health systems at the community, organization, practice, and patient levels.

Ensure Access to Affordable Health Care

Fundamental to the implementation of the Chronic Care Model is having a health care system that is designed to provide access to affordable care for all persons with chronic illnesses. According to a 2010 survey by the Commonwealth Fund (Collins et al., 2011), an estimated 52 million adults in America were uninsured at some point during 2010, up from 38 million in 2001. The prevalence of chronic illness is likely to be higher among those without insurance, especially since adults in families with low and moderate incomes are the most likely to be uninsured. In the 2010 survey, 54 percent of low-income adults (under $22,050 for a family of four) and 41 percent of moderate-income adults ($22,050 to $44,100 for a family of four) were uninsured for some time during the year, compared with 13 percent of adults with higher incomes.

Incentives to Improve Prevention and Control

Regardless of the design of a health care system, chronic disease prevention and control will not be routinely implemented across different settings unless all stakeholders have incentives to implement disease prevention and care. The challenge for policy makers is to understand the context in which care is being provided, identify key stakeholders, and determine what would motivate them to implement widespread disease prevention and coordinated care and then develop systems that provide those incentives (Singh, 2008).

One of the most fundamental aspects of the design of the health care system is how providers of chronic disease care are reimbursed for their services. Traditionally, there have been three ways to pay physicians and other health care professionals by either insurers or governments (e.g., Medicare, Medicaid): fee-for-service, capitation, and salary. All three have been used to pay providers at different levels in health care systems for the management of people with chronic illnesses, among other things. However, according to Busse and Mays (2008), none of these methods fully connects financial incentives to the overarching goal of quality care for patients with chronic illnesses, generating different perverse incentives for patient care.

Fee-for-service involves paying providers or health systems for the actual volume of services provided. This type of payment system is common in the United States and is an incentive to provide more care to more patients with chronic illnesses, since more care provides more income. Few incentives exist to prevent chronic diseases, and there is a potential for overuse of services. Nevertheless, patients with complex MCCs are embraced in a fee-for-service system.

Capitation systems, such as health maintenance organizations (HMOs), pay providers or health systems a fixed amount for a specified time period, regardless of the amount of services provided. Therefore, the incentives are to provide as little care as possible to patients with chronic illness, leading to a possible underuse of services. By providing incentives for delivery of less care, capitation also encourages health payers and providers to select healthier patients and exclude those with complex MCCs, who inherently require higher levels of health care. Some of these incentives may be modified in settings with multiple competing health systems, in which patients can choose to enroll with other providers (Busse and Mays, 2008) and providers have incentives to provide high-quality care in order to retain patients and income.

Providers working for a salary are guaranteed a specified income for a period of time, regardless of the amount of care provided to patients. Similarly, health systems, such as hospitals, may be provided a fixed budget to provide care to a defined population, such as the Veterans Administration or Indian Health Service hospitals. As a result, unlike fee-for-service and capitation payment systems, there are fewer incentives to over- or under-provide care to persons with chronic illnesses.

Pay-for-performance (P4P) is another alternative reimbursement strategy that attempts to address some of the limitations of fee-for-service models by shifting payment from one based solely on the quantity of services to one that is intended to reward quality or efficiency of care (Epstein, 2007). Over the past decade, P4P has been used increasingly in private health plans, as well as by the Centers for Medicare and Medicaid Services (CMS) (Guterman and Serber, 2007; Rosenthal et al., 2006). Most P4P designs have rewarded clinically high-quality care by an individual physician provider based on his or her ability to complete a relatively well-defined process of care (e.g., testing of HbA1c) on a predetermined minimum percentage (e.g., 70 percent) of that provider's own patients who meet criteria for having the process performed (e.g., diagnosed diabetes). Although not typically the focus, P4P could be used in an analogous fashion to reward care coordination, the collective care quality offered by a team of caregivers, or other innovations in chronic care delivery to achieve better outcomes of care.

Although promising conceptually, evaluation of the success of P4P used in isolation has yielded mixed results, making it clear that it is not a panacea for addressing the challenges of other payment designs. Findings of these studies suggest that P4P systems have the potential to provide incentives for the adoption of new behaviors by physicians, but that changes may be short-lived or decay as soon as the incentive is removed or reduced (Peterson et al., 2006; Scott et al., 2011). Also, payment for a clinical process of care, such as testing of HbA1c for patients with diabetes, can potentially increase the process without significant improvements in health outcomes (Scott et al., 2011). Another potential limitation is that P4P, in isolation, could lead some providers to avoid offering care to more challenging patient populations, who may be perceived to have barriers to completing visits or tests (Peterson et al., 2006). One strategy proposed to offset some of these limitations is to design blended payment systems that combine P4P with one or more forms of base payment, which are typically considered an advanced form of capitation (Davis, 2007; Miller, 2007). Conceptually, this works best if the capitation payment is risk-based, which essentially means that the reimbursement is adjusted for each patient's own complexity, which is determined by recent diagnoses, procedures, or pharmaceutical management. In other words, providers are paid more to manage complex patients than they are to manage healthy ones, and additional payments are added if the provider or care team is able to achieve beneficial processes of care or outcomes for some minimum percentage of all patients they serve. In theory, a blended payment scheme can avoid the limitations of capitation and P4P used in isolation and, if designed appropriately, can improve the delivery of evidence-based services and beneficial health outcomes. Although potentially promising, such strategies need to be subject to further evaluation before it is known whether they will prove feasible to implement and offer better outcomes for patients living with chronic illnesses.

Realigning Traditional Incentives

On October 20, 2011, the Centers for Medicare and Medicaid Services finalized new rules under the Affordable Care Act to help health care providers better manage care for Medicare patients through accountable care organizations (ACOs). Participation in an ACO is purely voluntary. ACOs produce incentives for health care providers to collaborate in treatment for an individual patient across multiple care settings that include doctors' offices, hospitals, and long-term care facilities. The Medicare Shared Savings Program will reward ACOs that minimize growth in health care costs while reaching performance standards on quality of care and making patients come first (CMS, 2011b).

The Affordable Care Act states that ACOs agree to be held accountable for three aims (IHI Triple Aim): (1) improving the experience of care for individuals, (2) reducing the rate of growth in health care spending, and (3) improving the health of populations. The final rule would set quality performance measures and a methodology for connecting quality and financial performance that will set high standards for delivering coordinated and patient-centered care by ACOs and stress continuous improvement regarding the better care for individuals, better health for populations, and lower growth in health care expenses (CMS, 2011b).

According to CMS, the final rule mandates that ACOs practice procedures and processes that promote evidence-based medicine and beneficiary engagement in their care, report quality measures to CMS with prompt feedback to providers, and invest continually in the workforce and team-oriented care. To guarantee better transparency, the final rule would further mandate ACOs to publicly report particular aspects of their program performance and operations (CMS, 2011b).

It is too early to determine the impact of the Affordable Care Act on the costs and quality of health care and on overall population health. Recent evidence from the Physician Group Practice Demonstration shows that there can be success in a pay-for-performance concept when it comes to improving the quality of care, coordinating services, and saving money in Medicare (CMS, 2011a). The 10 physician groups taking part in the demonstration project set out in 2005 to see if they could meet 32 performance measures and save money, which would earn them incentive payments. The performance measures tied to quality were phased in over 5 years.

By the 5th year of the demonstration, 7 of the 10 physician groups hit all 32 of the performance measures, and the other 3 groups made 30 of the 32 performance measures (CMS, 2011a). All 10 physician groups achieved benchmark performance on heart failure, coronary artery, and preventive care measures. Over the 5 years of the demonstration, the physician groups also increased their quality scores for chronic disease control for diabetes measures, heart failure, coronary artery disease, cancer screening, and hypertension. Each of the groups received incentive payments for both the savings they achieved for the Medicare program as well as quality improvements that have resulted in not only better health but also a better experience of care for patients (CMS, 2011a).

In contrast to these promising findings, some analysts suggest that, in the current environment, ACOs will have serious challenges to overcome, including concern about the economics and complexity of the final rule. Others are concerned about the downside risk, the financial penalties that teams of providers would face if they exceed spending targets set for them under the program (CMS, 2011b). In addition, since some health care providers earn more by increasing the volume of the services they provide, they may not see possible shared savings as enough to offset the revenue they would lose from the reduced use of their services. In addition, solo practitioners and small physician groups may lack the data systems and organizational structures needed to form ACOs.

Pay for Better Health Outcomes

Some have stated that rewarding health systems for better care and better clinical outcomes will not lead to significant improvements in overall population health (Kindig, 2006). Instead, systems could be designed to reward improvements in the overall health of entire populations. Such a "pay-for-population health performance" system would apply financial incentives to health outcomes that result from various sectors and agents working mostly separate from one another (Kindig, 2006). Kindig (2006) has suggested the formation of health outcome trusts, "a metaphor for local public-private partnerships with market-based incentives to integrate resources across determinants for better health outcomes."

Significant challenges must be met before such a population health improvement system could be implemented to improve the care for patients with chronic illnesses. There is no consensus on how to measure population health and its improvement. Despite success in developing financial incentives in the more defined settings (e.g., health care, education), it has not been determined how diverse systems could be integrated to coordinate the costs for population health investments and potential savings (Kindig, 2006).

THE COMMUNITY-BASED AND NON–HEALTH CARE SECTOR

The organizations in the community-based and non–health care sector include many volunteer organizations, such as the American Heart Association, the American Cancer Society, the Arthritis Foundation, the American Diabetes Association, and the American Lung Association; the community-level organizations that address the social, behavioral, and environmental aspects of people's lives also contribute to the prevention and treatment of chronic disease. These organizations can serve as important partners in providing prevention programs and policy advocacy.

Most clinical programs are developed with the focus on diagnosis and treatment in acute care settings, such as hospitals and ambulatory care settings (primary care practices or doctors' offices). This development has two implications. First, people are living longer with chronic illnesses and have better quality of life and functional capacity. Second, and probably more importantly, the concepts of self-care and self-management have become the hallmark of managing chronic illnesses (Bodenheimer et al., 2002). The consequences of these implications lead to the fact that people living with chronic illnesses now spend a significant amount of their time managing their own care with just a minuscule amount of time being spent at the hospital or in ambulatory care settings. If the gains in medical knowledge and advancement in the diagnosis and treatment of chronic illnesses are to be realized, then programs targeted at improving the care of people living with chronic illnesses must be implemented at community sites where they spend most of their time, without the burden of frequent office visits or trips to the hospital. This strategy is at the heart of translating evidence to practice (Westfall et al., 2007), and it provides sound rationale for implementation of public health interventions in community sites.

Approaches for Public Health Interventions in Community Sites

Community sites where people living with chronic illnesses spend most of their time include home, worksites, schools (children and teachers), faith-based organizations/settings, community-based organizations, and senior centers and assisted living arrangements (in case of the elderly). Recently, faith-based organizations have begun to play an increasing role in facilitating health care delivery via use of community/lay health workers (Duru et al., 2010; Faridi et al., 2010; Resnicow et al., 2001; Samuel-Hodge et al., 2009), and community-based organizations frequently serve as conduits linking persons living with chronic illnesses to health care in terms of access, and occasionally they may provide some lifestyle interventions (Perez et al., 2006). Others include public housing sites and community-based facilities such as the YMCA. By far the most evidence for wellness programs has been reported on worksites (Aldana et al., 2005; Anderson et al., 2009; Benedict and Arterburn, 2008; Burton and Connerty, 1998; Conn et al., 2009; Ni Mhurchu et al., 2010).

Worksites

For the purposes of this report, worksites are defined as places of work, regardless of type of employment. Because most adults spend many hours at work each week, worksites are ideal places to engage employees in programs targeted at improving lifestyle behaviors. Worksite wellness programs have grown tremendously in the past decade alone, and there is every indication for this trend to continue given its popularity not only with governmental agencies but also with a diverse set of employers and insurers. It should be noted that the worksite wellness programs discussed here are funded primarily by large employers, many of whom are self-insured. There is very limited data from small employers or businesses. The focus of worksite wellness programs is often improvement in lifestyle behaviors, including increasing levels of physical activity (Conn et al., 2009), adopting healthier diets (Ni Mhurchu et al., 2010), and engaging in self-management lifestyle behaviors, stress management, and smoking cessation. Evaluation of the effectiveness of these programs in several systematic reviews and meta-analyses suggests a robust and significant effect on improvement of targeted lifestyle behaviors (diet, weight loss, and physical activity) without focus on quality of life or other important health outcomes (Anderson et al., 2009; Ni Mhurchu et al., 2010). Recent examples of the implementation of programs targeted at reducing health risks in worksites include CDC's Steps Program, which is focused on helping worksites improve employee health. The CDC's Steps Program, currently in 40 U.S. communities, is targeted at reducing the burden of obesity and diabetes via improvement in three related health risk factors: physical inactivity, poor nutrition, and tobacco use and exposure. Some examples of the Steps Program include improving obesity management and reducing health care costs through worksite wellness programs; promoting healthy behaviors among school employees; and providing transit employees' access to exercise facilities, healthy foods, and health assessments to help them manage their weight (CDC, 2008).

The majority of the worksite programs did not target any particular illness, but a few of them evaluated the effect of wellness programs on cardiovascular risk reduction (Maron et al., 2008; Milani and Lavie, 2009; Racette et al., 2009). In a worksite study of Vanderbilt University employees with cardiovascular risk factors, a health risk appraisal (HRA) with disease management for worksite cardiovascular risk reduction was more effective in reducing cardiovascular risk scores in those who received an HRA without disease management (Maron et al., 2008). Another well-designed trial evaluated the efficacy and cost-effectiveness of a 6-month worksite health intervention consisting of health education, nutritional counseling, smoking cessation counseling, physical activity promotion, and selected physician referral versus usual care among 308 employees. Health risk status was determined at baseline and after the intervention program, and total medical claim costs were calculated for all participants during the year before and after intervention. Significant improvement was found in quality-of-life scores, body fat, high-density lipoprotein cholesterol, diastolic blood pressure, health habits, and total health risk. Of employees identified as high risk at baseline, more than half of them were downgraded to low-risk status, and the average employee annual claim costs decreased by almost half for the year after the intervention whereas control employees' costs stayed the same (Milani and Lavie, 2009).

There is very scant evidence of worksite programs targeted at people living with chronic illnesses, such as diabetes and arthritis. Although the feasibility of the Diabetes Prevention Program has been evaluated in a pre-post design (Aldana et al., 2005; Diabetes Prevention Program Group, 2002), there is limited evidence from well-controlled studies of its implementation in worksites. The only evidence of such programs was a large quasi-experimental study of an employer-sponsored Internet-based nutrition program for employees with cardiovascular risk factors, including diabetes (Sacks et al., 2009). In both programs, the interventions led to significant improvement in cardiovascular risk reduction and diabetes outcomes.

YMCA

The YMCA is one of the largest not-for-profit community service organizations in the nation, serving thousands of communities. Through its health and well-being programs, the YMCA plays a significant role in health promotion and chronic disease prevention. The largest program at the YMCA to date is the CDC's Pioneering Healthier Communities (PHC) program, which was created in collaboration with the YMCA to convene representatives from local government and the public health and private sectors. The focus of PHC is on changing the environment in a way that reduces community barriers for healthy living. Similar to worksite wellness programs, its effects on the quality of life and important health outcomes of people living with chronic illness are largely untested.

Faith-Based Organizations

There is growing evidence that wellness programs targeted at lifestyle behaviors in faith-based organizations are effective in improving weight loss and increasing intake of fruits and vegetable and levels of physical activity (Duru et al., 2010; Resnicow et al., 2001; Rucker-Whitaker et al., 2007), particularly for African Americans, given the central role that churches play in the lives of many. However, similar to worksite wellness programs, few of these interventions, often delivered by community health workers, target people living with chronic illness, such as diabetes and arthritis (Samuel-Hodge et al., 2009). One such program is the PREDICT project, which evaluated the effectiveness of a culturally appropriate, church-based diabetes self-management program among about 200 congregants with diabetes in 24 African American churches. At the end of the primary outcome assessment at 8 months, participants who were randomized to the intervention, consisting of 1 individual counseling visit, 12 group sessions, and monthly phone contacts, had lower HbA1c and higher diabetes knowledge and quality of life compared to those in the usual care who received standard educational pamphlets by mail (Samuel-Hodge et al., 2009).

Senior Centers

Similar to other community sites, the feasibility of interventions targeted at lifestyle behaviors among the physically active elderly in senior centers is well proven (Fernandez et al., 2008; Sarkisian et al., 2007). In recent years, multipurpose senior centers have proliferated across the country and constitute a source for community-based social, medical, geriatric programs to help older Americans retain their independence and a high quality of life. Some initiatives and programs include health and wellness education, including health screenings; senior fitness programs; outreach services, providing an array of services like transportation; meals and nutrition services; employment counseling; social networking opportunities; case management services; legal services; volunteer opportunities; and access to providers to render primary care services. However, the effectiveness of these programs on seniors living with chronic illnesses remains largely untested.

Community Health Centers

Community health centers have been the source of primary and mental health care for underserved communities since the 1970s. HHS (Hing and Hooker, 2011) reported that community health centers average 31.1 million visits annually, and the majority of these are by people who are poor or insured through public programs (Medicaid, State Children's Health Insurance Program). It is also of note that 21 percent of these health care visits are to nurse practitioners working in community health centers. Although nurse practitioners tend to see younger patients, nurse practitioners saw 39 percent of the patients with one or more chronic illnesses (Hing and Hooker, 2011).

Voluntary Health Agencies

Voluntary health agencies play a vital role in the prevention and treatment of chronic disease. These agencies tend to focus on a specific disease or group of diseases and contribute to prevention, management, and treatment in a variety of ways:

- Providing services to individuals and families affected by chronic illnesses
- Funding scientific research and promulgating scientific guidelines
- Educating professionals and the public
- Supporting quality improvement programs
- Advocating for laws, policies, and regulations that impact individuals and their families living with a particular illness

Thousands of voluntary health agencies exist in the United States. Table 6-1 describes the mission and a sample of the activities of just three voluntary health agencies: the American Cancer Society, the American Heart Association, and the Arthritis Foundation.

TABLE 6-1 Three Voluntary Health Agencies

Agency	Year Est.	Mission	Activities
American Cancer Society	1913	To eliminate "cancer as a major health problem by preventing cancer, saving lives, and diminishing suffering from cancer through research, education, advocacy, and service"	• Choose You, an initiative that encourages women to eat right, get active, quit smoking, and get regular health checks to fight cancer • Generation Fit, a program that promotes more physical activity and healthier eating for children between ages 11 and 18 • Meeting Well, a tool that helps companies organize healthy meetings and events • Cancer Survivors Network, a network that offers support to cancer survivors

TABLE 6-1 Continued

Agency	Year Est.	Mission	Activities
			• Cancer Prevention Study-3 (CPS-3), a prospective study of 300,000 people that aims to understand cancer prevention • American Cancer Society Cancer Action Network (ACS CAN), a cancer advocacy network
American Heart Association	1924	To "build healthier lives, free of cardiovascular diseases and stroke"	• Go Red for Women, an initiative designed to raise awareness about the impact of heart disease on women • Start! Movement, an initiative that promotes walking for a healthier lifestyle • Heart 360, an internet tool that gives people the ability to track their weight, physical activity, cholesterol, blood pressure, and other factors that contribute to heart health • Get With the Guidelines, a program to ensure consistent application of American Heart Association/American Stroke Association scientific guidelines in the in-patient setting • You're the Cure, a cardiovascular disease and stroke advocacy network
Arthritis Foundation	1948	To "improve lives through leadership in prevention, control and cure of arthritis and related diseases"	• Let's Move Together, a program that promotes physical activity to prevent and minimize arthritis problems • Arthritis Today, a magazine focused on issues related to arthritis • Arthritis Internet Registry, a study in which people with arthritis fill out questionnaires to advance arthritis science • Osteoarthritis, rheumatoid arthritis, and juvenile arthritis research

CONCLUSION

Patients spend a relatively minuscule amount of time at their physician's office; most time is spent at work and community-based settings like the YMCA, Senior Centers, faith-based organizations, and other recreation settings. This makes implementation of lifestyle interventions in these settings appealing especially given the proven efficacy of these interventions. These interventions mitigate the impact of chronic diseases on health outcomes for people living with chronic illnesses. Most of the literature related to population-based approaches to health improvement are not specifically focused on chronic disease and are limited in their evidence that these efforts produce the desired outcomes.

Although numerous studies have evaluated the impact of worksite wellness programs and lifestyle interventions on health outcomes, the efficacy of these studies is mixed and largely targeted at healthy employees, with only a handful of studies focused on people living with chronic illnesses. The few worksite programs that targeted people living with chronic illnesses were of short duration and small effect sizes. Also, the sustainability of worksite programs was not evaluated in these studies. Effective programs include those that targeted healthful behaviors rather than important health outcomes such as cardiovascular risk reduction or pain management.

Similarly, the literature reviewed on community-based programs reveals three important issues. First, there is ample evidence that wellness programs, like lifestyle interventions, are widely disseminated in community sites without adequate evaluation of their effect on quality of life and important health outcomes in persons living with chronic illnesses. Despite the scanty evidence that the interventions are targeted at people living with chronic illnesses, the implementation foundation for these programs does exist as reviewed in this chapter with regards to the YMCA, worksites, and faith-based organizations, especially when implemented by community health workers. For example, the YMCA has existing programs to target lifestyle interventions for cancer survivors, and it is increasingly involved with development of programs for other aging conditions such as arthritis. Given the above, there is a crucial need to utilize community sites as implementation platforms for interventions targeted at improving quality of life and other important health outcomes in people living with chronic illnesses. Second, there are little or no data on cost-effectiveness of health improvement programs at community sites other than worksites. Community-based programs tend to be sponsored by various stakeholders, which makes it difficult to assess their cost-effectiveness. Finally, reimbursement issues are also less well addressed, including the need for clarification regarding sponsors of community-based care. In addition, models to align population based public health interventions with health care are largely untested. The type of payment system can have a significant effect on the effectiveness of chronic disease prevention and control services in health care systems. Regardless of the type of payment system, however, few systems provide incentives for chronic disease prevention or improvements in the health outcomes in patients with chronic illnesses. For example, memberships for YMCA clubs or other exercise facilities may be steep for some segments of the population, making generalizability of wellness programs at such sites difficult to interpret.

There is a huge potential to leverage the infrastructure of wellness worksite programs and community-based sites like the YMCA and senior centers with regard to implementation of effective interventions and their sustainability. These organizations can serve as sites for community health workers to deliver evidence-based self-management interventions targeted at people living with chronic illnesses. In the context of the Frieden pyramid of the factors that affect health, ready access to community-based organizations equipped with well-trained staff that can counsel and educate people living with chronic illnesses on recommended lifestyle changes and self-management interventions would certainly yield a far greater public health impact than the individual approaches in health care settings would. Such effort would of course require an efficient delivery of information between health care and non–health care entities and an appropriate reimbursement incentive, which can potentially be incorporated into the patient-centered medical home model. This could motivate health payers and other third parties to offer payment to those community-based organizations that offer the program.

The discussion in this chapter continues to address the statement of task question presented in Chapter 4, specifically, which population-based interventions can help achieve outcomes that maintain or improve quality of life, functioning, and disability?

- What is the evidence on effectiveness of interventions on these outcomes?
- To what extent do the interventions that address these outcomes also affect clinical outcomes?
- To what extent can policy, environmental, and systems change achieve these outcomes?

RECOMMENDATIONS 13–15

The committee provides three recommendations.

Recommendation 13

The committee recommends that HHS agencies and state and local government public health agencies (GPHAs) evaluate existing (e.g., chronic care model, expanded chronic care model), emerging and/or new models of chronic disease care that promote collaboration among community-based organizations, the health care delivery system, employers and businesses, the media, and the academic community to improve living well with chronic illness.

- CDC and state and local GPHAs should serve convening and facilitating functions for developing and implementing emerging models.
- HHS agencies (e.g., the Health Resources and Services Administration, the Centers for Medicare and Medicaid Services, the Administration on Aging, CDC) and GPHAs should fund demonstration projects and evaluate these emerging models.
- Federal, private, and other payors should create new financing streams and incentives that support maintaining and disseminating emerging models that effectively address persons living well with chronic illness.

Recommendation 14

The committee recommends that CDC develop and promote, in partnership with organizations representing health care, public health, and patient advocacy, a set of evidenced-based policy goals and objectives specifically aimed at actions that decrease the burden of suffering and improve the quality of life of persons living with chronic illness.

Recommendation 15

The committee recommends that federal and state policy makers develop and implement pilot incentives programs for all employers, particularly low-wage employers, small businesses, and community-based organizations, to provide health promotion programs with known effectiveness for those living with chronic illness.

REFERENCES

Aldana, S.G., M. Barlow, R. Smith, F.G. Yanowitz, T. Adams, L. Loveday, J. Arbuckle, and M.J. LaMonte. 2005. The diabetes prevention program: A worksite experience. *Journal of the American Association of Occupational Health Nurses* 53(11):499–505; quiz 506–507.

Anderson, L.M., T.A. Quinn, K. Glanz, G. Ramirez, L.C. Kahwati, D.B. Johnson, L.R. Buchanan, W.R. Archer, S. Chattopadhyay, G.P. Kalra, D.L. Katz, and Task Force on Community Preventive Services. 2009. The effectiveness of worksite nutrition and physical activity interventions for controlling employee overweight and obesity: A systematic review. *American Journal of Preventive Medicine* 37(4):340–357.

Benedict, M.A., and D. Arterburn. 2008. Worksite-based weight loss programs: A systematic review of recent literature. *American Journal of Health Promotion* 22(6):408–416.

Bodenheimer, T., K. Lorig, H. Holman, and K. Grumbach. 2002. Patient self-management of chronic disease in primary care. *Journal of the American Medical Association* 288(19): 2469–2475.

Burton, W.N., and C.M. Connerty. 1998. Evaluation of a worksite-based patient education intervention targeted at employees with diabetes mellitus. *Journal of Occupational and Environmental Medicine* 40(8):702–706.

Busse, R., and N. Mays. 2008. Paying for chronic disease care. In *Caring for People with Chronic Conditions: A Health System Perspective*. Edited by E. Nolte and M. McKee. New York: Open University Press. Pp. 195–221.

Campaign for Tobacco-Free Kids. 2011. *Toll of Tobacco in the United States of America*. http://www.tobaccofreekids.org/research/factsheets/pdf/0072.pdf (accessed June 29, 2011).

Canadian Ministry of Health and Long-Term Care. 2007. *Preventing and Managing Chronic Disease: The Ontario Framework*. http://www.health.gov.on.ca/english/providers/program/cdpm/pdf/ framework_full.pdf (accessed October 6, 2011).

CDC (Centers for Disease Control and Prevention) (a). *CDC, Chronic Disease Prevention and Health Promotion, The American Recovery and Reinvestment Act*. http://www.cdc.gov/chronicdisease/recovery/ (accessed October 3, 2011).

CDC (b). *CDC's Arthritis Program History*. http://www.cdc.gov/arthritis/state_programs.htm (accessed June 28, 2011).

CDC (c). *CDC's Healthy Communities Program*. http://www.cdc.gov/healthycommunities program/communities/achieve/index.htm (accessed June 29, 2011).

CDC (d). *Diabetes Public Health Resource. About CDC's Division of Diabetes Translation*. http://www.cdc.gov/diabetes/about/index.htm (accessed September 21, 2011).

CDC (e). *National Breast and Cervical Cancer Early Detection Program (NBCCEDP)*. http://www.cdc.gov/cancer/NBCCEDP/ (accessed October 3, 2011).

CDC (f). *Racial and Ethnic Approaches to Community Health (REACH)*. http://www.cdc.gov/reach/about.htm (accessed October 3, 2011).

CDC (g). *Winnable Battles*. http://www.cdc.gov/winnablebattles/ (accessed July 4, 2011).

CDC. 2008. *The Steps Program in Action: Success Stories on Community Initiatives to Prevent Chronic Diseases*. Atlanta: U.S. Department of Health and Human Services. http://www.cdc.gov/steps/success_stories/pdf/SuccessStories.pdf (accessed October 11, 2011).

CMS (Centers for Medicare and Medicaid Services). 2011a. *Medicare Physician Group Practice Demonstration. Physician Groups Continue to Improve Quality and Generate Savings Under Medicare Physician Pay-for-Performance Demonstration*. Baltimore, MD. https://www.cms.gov/DemoProjectsEvalRpts/downloads/PGP_Fact_Sheet.pdf (accessed October 11, 2011).

CMS. 2011b. *Summary of Final Rule Provisions for Accountable Care Organizations Under the Medicare Shared Savings Program.* Baltimore, MD: Centers for Medicare and Medicaid Services. https://www.cms.gov/MLNProducts/downloads/ACO_Summary_Factsheet_ICN907404.pdf (accessed December 2, 2011).

Collins, J.L., J.S. Marks, and J.P. Koplan. 2009. Chronic disease prevention and control: Coming of age at the Centers for Disease Control and Prevention. *Preventing Chronic Disease: Public Health Research, Practice, and Policy* 6(3):A81. http://www.cdc.gov/pcd/issues/2009/jul/08_0171.htm (accessed June 27, 2011).

Collins, S.R., M.M. Doty, R. Robertson, and T. Garber. 2011. Help on the horizon: How the recession has left millions of workers without health insurance, and how health reform will bring relief. Findings from The Commonwealth Fund Biennial Health Insurance Survey of 2010. *The Commonwealth Fund.* http://www.commonwealthfund. org/~/media/Files/Publications/Fund%20Report/2011/Mar/1486_Collins_help_on_the_horizon_2010_biennial_survey_report_FINAL_v2.pdf (accessed October 10, 2011).

Compilation of Patient Protection and Affordable Care Act. As amended through May 1, 2010. 111th Cong., 2nd sess.

Conn, V.S., A.R. Hafdahl, P.S. Cooper, L.M. Brown, and S.L. Lusk. 2009. Meta-analysis of workplace physical activity interventions. *American Journal of Preventive Medicine* 37(4):330–339.

Davis, K. 2007. Paying for care episodes and care coordination. *New England Journal of Medicine* 356(11):1166–1168.

Diabetes Prevention Program Group. 2002. Reduction in the incidence of type 2 diabetes with lifestyle intervention or metformin. *New England Journal of Medicine* 346(6):393–403.

Diabetes Training and Technical Assistance Center (a). *CDC-Division of Diabetes Translation (DDT) Resource Archive.* http://www.dttac.org/resources/diabetes_translation.html (accessed September 7, 2011).

Dilley, J., B. Bekemeier, and J. Harris. (Unpublished). A Systematic Review of the Literature Describing Quality Improvement Interventions in Public Health Systems: Efforts to Connect the Dots Between Improving Public Health Practice and Improving Health.

Duru, O.K., C.A. Sarkisian, M. Leng, and C.M. Mangione. 2010. Sisters in motion: A randomized controlled trial of a faith-based physical activity intervention. *Journal of the American Geriatrics Society* 58(10):1863–1869.

Epstein, A.M. 2007. Pay for performance at the tipping point. *New England Journal of Medicine* 356:515–517.

Faridi, Z., K. Shuval, V.Y. Njike, J.A. Katz, G. Jennings, M. Williams, D.L. Katz, and PREDICT Project Working Group. 2010. Partners reducing effects of diabetes (PREDICT): A diabetes prevention physical activity and dietary intervention through African-American churches. *Health Education Research* 25(2):306–315.

Fernandez, S., K.L. Scales, J.M. Pineiro, A.M. Schoenthaler, and G. Ogedegbe. 2008. A senior center-based pilot trial of the effect of lifestyle intervention on blood pressure in minority elderly people with hypertension. *Journal of the American Geriatrics Society* 56(10):1860–1866.

Frieden, T.R. 2004. Asleep at the switch: Local public health and chronic disease. *American Journal of Public Health* 94(12):2059–2061.

Gostin, L.O., J.I. Boufford, and R.M. Martinez. 2004. The future of the public's health: Vision, values, and strategies. *Health Affairs* 23(4):96–107.

Guterman, S., and M.P. Serber. 2007. *Enhancing value in Medicare: Demonstrations and Other Initiatives to Improve the Program.* New York: The Commonwealth Fund. http://www.commonwealthfund.org/~/media/Files/Publications/Fund%20Report/2007/Feb/Enhancing%20Value%20in%20Medicare%20%20Demonstrations%20and%20Other%20Initiatives%20to%20Improve%20the%20Program/990_Guterman_enhancing_value_Medicare%20pdf.pdf (accessed October 10, 2011).

Halpin, H.A., M.M. Morales-Suárez-Varela, and J.M. Martin-Moreno. 2010. Chronic disease prevention and the new public health. *Public Health Reviews* 32(1):120–154.

Hayes, S.L., M.K. Mann, F.M. Morgan, H. Kitcher, M.J. Kelly, and A.L. Weightman. 2011. Collaboration between local health and local government agencies for health improvement (Review). *Cochrane Database of Systematic Reviews* 6.

Hing, E., and R.S. Hooker. 2011. *Community health centers: Providers, patients, and content of care*, NCHS data brief, no 65. Hyattsville, MD: National Center for Health Statistics. http://www.cdc.gov/nchs/data/databriefs/db65.pdf (accessed October 12, 2011).

Iliffe, S., and P. Lenihan. 2003. Integrating primary care and public health: Learning from the community-oriented primary care model. *International Journal of Health Services* 33(1):85–98.

IOM (Institute of Medicine). 1988. *The Future of Public Health*. Washington, DC: National Academy Press.

IOM. 2001. *Crossing the Quality Chasm: A New Health System for the 21st Century*. Washington, DC: National Academy Press.

IOM. 2002. *The Future of the Public's Health in the 21st Century*. Washington, DC: The National Academies Press.

IOM. 2010. *The Healthcare Imperative: Lowering Costs and Improving Outcomes: Workshop Series Summary*. Washington, DC: The National Academies Press.

IOM. 2011. *Leading Health Indicators for Healthy People 2020: Letter Report*. Washington, DC: The National Academies Press.

Katz, M.H. 2009. Structural interventions for addressing chronic health problems. *Journal of the American Medical Association* 302(6):683–685.

Kindig, D.A. 2006. A pay-for-population health performance system. *Journal of the American Medical Association* 296(21):2611–2613.

Madamala, K., K. Sellers, L.M. Beitsch, J. Pearsol, and P.E. Jarris, 2011. Structure and functions of state public health agencies in 2007. *American Journal of Public Health* 101(7):1179–1186.

Maron, D.J., B.L. Forbes, J.R. Groves, M.S. Dietrich, P. Sells, and A.G. DiGenio. 2008. Health-risk appraisal with or without disease management for worksite cardiovascular risk reduction. *Journal of Cardiovascular Nursing* 23(6):513–518.

Martin-Misener, R., and R. Valaitis. 2008. *A Scoping Literature Review of Collaboration Between Primary Care and Public Health. A Report to the Canadian Health Services Research Foundation*. http://www.swchc.on.ca/documents/MartinMisener-Valaitis-Review.pdf (accessed October 6, 2011).

McGinnis, J.M., and W.H. Foege. 1993. Actual causes of death in the United States. *Journal of the American Medical Association* 270(18):2207–2212.

Milani, R.V., and C.J. Lavie. 2009. Impact of worksite wellness intervention on cardiac risk factors and one-year health care costs. *American Journal of Cardiology* 104(10):1389–1392.

Miller, H.D. 2007. *Creating Payment Systems to Accelerate Value-Driven Health Care: Issues and Options for Policy Reform*. New York: The Commonwealth Fund. http://www.commonwealthfund.org/Publications/Fund-Reports/2007/Sep/Creating-Payment-Systems-to-Accelerate-Value-Driven-Health-Care--Issues-and-Options-for-Policy-Refor.aspx.

National Public Health Performance Standards (a). *National Public Health Performance Standards Program (NPHPSP)*. http://www.cdc.gov/od/ocphp/nphpsp (accessed July 4, 2011).

Ni Mhurchu, C., L.M. Aston, and S.A. Jebb. 2010. Effects of worksite health promotion interventions on employee diets: A systematic review. *BMC Public Health* 10:62.

Orza, M.J. 2010. High hopes: Public health approaches to reducing the need for health care. *National Health Policy Forum, George Washington University* 78. http://www.nhpf.org/library/background-papers/BP78_PublicHealthApproaches_09-27-10.pdf (accessed October 6, 2011).

Perez, M., S.E. Findley, M. Mejia, and J. Martinez. 2006. The impact of community health worker training and programs in NYC. *Journal of Health Care for the Poor and Underserved* 17(1 Supplemental):26–43.

Petersen, L.A., L.D. Woodard, T. Urech, C. Daw, and S. Sookanan. 2006. Does pay-for-performance improve the quality of health care? *Annals of Internal Medicine* 145(4):265–272.

Racette, S.B., S.S. Deusinger, C.L. Inman, T.L. Burlis, G.R. Highstein, T.D. Buskirk, K. Steger-May, and L.R. Peterson. 2009. Worksite Opportunities for Wellness (WOW): Effects on cardiovascular disease risk factors after 1 year. *Preventive Medicine* 49(2-3):108–114.

Resnicow, K., A. Jackson, T. Wang, A.K. De, F. McCarty, W.N. Dudley, and T. Baranowski. 2001. A motivational interviewing intervention to increase fruit and vegetable intake through black churches: results of the Eat for Life trial. *American Journal of Public Health* 91(10):1686–1693.

Rosenthal, M.B., B.E. Landon, S.L. Normand, R.G. Frank, and A.M. Epstein. 2006. Pay for performance in commercial HMOs. *New England Journal of Medicine* 355(18):1895–1902.

Rowan, M.S., W. Hogg, and P. Huston. 2007. Integrating public health and primary care. *Healthcare Policy* 3(1):e160–e181.

Rucker-Whitaker, C., S. Basu, G. Kravitz, M.K. Bushnell, and C.F. de Leon. 2007. A pilot study of self-management in African Americans with common chronic conditions. *Ethnicity and Disease* 17(4):611–616.

Sacks, N., H. Cabral, L.E. Kazis, K.M. Jarrett, D. Vetter, R. Richmond, and T.J. Moore. 2009. A web-based nutrition program reduces health care costs in employees with cardiac risk factors: Before and after cost analysis. *Journal of Medical Internet Research* 11(4):e43.

Samuel-Hodge, C.D., T.C. Keyserling, S. Park, L.F. Johnston, Z. Gizlice, and S.I. Bangdiwala. 2009. A randomized trial of a church-based diabetes self-management program for African Americans with type 2 diabetes. *The Diabetes Educator* 35(3):439–454.

Sarkisian, C.A., T.R. Prohaska, C. Davis, and B. Weiner. 2007. Pilot test of an attribution retraining intervention to raise walking levels in sedentary older adults. *Journal of the American Geriatrics Society* 55(11):1842–1846.

Scott, A., P. Sivey, D. Ait Ouakrim, L. Willenberg, L. Naccarella, J. Furler, and D. Young. 2011. The effect of financial incentives on the quality of health care provided by primary care physicians. *Cochrane Database Systematic Reviews* 7(9).

Singh, D. 2008. *How can chronic disease management programs operate across care settings and providers?* Health Systems and Policy Analysis. Policy Brief. Copenhagen, Denmark: World Health Organization. http://www.euro.who.int/__data/assets/pdf_file/0009/75474/E93416.pdf (accessed October 10, 2011).

Thacker, S.B., D.F. Stroup, V. Carande-Kulis, J.S. Marks, K. Roy, and J.L. Gerberding. 2006. Measuring the public's health. *Public Health Reports* 121(1):14–22.

Westfall, J.M., J. Mold, and L. Fagnan. 2007. Practice-based research—"Blue Highways" on the NIH roadmap. *Journal of the American Medical Association* 297(4):403–406.

Wisconsin Division of Public Health. 2010. *Healthiest Wisconsin 2010: A Partnership Plan to Improve the Health of the Public*. http://www.dhs.wisconsin.gov/statehealthplan/shp-pdf/pph0276phip.pdf (accessed October 4, 2011).

7

The Call for Action

Maintaining or enhancing quality of life for individuals living with chronic illnesses has not been given the attention it deserves by health care funders, health systems, policy makers, and public health programs and agencies. The social, economic, and functional impact of chronic illnesses on these individuals is not precisely or critically monitored in populations. Also, although many control programs exist for some of these conditions, they are not well evaluated, for either efficacy or population coverage. As the United States faces difficult economic times, the epidemic of chronic illness is increasing for many reasons: the aging of the adult population, as in other developed countries; the far from complete primary prevention of important illnesses, even when feasible; inadequate evidence on how to conduct effective public programs and interventions; inadequate public programmatic resources, even for effective, evidence-based programs; inadequate attention to chronic illness management by clinical health services charged with managing patients with chronic illnesses; and the failure to more effectively align clinical and public health services where synergies might be gained (Alliance for Health Reform, 2011). The chronic disease epidemic is steadily moving toward crisis proportions, and it is a global problem. This has been well documented, as a recent comprehensive study finds that noncommunicable diseases will cost the global economy $47 trillion by 2030 (Bloom et al., 2011).

This report addresses the following important areas:

- The economic consequences of chronic illnesses to individuals, families, the health care system, and the nation;
- The development and incorporation of conceptual models, created by the committee, as well as borrowing from the Centers for Disease Control and Prevention and sources, to provide a more detailed framework for the overall discussion and the major issues, including public health disease control, economics, and both clinical and public health interventions;
- A concerted approach to understanding the dimensions of prevention as they relate to chronic disease control in the community;
- A wide spectrum of chronic diseases, their clinical stages, their patterns and anticipated course, the common or cross-cutting burden and consequences of living with chronic illness, the populations that experience chronic illnesses disproportionately, the effect of comorbidity, and the adverse effects of clinical treatment. Appendix A, on depression and chronic medical illness, supports this discussion;
- A set of exemplar diseases, health conditions, and impairments for consideration to advance the next generation of chronic disease management programs from a public health perspective, with an explanation of the difficulties in determining a set of diseases that should be the focus for public health action;
- A detailed account of how to improve surveillance in order to better assess health-related quality of life and to plan, develop, implement, and evaluate public health policies, programs, and interventions relevant for individuals living with chronic illness;
- A discussion of the role of public health and community-based interventions for chronic disease management and control, along with examples and designation of venues in which evidence-based effective programs could be located. This discussion is supported by Appendix B, on new models of community-based care for people with chronic illness;
- A consideration of the importance of federal policy in enhancing chronic disease control, including an emphasis on the Affordable Care Act and related legislation, as well as exploring the Health in All Policies and the Health Impact Assessment approach, and how the execution of these laws and policies can be used to enhance public health strategies to improve living with chronic illness; and
- An assessment of the critical role of aligning public health and non–health care community organizations as a system change to better control chronic diseases and improve quality of life and health outcomes in patients living with them.

The overall goal of this report is to highlight the toll of all chronic illnesses on living well from a population health perspective; to discuss the deficits in chronic disease control; and to make recommendations to improve public health efforts to help individuals live better with chronic illness. However, there are many domains of chronic disease management from a public health perspective for which there is simply not enough research or program evaluations to draw definitive conclusions or make concrete recommendations. The committee examined and addressed several important dimensions of the difficulty of controlling chronic disease and makes recommendations on how to proceed. However, much more remains to be done. The committee provided seventeen recommendations without priority order or measured ranking, as all of them are believed to be equally important strategies and steps to undergird public health action to help individuals living with chronic illnesses.

Government public health agencies have the ability to take action to help people live better with chronic illness. They have the expertise to assess a public health problem, develop an appropriate program or policy, and ensure that programs and policies are effectively delivered and implemented. It is difficult, however, for state and local public health agencies to plan, develop, implement, evaluate, or sustain programs, policies, and strategies to manage and control chronic diseases when they are structurally deficient and lack the capacity at the system level to effectively take action. The availability of sufficient resources to fortify the operational infrastructure of government public health agencies is not abundant. Given the serious state of the U.S. economy, infrastructure difficulties, and the need to maximize the impact of public health efforts related to living well with chronic illness, the committee's recommendations are intended to respond to the statement of task, optimize efforts to better understand the burden and needs of people living with chronic illness, promote the creation and implementation of public health policies an emerging legislation, improve the dissemination of effective community-based interventions, improve preventive clinical guidelines for people with chronic illness, and promote the testing of an aligned health system to help people live well with chronic illness. We think that this report and the recommendations are rooted in a population-based approach and underscore the special attention needed and the importance of public health action and leadership in the management and control of chronic disease in support of living well.

REFERENCES

Alliance for Health Reform. 2011. *Preventing Chronic Disease: The New Public Health.* Washington, DC: Alliance for Health Reform. http://www.allhealth.org/publications/ Public_health/Preventing_Chronic_Disease_New_Public_Health_108.pdf (accessed December 18, 2011).

Bloom, D.E., E.T. Cafiero, E. Jané-Llopis, S. Abrahams-Gessel, L.R. Bloom, S. Fathima, A.B. Feigl, T. Gaziano, M. Mowafi, A. Pandya, K. Prettner, L. Rosenberg, B. Seligman, A. Stein, and C. Weinstein. 2011. *The Global Economic Burden of Non-communicable Diseases.* Geneva: World Economic Forum.

Appendix A

Improving Recognition and Quality of Depression Care in Patients with Common Chronic Medical Illnesses

Wayne J. Katon, M.D.[1]

INTRODUCTION

Delay of harmful effects of growing older has been called "compression of morbidity" (Fries, 1980), "successful aging" (Rowe and Kahn, 1987), and "healthy aging" (Guralnik and Kaplan, 1989). Both health promotion activities and enhanced management of chronic conditions have been suggested as ways to improve successful or healthy aging (Von Korff et al., 2011). Health promotion activities, such as exercise, healthy diet, weight loss, and cessation of smoking, are believed to potentially enhance successful aging. Given the high prevalence of chronic illness in aging populations, improving guideline-based management of the most common chronic illnesses, such as diabetes, heart disease, asthma and chronic obstructive pulmonary disease (COPD), cancer, and depression, would also have a major public health impact in improving successful aging (Mor, 2005). Depression is unique in that it is as common in the general population as these other chronic conditions but also occurs in high prevalence as a comorbid condition (Katon, 2011). Effective treatment of comorbid depression has been found to reduce functional impairment in patients with diabetes (Ell et al., 2010; Williams et al., 2004), heart disease (Lesperance et al., 2007; Rollman et al., 2009), arthritis (Lin et al., 2003), and chronic pain (Kroenke et al., 2009). However, there are major gaps in the recognition and quality

[1]Professor and Vice-Chair, Department of Psychiatry & Behavioral Sciences, Box 356560, University of Washington School of Medicine, Seattle, Washington.

of treatment of depression in aging populations with chronic medical illness (Katon et al., 2004a).

Patients with chronic medical illness have been found to have two- to threefold higher rates of major depression compared with age- and gender-matched primary care controls (Katon, 2011). Rates of depression among primary care patients are between 5 and 10 percent (Katon and Schulberg, 1992), whereas prevalence rates of depression in patients with chronic medical illnesses, such as diabetes and coronary artery disease, have been estimated to be 12 to 18 percent (Ali et al., 2006) and 18 to 23 percent, respectively (Schleifer et al., 1989; Spijkerman et al., 2005). Rates of depression in complex multicondition aging populations may be as high as 25 percent (McCall et al., 2002).

Studies have suggested that there is a bidirectional relationship between depression and such chronic medical illnesses as diabetes, heart disease, and COPD (Figure A-1) (Katon, 2011). Depression often develops in the teen-age years or early adulthood. Predisposing factors to depression include genetic factors as well as experiencing childhood adversities, such as the loss of one or both parents, neglect, and abuse (Kendler et al., 2002). Stressful life events in people with these vulnerabilities often precipitate depressive episodes (Caspi et al., 2003). Exposure to childhood adversity also often leads to problems with maladaptive attachment patterns in adult relationships, resulting in lack of social support and problems with interpersonal relationships (Bifulco et al., 2002). Lack of support and interpersonal problems may precipitate and prolong depressive episodes (Bifulco et al., 2002).

Depression in adolescence and early adulthood is associated with three health behaviors that have been estimated to cause 40 percent of premature mortality in the United States: obesity, smoking, and sedentary lifestyle (Katon et al., 2010c). Psychobiological changes that have been shown to be associated with depression, such as increased cortisol levels, sympathetic nervous system dysregulation, and increased proinflammatory factors, are likely to add to maladaptive health factors in increasing the risk of premature development of chronic illness (Katon, 2011).

Once chronic illness develops, comorbid depression is associated with poor self-care (DiMatteo et al., 2000; Lin et al., 2004) and increased risk of adverse outcomes (Lin et al., 2009; van Melle et al., 2004). As Figure A-1 shows, patients with comorbid depression and chronic medical illness often have problems collaborating with physicians and are less likely to adhere to self-care regimens (diet, cessation of smoking, exercise, and taking medications as prescribed) (Katon, 2011). These maladaptive patterns lead to a higher risk of medical complications, increased symptom burden, and worsening function, which can then in turn precipitate or worsen depressive episodes.

Extensive epidemiological data have shown that, after controlling for

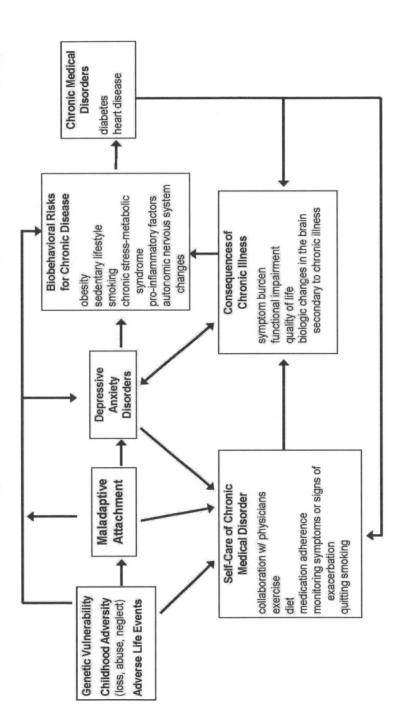

FIGURE A-1 Bidirectional interaction between depression and chronic medical disorders.
SOURCE: Adapted and reprinted from *Biological Pyschiatry*, 54, Wayne J. Katon, Clinical health services and relationship between major depression, depressive symptoms, and general medical illness, 216–226, 2003, with permission from Elsevier.

sociodemographic factors and severity of medical illness, patients with comorbid depression and chronic medical illnesses, such as diabetes, coronary heart disease (CHD), COPD/asthma, and cancer, also have a higher medical symptom burden (Katon et al., 2007), additive functional impairment (Von Korff et al., 2005), higher medical costs (Simon et al., 2005; Sullivan et al., 2002), increased complication and hospitalization rates (Davydow et al., 2011; Lin et al., 2010; van Melle, et al., 2004), and increased mortality (Egede et al., 2005; Katon et al., 2005b; Lin et al., 2009, 2010; van Melle et al., 2004; Zhang et al., 2005). Figure A-2 describes the results of comorbid depression on diabetes symptom burden from a 5-year prospective study of approximately 4,800 predominately type 2 diabetes patients enrolled in a large health care system in Washington state. After controlling for sociodemographic factors and severity of medical illness, comorbid major depression in these patients was a stronger predictor of 10 symptoms on a diabetes symptom scale than was number of diabetes complications or HbA1c level (Ludman et al., 2004). In addition, in this cohort of approximately 4,800 patients with diabetes, comorbid depression was associated with more than additive functional impairment (Von Korff et al., 2005), and approximately 50 to 70 percent higher medical costs (Simon et al., 2005). Over the 5-year period, after controlling for sociodemographic factors and the baseline severity of medical illness, patients with comorbid depression and diabetes compared with those with diabetes alone had a 24 percent greater risk of macrovascular complications (Lin et al., 2010), a 36 percent greater risk of microvascular complications (Lin et al., 2010), a twofold increased risk of incident foot ulcers (Williams et al., 2010), a twofold increased risk of dementia (Katon et al., 2010b), and a 50 percent greater risk of mortality (Katon et al., 2005b; Lin et al., 2009), as seen in Table A-1.

In considering ways to improve diagnosis and treatment of people with depression and chronic illnesses, it is important to recognize that these are often aging populations. The prevalence of chronic medical illness increases with each decade of life, and approximately 40 percent of Medicare beneficiaries have two or more chronic medical illnesses (Hoffman et al., 1996). Aging populations with depression have been found to be significantly less likely to utilize mental health services compared with younger depressed patients (Unützer et al., 2000). This is likely to be due to increased stigma regarding mental illness in aging populations, less access due to insurance issues (i.e., many private mental health specialists do not accept Medicare payments), decreased mobility due to chronic medical illnesses and functional decline, and less knowledge about mental illness in this population (Unützer et al., 2000; Van Citters and Bartels, 2004). Among the patients whose depression is recognized in primary care, few receive guideline-level pharmacotherapy or psychotherapy (Druss, 2004; Katon et al., 2004a).

Relationship of Major Depression to Diabetes Symptoms – Odds Ratios

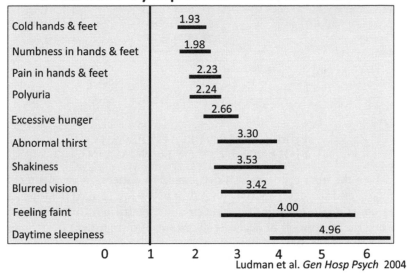

Ludman et al. *Gen Hosp Psych* 2004

Relationship of Diabetes Complications (≥2) to Diabetes Symptoms – Odds Ratios

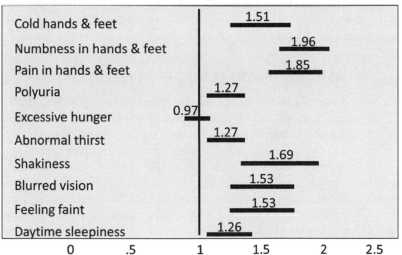

FIGURE A-2 Relationship of depression and diabetes symptoms.
SOURCE: Ludman et al., 2004.

TABLE A-1 Relationship of Depression and Diabetes Symptoms

	Minor Depression	Major Depression
Microvascular Complications	1.05 (0.83, 1.33)	1.33 (1.08, 1.65)
Macrovascular Complications	1.32 (0.99, 1.75)	1.38 (1.08, 1.78)
Mortality (All Cause[s])	1.23 (0.94, 1.61)	1.53 (1.19, 1.96)
Foot Ulcers	1.32 (0.74, 2.35)	1.99 (1.22, 3.24)
Dementia	—	2.69 (1.77, 4.07)

SOURCE: Katon, 2011.

PUBLIC HEALTH PLATFORMS TO ENHANCE CARE OF DEPRESSION

Given the high prevalence of depression in patients with chronic medical illness and the decreased likelihood of accessing mental health services, it is important to consider possible "public health platforms" that could improve the likelihood of accurate diagnosis and treatment of people with depression and chronic medical illness.

Because of the lack of access to traditional mental health services in aging medically ill populations, several recent reports have advocated either developing community-based outreach mental services for frail elderly with multiple chronic illnesses or integrating mental health services into primary care. These recent publications include the surgeon general's report on mental health (HHS, 1999), the report by the Administration on Aging (2001), and the summary of the subcommittee of the President's New Freedom Commission on Mental Health (Bartels, 2003).

COMMUNITY-BASED PUBLIC HEALTH PLATFORMS

A recent meta-analysis that evaluated face-to-face psychological services for adults ages 65 and older with mental illness identified 14 studies, including 5 randomized controlled trials (Van Citters and Bartels, 2004). An interesting finding from this systematic review compared studies that used "gatekeeper models" of recruitment, such as meter readers, building supervisors, or utility workers, with those using medical or social work personnel. Those using gatekeepers tended to identify more socially isolated elderly, such as those living alone and people more often widowed or divorced (Van Citters and Bartels, 2004). However, individuals identified by either gatekeepers or medical/mental health personnel had similar mental and physical health services needs.

Of the 14 studies reviewed in this meta-analysis, 2 found support for using gatekeepers, such as utility workers, to identify socially isolated aging populations with mental illness (Florio and Raschko, 1998; Florio et al., 1998). Other researchers are piloting work with community-based organizations to educate and screen populations for depression, such as churches or adult day care centers (Chung et al., 2010). In all, 12 studies (of which only 5 were randomized controlled trials) found that home- and community-based treatment of psychiatric symptoms were associated with improved psychological status (Van Citters and Bartels, 2004). All five randomized trials (and a more recent sixth trial) reported home-based interventions were associated with improved depressive symptoms, and one reported improved overall psychological symptoms (Banerjee et al., 1996; Blanchard et al., 2002; Ciechanowski et al., 2004; Llewellyn-Jones et al., 1999; Rabins et al., 2000). This review will focus on the evidence from the randomized controlled trials, which focused on depression in socially isolated, often medically frail elderly.

Many communities have developed visiting home-based services for aging patients with disabilities that limit mobility. These services are often provided by either social workers or nurses. These frail elderly have been found to have a high prevalence of major depression due to social isolation, chronic pain, and lack of access to medical and mental health services (McCall et al., 2002).

Research has shown that depression screening that is connected to an organized treatment program, increasing exposure to evidenced-based depression treatment, can significantly improve outcomes of these patients (Banerjee et al., 1996; Blanchard et al., 2002; Ciechanowski et al., 2004; Llewellyn-Jones et al., 1999; Rabins et al., 2000).

A recent study randomized 138 patients ages 60 and over with minor depression or dysthmia to the Program to Encourage Active, Rewarding Lives for Seniors (PEARLS) or usual care (Ciechanowski et al., 2004). The PEARLS intervention consisted of problem-solving treatment, social and physical activation, and potential recommendations to patients' physicians regarding antidepressant medications (Ciechanowski et al., 2004). The intervention was provided by social workers who were supervised by psychiatrists employed by Aging and Disability Services, a county-funded home visiting program for frail elderly. Social workers screened clients with the Patient Health Questionnaire-2 (PHQ-2) during routine in-home visits or during telephone calls. Positive scores then led to screening with a structured psychiatric interview, and clients with either minor depression or dysthmia were offered randomization to the study intervention compared with usual care. This intervention significantly increased the percentage of patients with at least a 50 percent decrease in depressive symptoms or remission of depressive symptoms (Ciechanowski et al., 2004). Intervention patients compared with usual care controls also were found to have greater improvement in health-related quality of life and emotional well-being.

This home-based PEARLS program was also recently tested in 80 patients with comorbid depression and epilepsy (Ciechanowski et al., 2010). Patients with epilepsy have extremely high rates of depression and markedly higher rates of suicide compared with other medical populations (Ciechanowski et al., 2010). The PEARLS intervention was delivered by master's-level counselors and compared with usual primary care and was found to significantly decrease depressive symptoms and suicidality over a 12-month period (Ciechanowski et al., 2010).

Rabins et al., examined in a randomized controlled trial the effect of a multidisciplinary care protocol and nurse-based outreach to 298 seniors living in public housing (Rabins et al., 2000). Among the six housing sites, residents in three buildings were randomized to receive the intervention and three buildings were randomized to usual care. The intervention group had significantly more improvement in overall general psychological symptoms as well as depression symptoms compared with controls (Rabins et al., 2000). The intervention had two key components: (1) identification of potential patients by gatekeepers (managers, social workers, janitors) and (2) evaluation and treatment by a psychiatric nurse supervised by a psychiatrist. A limitation of this protocol was the lack of a standardized treatment.

Llewellyn-Jones and colleagues examined the effect of a multidisciplinary treatment program provided primarily by a general practitioner in 220 elderly people living in a residential facility (Llewellyn-Jones et al., 1999). The intervention group had significantly greater improvement in depressive symptoms compared with controls (Llewellyn-Jones et al., 1999). The shared care intervention program involved multidisciplinary consultation and collaboration, training of several practitioners and caretakers in detection and management of depression, and depression-related health education and activity programs for residents. The control group received routine care.

Blanchard and colleagues tested a screening and multidisciplinary multimodal intervention in 96 elderly people living at home with minor or major depression (Blanchard et al., 2002). The intervention involved a psychiatrist interview, presentation of results to a multidisciplinary geriatric psychiatry team, and a nurse interventionist working closely with a general practitioner to implement recommendations made by the team (Blanchard et al., 2002). Controls received standard or usual care. The intervention group showed greater improvement in depressive symptoms than controls at 3 months. Limitations include lack of control for baseline factors and a lag between initial assessment and the start of the intervention.

Banerjee and colleagues tested a home-based intervention for depression with 69 people ages 65 and over who received home care and were depressed (Banerjee et al., 1996). Members of the intervention group received a package of care that was developed by a community psychogeriatric team and implemented by one psychiatrist. Controls received care as usual by a general practitioner. Patients in the intervention group were significantly more likely to have recovered from depression at 6 months compared with controls (Banerjee et al., 1996).

The home-based programs for frail elderly that utilized nurses as case managers and/or geriatric multidisciplinary teams often also evaluated medical conditions and geriatric risk factors, such as potential for falls and poor nutrition.

PRIMARY CARE PLATFORMS

Large observational studies have found that severity of medical illness was a predictor of chronicity of depression symptoms in aging populations with chronic medical illness (Kennedy et al., 1991). Therefore, a key research question is whether evidenced-based psychotherapeutic and pharmacological treatment approaches that have been found to be efficacious in depressed patients without chronic medical illness would be as effective in those with depression and comorbid conditions, such as diabetes, CHD, or cancer.

Several systematic reviews have found that antidepressants are more effective than placebo in patients with depression and chronic medical illness (Gill and Hatcher 2000; van der Feltz-Cornelis et al., 2010). Systematic reviews have also found that evidence-based psychotherapies, such as cognitive behavioral therapy, were more effective than supportive, nonspecific theories in treatment of depression in patients with comorbid medical illness (van der Feltz-Cornelis et al., 2010). Most of these trials of antidepressant medication or psychotherapy were small, with fewer than 100 patients, and they often selected patients with less severe medical illness and limited psychiatric comorbidities (Gill and Hatcher, 2000; van der Feltz-Cornelis et al., 2010).

A key question has been how to deliver evidence-based depression treatment to the large populations of patients with chronic conditions across a range of severity. Since most patients with comorbid depression and chronic medical illness are seen by primary care physicians and/or medical specialists, integrating depression services into these systems of care is a logical way to deliver mental health services to larger populations.

Collaborative care models have been shown to be effective in improving the quality of depression care and depression outcomes compared with usual primary care in a wide range of primary care populations, from adolescent (Asarnow et al., 2005) through geriatric populations (Unützer et al., 2002). Collaborative care programs integrate an allied health professional, such as a nurse or social worker, into primary care to support behavioral and pharmacological treatments initiated by primary care providers (Gilbody et al., 2006). These allied health professionals are trained to provide patient education about common mental disorders, proactively track clinical symptoms using such rating scales as the Patient Health Questionnaire-9 (PHQ-9), support adherence to medications, and provide brief evidence-based forms of psychotherapy, such as problem-solving, cognitive behavioral, or interpersonal therapy (Gilbody et al., 2006). Collaborative care teams also usually include a consulting psychiatrist who provides caseload-focused supervision for a panel of patients treated in primary care. The psychiatrist advises primary care providers about diagnostic and therapeutic approaches if patients are not improving with initial treatments, and they may provide in-person consultation for selected patients with persistent symptoms or diagnostic complexity. Collaborative care models have been tested in over 40 primary care–based randomized controlled trials and have been shown to be more effective than usual primary care in improving quality of depression care and depression and functional outcomes for up to 2 years (Gilbody et al., 2006).

In recent years collaborative care approaches have also been tested in patients with depression and chronic medical illness. Three collaborative care trials have been completed in primary care patients with comorbid depression and diabetes (Ell et al., 2010; Katon et al., 2004b; Williams et al., 2004). In each of these trials, intervention patients were provided with a psychiatrically supervised case manager who offered an initial choice of problem-solving treatment (PST) or antidepressant medication (Ell et al., 2010; Katon et al., 2004b; Williams et al., 2004). Patients were treated with stepped care principles so if they did not respond to therapy, a medication could be added, or if they did not respond to an initial medication, another medication could be tried or PST could be added. Collaborative care was shown to improve quality of depression care, depression outcomes, functioning, and patient satisfaction with care compared with usual care (Ell et al., 2010; Katon et al., 2004b; Williams et al., 2004). Moreover, collaborative care compared with usual care was shown to be associated with savings in total medical costs in each of these three randomized controlled trials (Hays et al., 2011; Katon et al., 2006; Simon et al., 2007).

The IMPACT trial randomized 1,801 aging patients with major depression and/or dysthymia from 8 health care organizations to collaborative care and usual care. These patients had a mean of four chronic medical illnesses. Compared with usual primary care, collaborative care was associated with improved quality of depressive care and functional and depression outcomes over a 2-year period (Katon et al., 2005a). In IMPACT, the cost of collaborative care was offset by savings in medical costs over a 2-year period (Katon et al., 2005a). In one of the above diabetes depression collaborative care trials and in the IMPACT trial, long-term costs were examined and showed continued cost savings for up to

5 years compared with usual primary care (Katon et al., 2008a; Unützer et al., 2008).

Two trials of collaborative care have also been shown to improve quality of care and outcomes in cardiac patients compared with usual care. Rollman and colleagues tested a telephone-based depression collaborative care model delivered by nurses working with patients' primary care providers to enhance antidepressant medication treatment, patient education, and behavioral activation (Rollman et al., 2009). In 302 postcoronary bypass graft patients with comorbid depression, this intervention was associated with significant improvements in depression symptoms and mental health functioning over an 8-month period compared with usual care (Rollman et al., 2009). Davidson and colleagues tested a depression collaborative care model that gave patients a choice of starting treatment with pharmacotherapy or problem-solving treatment in 157 patients persistently depressed for 3 months after an acute coronary event (Davidson et al., 2010). Collaborative care compared with usual primary care was shown to significantly improve depressive symptoms over a 1-year period (Davidson et al., 2010).

Four collaborative care trials have also been tested in patients with comorbid depression and cancer (Ell et al., 2008; Fann et al., 2009; Kroenke et al., 2010; Strong et al., 2008). Fann and colleagues examined results from the 215 patients with depression and cancer enrolled in the IMPACT trial (Fann et al., 2009). Patients randomized to collaborative care had significant improvements in depressive symptoms and functioning and enhanced quality of life compared with those randomized to usual care (Fann et al., 2009). Strong and colleagues randomized 200 patients with comorbid depression and cancer to collaborative care and usual care (Strong et al., 2008). Collaborative care involved a nurse-delivered intervention that included a choice of either problem-solving treatment or antidepressant medication provided by the patient's primary care physician. Patients in the intervention group have improved depression, anxiety, and fatigue outcomes compared with usual care over a 12-month period (Strong et al., 2008).

Kroenke and colleagues tested a collaborative care approach for 405 patients with cancer with either comorbid depression, significant persistent pain, or both (Kroenke et al., 2010). The intervention was a telephone-based care management program that provided education about pain and depression, and a stepped medication algorithm for both pain and depression based on patient symptoms measured on standard scales (Kroenke et al., 2010). Nurses were supervised weekly by both pain and psychiatric specialists and medication recommendations were communicated by nurse managers to patients' primary care physicians. Intervention patients had significant decreases in both pain and depressive symptoms compared with usual care controls over a 12-month period.

Ell and colleagues randomized 472 low-income, predominately Hispanic patients with cancer and comorbid major depression or dysthymia to a collaborative care intervention and usual care (Ell et al., 2008). Intervention patients had up to 12 months of access to a depression clinical specialist (supervised by a psychiatrist) who provided education, structured psychotherapy, and maintenance/relapse prevention support (Ell et al., 2008). The supervising psychiatrist prescribed antidepressant medication for patients preferring medication initially or for those not responding to psychotherapy. Intervention patients had significantly greater quality of depression care and had improved depressive and functional outcomes over 12 months compared with usual care patients (Ell et al., 2008).

A recent study examined the effectiveness of collaborative care for 249 patients with human immunodeficiency virus (HIV) and comorbid depression (Pyne et al., 2011). An off-site HIV depression team (a registered nurse depression care manager, a pharmacist, and a psychiatrist) provided depression care for 12 months backed by a web-based discussion support system (Pyne et al., 2011). Intervention patients were found to have significantly more depression-free days and less HIV symptom severity over a 12-month period compared with usual care controls (Pyne et al., 2011).

Although quality improvement trials have shown that care management approaches aimed at improving care of single illnesses, such as depression, diabetes, and coronary heart disease, can improve outcomes, many patients have multiple chronic illnesses, and these patients have the most problems with quality of care and adverse outcomes and are very costly to medical systems. For example, among Medicare beneficiaries with diabetes, depression or congestive heart failure, approximately 60 to 70 percent have three or more other chronic medical conditions (Partnership for Solutions National Program Office, 2001). Patients with three or more chronic conditions (approximately 32 percent of Medicare beneficiaries aged 65 to 69 have three or more conditions increasing to 52 percent in the 80 to 84 year subgroup) (Schafer et al., 2010) have been found to account for approximately 89 percent of Medicare costs (Partnership for Solutions National Program Office, 2001). A new multicondition collaborative care intervention program has been shown to improve depression, glucose, blood pressure and low-density lipoprotein cholesterol, and functional outcomes compared with usual care in patients with poorly controlled diabetes and/or coronary heart disease and comorbid depression (Katon et al., 2010a). This program trained diabetes nurses to enhance treatment of diabetes, coronary heart disease, and depression and provided weekly supervision of nurses by both a psychiatrist and a primary care physician (Katon et al., 2010a). Cost-effectiveness analysis from this new multi-condition collaborative care study also found a high likelihood of total outpatient cost savings over a 2-year period (Katon et al., unpublished).

Two other models of care have also been tested in older patients with multiple chronic illnesses. Neither of these trials required the patients to have comorbid depression, but they did include intervention components that could be used to address depression if present. The GRACE model tested a home-based care management intervention by a nurse practitioner and a social worker who collaborated with the primary care physician and a geriatrics interdisciplinary team (Counsell et al., 2007). This intervention was guided by 12 core protocols for common geriatric conditions. A randomized trial that included 951 adults ages 65 years or older showed that, compared with usual primary care, the GRACE intervention was associated with improvements in general health, vitality, social functioning, and mental health but not activities of daily living or mortality (Counsell et al., 2007). The guided care model tested the effect of a nurse working in partnership with the patient's primary care physician for patients with multiple chronic conditions (Boult et al., 2011). The intervention included comprehensive geriatric assessment, evidence-based care planning, monitoring of symptoms and adherence, transitional care, coordination of health care professionals, support for self-management, support for family caregivers, and enhanced access to community services (Boult et al., 2011). Guided care was found to reduce home health care but had little effect on the use of other health services and did not improve patient functional outcomes compared with usual primary care (Boult et al., 2011).

Based on the above successful trials, the American Diabetes Association and the American Heart Association have recently recommended screening for depression by medical systems of care. However, studies have shown that screening for depression alone does not improve outcomes; screening must be connected with organized approaches to care to improve outcomes.

COMMUNITY-BASED ALTERNATIVE APPROACHES TO DEPRESSION

Many community organizations offer aerobics and other exercise classes as well as classes on yoga, meditation, and other potentially therapeutic modalities. Although these types of interventions are generally accepted as helping psychological well-being in relatively healthy populations, it is less clear that these treatments are effective for clinical depression. There is an emerging literature describing exercise interventions for depression and several recent systematic reviews, but the research is much more limited on the effectiveness of yoga and meditation.

Exercise could potentially have a therapeutic effect on depression because of beneficial effects on neurogenesis, endorphins, and serotonin drive (Krogh et al., 2011). A recent Cochrane review of exercise as a treatment for depression found that many studies had significant methodological flaws; when analyses were restricted to more robust trials, there was a moderate but nonsignificant beneficial effect of exercise compared with nonexercise control groups (Mead et al., 2008). A critique of these studies is that, although many of the enrolled patients had mild depression based on a depression rating scale score, most would not meet criteria for major depression or dysthymia. A more recent systematic review included only studies in which a clinical diagnosis of depression was made. That review found a short-term mild significant effect of exercise on depression compared with nonexercise control groups (Krogh et al., 2011). However, there was limited evidence of a beneficial long-term effect, with the trials lasting more than 10 weeks no longer showing significant effects.

A key critique of exercise trials has been the potential lack of generalizability to populations of depressed patients. Symptoms of depression, such as lack of motivation and energy, will probably limit the ability of many patients to enroll in these studies. Thus, even if exercise has a modest effect in ameliorating symptoms of depression, it is likely to have only mild effects on decreasing prevalence of serious depression in populations.

Several small trials have suggested that yoga and meditation may have beneficial effects on depression. These trials need replication in larger numbers of patients meeting criteria for major depression or dysthymia.

HEALTH POLICY CHANGES THAT COULD IMPROVE QUALITY AND OUTCOMES OF DEPRESSION CARE

Berwick has emphasized that major organizational changes will be necessary for medical care systems to adapt existing primary care and medical specialty services to optimize care of patients with chronic illnesses, such as depression or diabetes (Berwick et al., 2003). These changes include investing in clinical information systems, such as registries to help track the quality and outcomes of care in specific populations; linking these systems to medical records; and designing decision support systems that will develop and implement treatment guidelines in a timely manner (Berwick et al., 2003). Organizational changes will also be needed to create delivery systems, such as depression management teams to implement more frequent systematic follow-up and monitoring of outcomes, promote integration of mental health specialty care into primary care, and develop self-management tool-kits for patients and providers.

Economic incentives and regulatory changes will be needed to implement these costly changes in care. As Berwick has emphasized, "For most organizations, investment on this scale is a strategic issue and will only be undertaken if the market—employers and government purchasers, principally and consumers secondarily—permits and rewards these strategies" (Berwick et al., 2003).

Key "demand side" levers include increasing community, consumer, and employer demand for integrating evidence-based changes in systems of care, aligning financial models of care to defray the costs of reorganizing health services to provide "collaborative care, and developing new Health Plan Employer Data Information Set (HEDIS) depression performance criteria that evidence suggests are linked with improved outcomes" (Katon and Seelig, 2008b). Increasing demand will necessitate education of consumer groups, employers, and insurers about cost-effective models to improve depression care, including information on how these models may decrease overall medical costs in patients with comorbid medical illnesses, such as diabetes (Katon and Seelig, 2008b). Katon and Selig have reported that "several of the research groups involved in dissemination of collaborative care are working with consumer groups, such as the American Association of Retired Persons (AARP), and the Depression and Bipolar Support Alliance, to lobby insurers to develop payment systems for collaborative care" (Katon and Seelig, 2008b). An innovative approach would be to have insurers help pay for the cost of training and changes in systems of care to help defray initial investment costs, since health insurers are likely to realize cost savings with collaborative care programs. Employers have also recognized the adverse impact of poor quality of care of chronic illnesses like depression on the workforce in terms of decreased productivity, absenteeism, and disability (Stewart et al., 2003). Recent research suggests that employed patients with depression who have poor adherence to acute and continuation phase antidepressant treatment were 39 and 46 percent more likely, respectively, to file short-term disability claims (Burton et al., 2007). Wang and colleagues have shown that an innovative program combining depression screening with telephone-based collaborative depression care improved both depression outcomes and work productivity compared with usual care when implemented in a large corporation (Wang et al., 2007). Based on research demonstrating the effectiveness of collaborative care, the National Business Group on Health has recently strongly recommended implementation of payment for evidence-based collaborative care programs for depression (Finch and Phillips, 2005).

In primary care systems, quality improvement efforts to integrate depression collaborative care programs have been hindered by lack of billing codes for the depression care manager in-person and telephone visits and time for caseload supervision by a psychiatrist. Development of Medicare billing codes for these crucial components of collaborative care could enhance dissemination efforts of this evidence-based model. The six major insurers in Minnesota are collaborating in a quality improvement project (DIAMOND program) for depression in primary care and have developed payment models for the above components of collaborative care; early reports suggest high levels of patient recovery similar to randomized trials of collaborative care (Korsen and Pietruszewski, 2009).

Changes in health insurance that provide higher payments for enhanced outcomes of populations with chronic illnesses such as depression could also enhance dissemination of collaborative care. Most collaborative care trials have enhanced clinical response to depression treatment (percentage of patients with at least 50 percent decrease in depressive symptoms) by 15 to 30 percent (Gilbody et al., 2006). However, lack of financial incentives for clinical improvement as well as difficulty billing for the mental health services utilized in collaborative care has made investment in integrating depression care managers and supervising psychiatrists difficult for systems of care.

Another key policy change that could enhance dissemination of collaborative care is to develop HEDIS performance criteria that research suggests are "tightly linked" to enhanced outcomes (Kerr et al., 2001). The current criteria include documenting the percentage of patients receiving at least 3 visits in the 90 to 120 days after diagnosis and initiation of treatment in primary care as well as the percentage of patients adhering to antidepressant medications at 3 and 6 months (Druss, 2004; NCQA, 2000). These criteria have not been shown by researchers to be linked to enhanced outcomes. Moreover only 20 percent of patients across multiple systems of care actually receive the three visits that HEDIS criteria suggest are important (Druss, 2004). Many patients who are taking their antidepressant at 6 months are still on the small dosage that was started, which makes few patients better. Most patients need upward titration of medication based on measurement of depressive symptom response, and they often need a second or third medication trial before an optimum type and dosage of antidepressant is found. A performance criterion tightly linked to outcomes could be the percentage of patients with less than a 50 percent decrease in symptoms 12 weeks after initiating antidepressant treatment who receive intensification of depression treatment, such as increased dosage of medication, change to a second medication, or referral for a mental health consultation. Payments to health organizations that report improvement in percentage of patients with at least a 50 percent improvement in their initial level of depressive symptoms at 3 and 6 months could also increase motivation for systems of care to integrate evidence-based models of care.

PREVENTION OF DEPRESSION IN PATIENTS WITH CHRONIC MEDICAL ILLNESSES

Preventive interventions to decrease incidence of depression in patients with chronic medical illness have been developed in recent years. Rovner and colleagues tested the effect of problem-solving therapy (PST) in patients with macular degeneration in one eye and a recent change in vision due to macular disease in the other eye (Rovner et al., 2007). The rationale for this study was data suggesting high rates of depression in patients who developed this irreversible disease. Patients randomized to PST and usual care were found to have significantly lower incidence of depression and were less likely to have decreased function (Rovner et al., 2007). de Jonge and colleagues tested a multifaceted nurse intervention aimed at preventing depression in 100 patients with diabetes or rheumatological disease (de Jonge et al., 2009). At 1-year follow-up, lower rates of incident depression were found in intervention versus usual care patients (36 versus 63 percent) (de Jonge et al., 2009). Pitceathly and colleagues tested a brief psychological intervention versus usual care in a large sample of patients recently diagnosed with cancer (Pitceathly et al., 2009). Although at 12 months there were no intervention versus control differences in incident depression in the overall group (intent-to-treat analysis), among patients with a high risk of depression, a significant intervention effect was found (Pitceathly et al., 2009). Robinson and colleagues tested antidepressants versus PST versus placebo to prevent depression in 176 patients with a recent stroke (Robinson et al., 2008). Over the 12-month period, patients receiving placebo were more likely to develop depression compared with those receiving antidepressants or PST (Robinson et al., 2008).

The above studies are promising, but more studies are needed. A key question will be to determine whether it is cost-effective to provide preventive interventions to only high-risk groups, such as those with a prior history of anxiety and/or depression. Our research group has found in a 5-year longitudinal study of approximately 3,000 patients with type 2 diabetes that over 80 percent who were depressed at 5-year follow-up either had minor or major depression at baseline (Katon et al., 2009). These data and the results of the above studies suggest preventive treatment of high-risk populations may be most cost-effective.

COMMUNITY APPROACHES TO IMPROVING TREATMENT OF DEPRESSION

One exciting community-based effort that could be implemented to disseminate collaborative care would be for the Center for Medicare and Medicaid Innovations to develop a dissemination project to test the cost-effectiveness of collaborative care in a large region of the United States. Given the evidence that depression increases medical costs by 50 to 100 percent and that collaborative care often is associated with total medical cost savings, this would seem like a logical next step to decrease Medicare and Medicaid costs. This project could build on the effective training model used in the DIAMOND project that has improved quality and outcomes of depression care among primary care patients in Minnesota (Korsen and Pietruszewski, 2009).

A second exciting community-based project would involve testing methods to improve mental health care for patients in federally qualified primary care clinics and the medical care of patients with chronic mental illness enrolled in community mental health systems. Funding from the Substance Abuse and Mental Health Services Administration has helped stimulate new models of care with funding for demonstration projects for these two systems to enhance coordination of mental health and physical health care. This funding has led to unique partnerships in which primary care physicians and advanced registered nurse practitioners from federally funded primary care clinics have established clinics in community mental health centers, and, in turn, mental health practitioners from community mental health centers have established clinics in federally funded primary care clinics.

CONCLUSION

In summary, depression and chronic medical illnesses are associated with functional decline in aging populations. Depression is two to three times more common in people with chronic conditions (Katon, 2011), but there are major gaps in recognition and quality of care for this affective illness. Interventions have been developed and integrated into both community-based public health platforms and primary care platforms and have been shown in randomized controlled trials to improve depression and functional outcomes. Several of the primary care–based collaborative care intervention programs have also shown a high likelihood of total medical cost savings over a 2-year period. Key changes in reimbursement for these new models of care will need to be completed to enhance dissemination effects.

REFERENCES

Ali, S., M.A. Stone, J.L. Peters, M.J. Davies, and K. Khunti. 2006. The prevalence of co-morbid depression in adults with Type 2 diabetes: A systematic review and meta-analysis. *Diabetic Medicine* 23(11):1165–1173.

AoA (Administration on Aging). 2001. *Older Adults and Mental Health: Issues and Opportunities.* Washington, DC: Department of Health and Human Services.

Asarnow, J.R., L.H. Jaycox, N. Duan, A.P. LaBorde, M.M. Rea, P. Murray, M. Anderson, C. Landon, L. Tang, and K.B. Wells. 2005. Effectiveness of a quality improvement intervention for adolescent depression in primary care clinics: A randomized controlled trial. *Journal of American Medical Association* 293(3):311–319.

Banerjee, S., K. Shamash, A.J. Macdonald, and A.H. Mann. 1996. Randomised controlled trial of effect of intervention by psychogeriatric team on depression in frail elderly people at home. *British Medical Journal* 313(7064):1058–1061.

Bartels, S. J. 2003. Improving system of care for older adults with mental illness in the United States. Findings and recommendations for the President's New Freedom Commission on Mental Health. *American Journal of Geriatric Psychiatry* 11(5):486–497.

Berwick, D.M., B. James, and M.J. Coye. 2003. Connections between quality measurement and improvement. *Medical Care* 41(1 Supplemental):I30–I38.

Bifulco, A., P.M. Moran, C. Ball, and A. Lillie. 2002. Adult attachment style. II: Its relationship to psychosocial depressive-vulnerability. *Social Psychiatry and Psychiatric Epidemiology* 37(2):60–67.

Blanchard, E.B., L. Keefer, A. Payne, S.M. Turner, and T.E. Galovski. 2002. Early abuse, psychiatric diagnoses and irritable bowel syndrome. *Behaviour Research Therapy* 40(3): 289–298.

Boult, C., L. Reider, B. Leff, K.D. Frick, C.M. Boyd, J.L. Wolff, K. Frey, L. Karm, S.T. Wegener, T. Mroz, and D.O. Scharfstein. 2011. The effect of guided care teams on the use of health services: Results from a cluster-randomized controlled trial. *Archives of Internal Medicine* 171(5):460–466.

Burton, W.N., C.Y. Chen, D.J. Conti, A.B. Schultz, and D.W. Edington. 2007. The association of antidepressant medication adherence with employee disability absences. *American Journal of Managed Care* 13(2):105–112.

Caspi, A., K. Sugden, T.E. Moffitt, A. Taylor, I.W. Craig, H. Harrington, J. McClay, J. Mill, J. Martin, A. Braithwaite, and R. Poulton. 2003. Influence of life stress on depression: Moderation by a polymorphism in the 5-HTT gene. *Science* 301(5631):386–389.

Chung, B., L. Jones, E.L. Dixon, J. Miranda, K. Wells; Community Partners in Care Steering Council. 2010. Using a community partnered participatory research approach to implement a randomized controlled trial: Planning community partners in care. *Journal of Health Care for the Poor and Underserved* 21(3):780–795.

Ciechanowski, P., E. Wagner, K. Schmaling, S. Schwartz, B. Williams, P. Diehr, J. Kulzer, S. Gray, C. Collier, and J. LoGerfo. 2004. Community-integrated home-based depression treatment in older adults: A randomized controlled trial. *Journal of American Medical Association* 291(13):1569–1577.

Ciechanowski, P., N. Chaytor, J. Miller, R. Fraser, J. Russo, J. Unützer, and F. Gilliam. 2010. PEARLS depression treatment for individuals with epilepsy: A randomized controlled trial. *Epilepsy & Behavior* 19(3):225–231.

Counsell, S.R., C.M. Callahan, D.O. Clark, W. Tu, A.B. Buttar, T.E. Stump, and G.D. Ricketts. 2007. Geriatric care management for low-income seniors: A randomized controlled trial. *Journal of American Medical Association* 298(22):2623–2633.

Davidson, K.W., N. Rieckmann, L. Clemow, J.E. Schwartz, D. Shimbo, V. Medina, G. Albanese, I. Kronish, M. Hegel, and M.M. Burg. 2010. Enhanced depression care for patients with acute coronary syndrome and persistent depressive symptoms: Coronary psychosocial evaluation studies randomized controlled trial. *Archives of Internal Medicine* 170(7):600–608.

Davydow, D.S., J.E. Russo, E. Ludman, P. Ciechanowski, E.H. Lin, M. Von Korff, M. Oliver, and W.J. Katon. 2011. The association of comorbid depression with intensive care unit admission in patients with diabetes: A prospective cohort study. *Psychosomatics* 52(2):117–126.

de Jonge, P., F.B. Hadj, D. Boffa, C. Zdrojewski, Y. Dorogi, A. So, J. Ruiz, and F. Stiefel. 2009. Prevention of major depression in complex medically ill patients: Preliminary results from a randomized, controlled trial. *Psychosomatics* 50(3):227–233.

DiMatteo, M.R., H.S. Lepper, and T.W. Croghan. 2000. Depression is a risk factor for noncompliance with medical treatment: Meta-analysis of the effects of anxiety and depression on patient adherence. *Archives of Internal Medicine* 160(14):2101–2107.

Druss, B.G. 2004. A review of HEDIS measures and performance for mental disorders. *Managed Care* 13(6 Supplemental Depression):48–51.

Egede, L.E., P.J. Nietert, and D. Zheng. 2005. Depression and all-cause and coronary heart disease mortality among adults with and without diabetes. *Diabetes Care* 28(6):1339–1345.

Ell, K., B. Xie, B. Quon, D.I. Quinn, M. Dwight-Johnson and P.J. Lee. 2008. Randomized controlled trial of collaborative care management of depression among low-income patients with cancer. *Journal of Clinical Oncology* 26(27):4488–4496.

Ell, K., W. Katon, B. Xie, P.J. Lee, S. Kapetanovic, J. Guterman, and C.P. Chou. 2010. Collaborative care management of major depression among low-income, predominantly Hispanic subjects with diabetes: A randomized controlled trial. *Diabetes Care* 33(4):706–713.

Fann, J.R., M.Y. Fan, and J. Unützer. 2009. Improving primary care for older adults with cancer and depression. *Journal of General Internal Medicine* 24(Suppl 2):S417–S424.

Finch, R.A., and K. Phillips. 2005. An employer's guide to behavioral health services: A roadmap and recommendations for evaluating, designing, and implementing behavioral health services. *Center for Prevention and Health Services, National Business Group on Health*. Washington, DC.

Florio, E.R., and R. Raschko. 1998. The gatekeeper model: Implications for social policy. *Journal of Aging and Social Policy* 10(1):37–55.

Florio, E.R., J.E. Jensen, M. Hendryx, R. Raschko, and K. Mathieson. 1998. One-year outcomes of older adults referred for aging and mental health services by community gatekeepers. *Journal of Case Management* 7(2):74–83.

Fries, J.F. 1980. Aging, natural death, and the compression of morbidity. *New England Journal of Medicine* 303(3):130–135.

Gilbody, S., P. Bower, J. Fletcher, D. Richards, and A.J. Sutton. 2006. Collaborative care for depression: a cumulative meta-analysis and review of longer-term outcomes. *Archives of Internal Medicine* 166(21):2314–2321.

Gill, D., and S. Hatcher. 2000. Antidepressants for depression in medical illness. *Cochrane Database Systematic Reviews* (4):CD001312.

Guralnik, J.M., and G.A. Kaplan. 1989. Predictors of healthy aging: Prospective evidence from the Alameda County study. *American Journal of Public Health* 79(6):703–708.

Hays, J., W. Katon, K. Ell, P.J. Lee, and J.J. Guterman. 2011. *Cost effectiveness analysis of collaborative care management for major depression among low-income, predominately Hispanics with diabetes: assessment in psychiatry*. Tenth Workshop on Costs and Assessment in Psychiatry. Venice, Italy: Mental Health Policy and Economics. March 14.

HHS (U.S. Department of Health and Human Services). 1999. *Mental Health: A Report of the Surgeon General*. Washington, DC: Office of the Surgeon General, U.S. Public Health Service, U.S. Department of Health and Human Services.

Hoffman, C., D. Rice, and H.Y. Sung. 1996. Persons with chronic conditions. Their prevalence and costs. *Journal of American Medical Association* 276(18):1473–1479.

Katon, W.J. 2003. Clincial health services and relationship between major depression, depressive symptoms, and general medical illness. *Biological Pyschiatry* 54:216–226.

Katon, W.J. 2011. Epidemiology and treatment of depression in patients with chronic medical illness. *Dialogues in Clinical Neuroscience* 13(1):7–23.

Katon, W., and H. Schulberg. 1992. Epidemiology of depression in primary care. *General Hospital Psychiatry* 14(4):237–247.

Katon, W.J., G. Simon, J. Russo, M. Von Korff, E.H. Lin, E. Ludman, P. Ciechanowski, and T. Bush. 2004a. Quality of depression care in a population-based sample of patients with diabetes and major depression. *Medical Care* 42(12):1222–1229.

Katon, W.J., M. Von Korff, E.H. Lin, G. Simon, E. Ludman, J. Russo, P. Ciechanowski, E. Walker, and T. Bush. 2004b. The Pathways Study: A randomized trial of collaborative care in patients with diabetes and depression. *Archives of General Psychiatry* 61(10):1042–1049.

Katon, W.J., M. Schoenbaum, M.Y. Fan, C.M. Callahan, J. Jr. Williams, E. Hunkeler, L. Harpole, X.H. Zhou, C. Langston, and J. Unützer. 2005a. Cost-effectiveness of improving primary care treatment of late-life depression. *Archives of General Psychiatry* 62(12):1313–1320.

Katon, W.J., C. Rutter, G. Simon, E.H. Lin, E. Ludman, P. Ciechanowski, L. Kinder, B. Young, and M. Von Korff. 2005b. The association of comorbid depression with mortality in patients with type 2 diabetes. *Diabetes Care* 28(11):2668–2672.

Katon, W., J. Unützer, M.Y. Fan, J.W. Jr. Williams, M. Schoenbaum, E.H. Lin, and E.M. Hunkeler. 2006. Cost-effectiveness and net benefit of enhanced treatment of depression for older adults with diabetes and depression. *Diabetes Care* 29(2):265–270.

Katon, W., E.H. Lin, and K. Kroenke. 2007. The association of depression and anxiety with medical symptom burden in patients with chronic medical illness. *General Hospital Psychiatry* 29(2):147–155.

Katon, W.J., J.E. Russo, M. Von Korff, E.H. Lin, E. Ludman, and P.S. Ciechanowski. 2008a. Long-term effects on medical costs of improving depression outcomes in patients with depression and diabetes. *Diabetes Care* 31(6):1155 1159.

Katon, W.J., and M. Seelig 2008b. Population-based care of depression: Team care approaches to improving outcomes. *Journal of Occupation and Environmental Medicine* 50(4):459–467.

Katon, W., J. Russo, E.H. Lin, S.R. Heckbert, P. Ciechanowski, E.J. Ludman, and M. Von Korff. 2009. Depression and diabetes: Factors associated with major depression at five-year follow-up. *Psychosomatics* 50(6):570–579.

Katon, W.J., E.H. Lin, M. Von Korff, P. Ciechanowski, E.J. Ludman, B. Young, D. Peterson, C.M. Rutter, M. McGregor, and D. McCulloch. 2010a. Collaborative care for patients with depression and chronic illnesses. *New England Journal of Medicine* 363(27): 2611–2620.

Katon, W.J., E.H. Lin L.H. Williams, P. Ciechanowski, S.R. Heckbert, E. Ludman, C. Rutter, P.K. Crane, M. Oliver, and M. Von Korff. 2010b. Comorbid depression is associated with an increased risk of dementia diagnosis in patients with diabetes: A prospective cohort study. *Journal of General Internal Medicine* 25(5):423–429.

Katon, W., L. Richardson, J. Russo, C.A. McCarty, C. Rockhill, E. McCauley, J. Richards, and D.C. Grossman. 2010c. Depressive symptoms in adolescence: The association with multiple health risk behaviors. *General Hospital Psychiatry* 32(3):233–239.

Katon, W.J., J. Russo, and E. Lin. Unpublished. Cost-effectiveness of a multi-condition collaborative care intervention: A randomized controlled trial. *Archives of General Psychiatry*.

Kendler, K., C. Gardner, and C.A. Prescott. 2002. Toward a comprehensive developmental model for major depression in women. *American Journal of Psychiatry* 159(7):1133–1145.

Kennedy, G.J., H.R. Kelman, and C. Thomas. 1991. Persistence and remission of depressive symptoms in late life. *American Journal of Psychiatry* 148(2):174–178.

Kerr, E.A., S.L. Krein, S. Vijan, T.P. Hofer, and R.A. Hayward. 2001. Avoiding pitfalls in chronic disease quality measurement: A case for the next generation of technical quality measures. *American Journal of Managed Care* 7(11):1033–1043.

Korsen, N., and P. Pietruszewski. 2009. Translating evidence to practice: Two stories from the field. *Journal of Clinical Psychology in Medical Settings* 16(1):47–57.

Kroenke, K., M.J. Bair, T.M. Damush, J. Wu, S. Hoke, J. Sutherland, and W. Tu. 2009. Optimized antidepressant therapy and pain self-management in primary care patients with depression and musculoskeletal pain: A randomized controlled trial. *Journal of American Medical Association* 301(20):2099–2110.

Kroenke, K., D. Theobald, J. Wu, K. Norton, G. Morrison, J. Carpenter, and W. Tu. 2010. Effect of telecare management on pain and depression in patients with cancer: A randomized trial. *Journal of American Medical Association* 304(2):163–171.

Krogh, J., M. Nordentoft, J.A. Sterne, and D.A. Lawlor. 2011. The effect of exercise in clinically depressed adults: Systematic review and meta-analysis of randomized controlled trials. *Journal of Clinical Psychiatry* 72(4):529–538.

Lesperance, F., N. Frasure-Smith, D. Koszycki, M.A. Laliberté, L.T. van Zyl, B. Baker, J.R. Swenson, K. Ghatavi, B.L. Abramson, P. Dorian, and M.C. Guertin; CREATE Investigators. 2007. Effects of citalopram and interpersonal psychotherapy on depression in patients with coronary artery disease: The Canadian Cardiac Randomized Evaluation of Antidepressant and Psychotherapy Efficacy (CREATE) trial. *Journal of American Medical Association* 297(4):367–379.

Lin, E.H., W. Katon, M. Von Korff, L. Tang, J.W. Jr. Williams, K. Kroenke, E. Hunkeler, L. Harpole, M. Hegel, P. Arean, M. Hoffing, R. Della Penna, C. Langston, and J. Unützer; IMPACT Investigators. 2003. Effect of improving depression care on pain and functional outcomes among older adults with arthritis: A randomized controlled trial. *Journal of American Medical Association* 290(18):2428–2429.

Lin, E.H., W. Katon, M. Von Korff, C. Rutter, G.E. Simon, M. Oliver, P. Ciechanowski, E.J. Ludman, T. Bush, and B. Young. 2004. Relationship of depression and diabetes self-care, medication adherence, and preventive care. *Diabetes Care* 27(9):2154–2160.

Lin, E.H., S.R. Heckbert, C.M. Rutter, W.J. Katon, P. Ciechanowski, E.J. Ludman, M. Oliver, B.A. Young, D.K. McCulloch, and M. Von Korff. 2009. Depression and increased mortality in diabetes: Unexpected causes of death. *Annals of Family Medicine* 7(5):414–421.

Lin, E.H., C.M. Rutter, W. Katon, S.R. Heckbert, P. Ciechanowski, M.M. Oliver, E.J. Ludman, B.A. Young, L.H. Williams, D.K. McCulloch, and M. Von Korff. 2010. Depression and advanced complications of diabetes: A prospective cohort study. *Diabetes Care* 33(2):264–269.

Llewellyn-Jones, R.H., K.A. Baikie, H. Smithers, J. Cohen, J. Snowdon, and C.C. Tennant. 1999. Multifaceted shared care intervention for late life depression in residential care: Randomised controlled trial. *British Medical Journal* 319(7211):676–682.

Ludman, E. J., W. Katon, J. Russo, M. Von Korff, G. Simon, P. Ciechanowski, E. Lin, T. Bush, E. Walker, and B. Young. 2004. Depression and diabetes symptom burden. *General Hospital Psychiatry* 26(6):430–436.

McCall, N.T., P. Parks, K. Smith, G. Pope, and M. Griggs. 2002. The prevalence of major depression or dysthymia among aged Medicare Fee-for-Service beneficiaries. *International Journal of Geriatric Psychiatry* 17(6):557–565.

Mead, G.E., W. Morley, P. Campbell, C.A. Greig, M. McMurdo, and D.A. Lawlor. 2008. Exercise for depression. *Cochrane Database Systematic Reviews* (4):CD004366.

Mor, V. 2005. The compression of morbidity hypothesis: A review of research and prospects for the future. *Journal of the American Geriatrics Society* 53(9 Suppl):S308–S309.

NCQA (National Center for Quality Assurance). 2000. *The State of Managed Care Quality 2000.* Washington, DC: National Center for Quality Assurance.

Partnership for Solutions National Program Office. 2001. *Chronic Conditions: Making the Case for Ongoing Care.* Robert Wood Johnson Foundation.

Pitceathly, C., P. Maguire, I, Fletcher, M. Parle, B. Tomenson, and F. Creed. 2009. Can a brief psychological intervention prevent anxiety or depressive disorders in cancer patients? A randomised controlled trial. *Annals of Oncology* 20(5):928–934.

Pyne, J.M., J.C. Fortney, G.M. Curran, S. Tripathi, J.H. Atkinson, A.M. Kilbourne, H.J. Hagedorn, D. Rimland, M.C. Rodriguez-Barradas, T. Monson, K.A. Bottonari, S.M. Asch, and A.L. Gifford. 2011. Effectiveness of collaborative care for depression in human immunodeficiency virus clinics. *Archives of Internal Medicine* 171(1):23–31.

Rabins, P.V., B.S. Black, R. Roca, P. German, M. McGuire, B. Robbins, R. Rye, and L. Brant. 2000. Effectiveness of a nurse-based outreach program for identifying and treating psychiatric illness in the elderly. *Journal of American Medical Association* 283(21):2802–2809.

Robinson, R.G., R.E. Jorge, D.J. Moser, L. Acion, A. Solodkin, S.L Small, P. Fonzetti, M. Hegel, and S. Arndt. 2008. Escitalopram and problem-solving therapy for prevention of poststroke depression: A randomized controlled trial. *Journal of American Medical Association* 299(20):2391–2400.

Rollman, B.L., B.H. Belnap, M.S. LeMenager, S. Mazumdar, P.R. Houck, P.J. Counihan, W.N. Kapoor, H.C. Schulberg, and C.F. Reynolds III. 2009. Telephone-delivered collaborative care for treating post-CABG depression: A randomized controlled trial. *Journal of American Medical Association* 302(19):2095–2103.

Rovner, B.W., R.J. Casten, M.T. Hegel, B.E. Leiby, and W.S. Tasman. 2007. Preventing depression in age-related macular degeneration. *Archives of General Psychiatry* 64(8):886–892.

Rowe, J.W., and R.L. Kahn 1987. Human aging: Usual and successful. *Science* 237(4811): 143–149.

Schafer, I., E.C. von Leitner, G. Schön, D. Koller, H. Hansen, T. Kolonko, H. Kaduszkiewicz, K. Wegscheider, G. Glaeske, and H. van den Bussche. 2010. Multimorbidity patterns in the elderly: a new approach of disease clustering identifies complex interrelations between chronic conditions. *PLoS One* 5(12):e15941.

Schleifer, S.J., M.M. Macari-Hinson, D.A. Coyle, W.R Slater, M. Kahn, R. Gorlin, and H.D. Zucker. 1989. The nature and course of depression following myocardial infarction. *Archives of Internal Medicine* 149(8):1785–1789.

Simon, G.E., W.J. Katon, E.H. Lin, E. Ludman, M. VonKorff, P. Ciechanowski, and B.A. Young. 2005. Diabetes complications and depression as predictors of health care costs. *General Hospital Psychiatry* 27(5):344–351.

Simon, G.E., W.J. Katon, E.H. Lin, C. Rutter, W.G. Manning, M. Von Korff, P. Ciechanowski, E.J. Ludman, and B.A. Young. 2007. Cost-effectiveness of systematic depression treatment among people with diabetes mellitus. *Archives of General Psychiatry* 64(1):65–72.

Spijkerman, T., P. de Jonge, R.H. van den Brink, J.H. Jansen, J.F. May, H.J. Crijns, and J. Ormel. 2005. Depression following myocardial infarction: First-ever versus ongoing and recurrent episodes. *General Hospital Psychiatry* 27(6):411–417.

Stewart, W.F., J.A. Ricci, E. Chee, S.R. Hahn, and D. Morganstein. 2003. Cost of lost productive work time among US workers with depression. *Journal of American Medical Association* 289(23):3135–3144.

Strong, V., R. Waters, C. Hibberd, G. Murray, L. Wall, J. Walker, G. McHugh, A. Walker, and M. Sharpe. 2008. Management of depression for people with cancer (SMaRT oncology 1): A randomised trial. *Lancet* 372(9632):40–48.

Sullivan, M., G. Simon, J. Spertus, and J. Russo. 2002. Depression-related costs in heart failure care. *Archives of Internal Medicine* 162(16):1860–1866.

Unützer, J., G. Simon, T.R. Belin, M. Datt, W. Katon, and D. Patrick. 2000. Care for depression in HMO patients aged 65 and older. *Journal of American Geriatrics Society* 48(8):871–878.

Unützer, J., W. Katon, C.M. Callahan, J.W. Jr. Williams, E. Hunkeler, L. Harpole, M. Hoffing, R.D. Della Penna, P.H. Noël, E.H. Lin, P.A. Areán, M.T. Hegel, L. Tang, T.R. Belin, S. Oishi, and C. Langston; IMPACT Investigators. Improving Mood-Promoting Access to Collaborative Treatment. 2002. Collaborative care management of late-life depression in the primary care setting: A randomized controlled trial. *Journal of American Medical Association* 288(22):2836–2845.

Unützer, J., W.J. Katon, M.Y. Fan, M.C. Schoenbaum, E.H. Lin, R.D. Della Penna, and D. Powers. 2008. Long-term cost effects of collaborative care for late-life depression. *American Journal of Managed Care* 14(2):95–100.

Van Citters, A.D., and S.J. Bartels. 2004. A systematic review of the effectiveness of community-based mental health outreach services for older adults. *Psychiatric Services* 55(11):1237–1249.

van der Feltz-Cornelis, C.M., J. Nuyen, C. Stoop, J. Chan, A.M. Jacobson, W. Katon, F. Snoek, and N. Sartorius. 2010. Effect of interventions for major depressive disorder and significant depressive symptoms in patients with diabetes mellitus: A systematic review and meta-analysis. *General Hospital Psychiatry* 32(4):80–395.

van Melle, J.P., P. de Jonge, T.A. Spijkerman, J.G. Tijssen, J. Ormel, D.J. van Veldhuisen, R.H. van den Brink, and M.P. van den Berg. 2004. Prognostic association of depression following myocardial infarction with mortality and cardiovascular events: A meta-analysis. *Psychosomatic Medicine* 66(6):814–822.

Von Korff, M., W. Katon, E.H. Lin, G. Simon, E. Ludman, M. Oliver, P. Ciechanowski, C. Rutter, and T. Bush. 2005. Potentially modifiable factors associated with disability among people with diabetes. *Psychosomatic Medicine* 67(2):233–240.

Von Korff, M., W.J. Katon, E.H. Lin, P. Ciechanowski, D. Peterson, E.J. Ludman, B. Young, and C.M. Rutter. 2011. Functional outcomes of multi-condition collaborative care and successful aging. *British Medical Journal* 343:d6612.

Wang, P.S., G.E. Simon, J. Avorn, F. Azocar, E.J. Ludman, J. McCulloch, M.Z. Petukhova, and R.C. Kessler. 2007. Telephone screening, outreach, and care management for depressed workers and impact on clinical and work productivity outcomes: A randomized controlled trial. *Journal of American Medical Association* 298(12):1401–1411.

Williams, J.W., Jr., W. Katon, E.H. Lin, P.H. Nöel, J. Worchel, J. Cornell, L. Harpole, B.A. Fultz, E. Hunkeler, V.S. Mika, and J. Unützer; IMPACT Investigators. 2004. The effectiveness of depression care management on diabetes-related outcomes in older patients. *Annals of Internal Medicine* 140(12):1015–1024.

Williams, L.H., C.M. Rutter, W.J. Katon, G.E. Reiber, P. Ciechanowski, S.R. Heckbert, E.H. Lin, E.J. Ludman, M.M. Oliver, B.A. Young, and M. Von Korff. 2010. Depression and incident diabetic foot ulcers: A prospective cohort study. *American Journal of Medicine* 123(8):748–754.

Zhang, X., S.L. Norris, E.W. Gregg, Y.J. Cheng, G. Beckles, and H.S. Kahn. 2005. Depressive symptoms and mortality among persons with and without diabetes. *American Journal of Epidemiology* 161(7):652–660.

Appendix B

New Models of Comprehensive Health Care for People with Chronic Conditions

Chad Boult, M.D., M.P.H., M.B.A.[1]
Erin K. Murphy, M.P.P.[2]

SUMMARY

This paper focuses on one of this report's primary goals: "identifying which population-based interventions can help achieve outcomes that maintain or improve quality of life, functioning, and disability" for adults who have chronic illnesses. It has several goals:

- Identify new models of comprehensive health care that have been reported to improve the functional autonomy or overall quality of chronically ill people's lives.
- Describe the goals, target populations, and operational features of these models.
- Recommend public health initiatives that would support the refinement and spread of the identified new models of comprehensive health care for chronically ill persons.

In composing this manuscript, we completed:

- Electronic searches of the scientific literature (1987–2011) to identify models of comprehensive health care that have produced sig-

[1]Professor of Public Health, Johns Hopkins Bloomberg School of Public Health, Johns Hopkins University, Baltimore, Maryland.
[2]Doctoral Student, Johns Hopkins Bloomberg School of Public Health, Johns Hopkins University, Baltimore, Maryland.

nificant improvements in the functional autonomy or quality of life of chronically ill persons.

- Tabulation of the statistically significant findings of these studies and the models' relationships to community-based services, such as whether medical and community-based services were coordinated or not.
- Internet searches for reports posted between June 1, 2008, and June 30, 2011, to obtain information about other promising models of chronic care, research about which has not yet been peer-reviewed or published in scientific journals.

From among 15 models of comprehensive care that have been shown to improve life significantly for chronically ill persons, we identified 6 that integrate medical and community-based care:

- Transitional care
- Caregiver education and support
- Chronic disease self-management
- Interdisciplinary primary care
- Care/case management
- Geriatric evaluation and management

In the future, other new models of comprehensive care may also be shown to improve functional autonomy and quality of life.

Public health initiatives that seek to improve the functional autonomy and quality of life of persons with chronic conditions should:

- Explore opportunities to collaborate with organizations that pay for (i.e., insurers) or participate in (i.e., providers) these six successful new models of comprehensive chronic care.
- Use mass media to communicate public messages to chronically ill persons, their families, their health care providers and their local community agencies about the importance of integrating medical and community-based care.
- Evaluate longitudinally the effects of collaborations between medical and community-based care providers on the functional autonomy and quality of life of Americans living with chronic conditions.

INTRODUCTION

Throughout 2011, the American baby boom generation began reaching age 65. The population ages 65 and older will swell to 40 million in 2011, nearly 55 million by 2020, and more than 70 million by 2030 (CMS, 2009; IOM, 1978, 1987, 2001; Salsberg and Grover, 2006; Shea et al., 2008; U.S. Census Bureau, 2004; Wenger et al., 2003; Wolff et al., 2002). Many older persons, especially the "oldest old," have chronic conditions and disability, so as the population of older Americans expands, the absolute number with chronic conditions and disability will also rise. Unless scientists make unprecedented breakthroughs in preventing or curing chronic conditions soon, the United States will face growing pandemics of chronic disease and disability throughout the next several decades.

America's providers of health care and supportive services have not yet developed the capacity to provide high-quality, comprehensive chronic care. Its hospitals, nursing homes, physicians, clinics, and community-based service agencies still operate as uncoordinated "silos" (IOM, 2001), much of the physician workforce is inadequately trained in chronic care (Salsberg and Grover, 2006), and the quality and efficiency of chronic care remain "far from optimal" (IOM, 2001; Salsberg and Grover, 2006; Wenger et al., 2003). In a recent study of health care in seven developed nations, the United States was first (by far) in health care spending but sixth in the quality of care and last in care efficiency, equity, and access (tie). The United States was also last in enabling long, healthy, productive lives for its citizens (Davis et al., 2010).

A successful, long-term, population-based approach to reducing the prevalence and the consequences of chronic illness in the United States would include (a) the primary prevention of chronic diseases, (b) secondary prevention by screening and treatment of preclinical chronic conditions, and (c) tertiary prevention of disability and suffering by effectively treating chronic conditions that are already clinically manifest. Primary preventive initiatives might seek to reduce the incidence of chronic conditions by altering social, cultural, and environmental influences on the population's diet, physical activity, and exposure to toxins (e.g., tobacco) and infection (e.g., HIV/AIDS). Secondary and tertiary preventive initiatives would seek to treat chronic diseases promptly and effectively through the coordinated efforts of multiple health care providers and community-based supportive services. The ultimate goal of this paper is to identify opportunities for public health agencies to promote such coordination of "medical" and "social" resources to limit the functional and quality of life consequences often borne by Americans with chronic conditions.

Two overlapping conceptual models help to explicate the complex interacting factors that must be addressed to control the effects of chronic disease in the U.S. population. Not only does the Chronic Care Model (Bodenheimer et al., 2002) focus mostly on improving the ability of the health care delivery system (and its patients and families) to treat chronic illnesses, but it also acknowledges the importance of integrating the deliv-

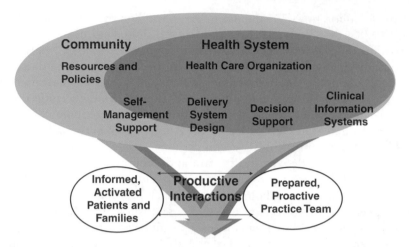

Improved Outcomes

FIGURE B-1 Chronic Care Model.
SOURCE: Reproduced with permission of Wolters Kluwer Law & Business from
Wagner, E.H., et al. A survey of leading chronic disease management programs: Are
they consistent with the literature? *Managed Care Quarterly* 7(3):58, 1999.

ery system with community-based resources and policies. The Expanded
Chronic Care Model (Barr et al., 2003) subsumes the Chronic Care Model,
but it has a broader perspective. It illuminates the importance of reducing
the occurrence of chronic conditions by addressing societal influences on
diet, exercise, and other determinants of health. The original, more nar-
rowly focused, Chronic Care Model is better aligned with the secondary
and tertiary preventive orientation of this paper (Figure B-1).

Methods

To identify promising new models of comprehensive chronic care, we
completed three processes:

- MEDLINE searches of the scientific literature (1987–2011) to
  identify comprehensive models that have, in high-quality studies,
  produced significant improvements in the functional autonomy or
  quality of life of chronically ill persons. We considered a model to
  be comprehensive if it addresses multiple health-related needs of
  adults, that is, the model provides care for several chronic conditions, for several aspects of one condition, or for persons receiving
  care from several health care providers. We excluded models that

addressed a single treatment for one condition, such as innovations in conducting cataract surgery or managing one medication. We rated study designs as of high quality if they were clinical trials, randomized controlled trials, controlled clinical trials, systematic reviews, or meta-analyses. To cover this 24-year span, we extended two literature searches that we had conducted previously. The first, conducted in 2007, had identified promising models to help inform the Institute of Medicine's 2008 recommendations for reshaping the U.S. workforce of health professionals to better care for the aging American population (IOM, 2008). The second, conducted in mid-2008, was an update of the 2007 search (Boult et al., 2009). For purposes of this report, we extended our previous searches to include information available through June 2011.

- Tabulation of the statistically significant findings of these studies and the models' relationships to community-based services (i.e., whether medical and community-based services were coordinated or not). Because of the considerable heterogeneity of target populations and care processes included in the identified models—and the methods used to study them—we were not able to conduct meta-analyses or systematic reviews of the models' positive and negative effects.

- Internet searches for reports posted between June 1, 2008, and June 30, 2011, to obtain information about other promising models of chronic care, research about which has not yet been peer-reviewed or published in scientific journals.

PROMISING MODELS OF COMPREHENSIVE CHRONIC CARE

Numerous new models of care for people with chronic conditions have been proposed, created, tested, and promoted in recent years. Some are primarily innovations in paying for care—such as capitated models, like Medicare Advantage and Special Needs Plans; shared savings models, like accountable care organizations; and pay-for-performance models. Such financial models are designed to drive improvements in the delivery, quality, and outcomes of care, but they do not specify how care should be provided. Other new models are primarily innovations in the provision of care, many of which also require changes in payment in order to be financially sustainable.

Our searches and this report focus on the latter, that is, on new models of providing care for people with chronic health conditions, emphasizing those that credible scientific evidence suggests can improve patients' quality of life or functional autonomy. The following two sections describe 17 new models that address some or all components of the Chronic Care

Model and appear promising. A brief description of each model outlines its goals, target population, methods of operation, and the currently available evidence of its effectiveness in improving quality of life and functional autonomy—as well as in reducing the use and cost of health services. Innovative models that reduce the cost of health care (or at least do not increase it) are inherently more likely than those that incur additional costs to be adopted widely in today's cost-conscious environment. When appropriate, we note how these models incorporate community-based services.

The first section (A) describes 15 new models in which credible scientific evidence published in peer-reviewed journals has shown statistically significant improvements in chronically ill patients' functional autonomy or quality of life. A table that summarizes this evidence follows section A. The second section (B) describes new two new models that may improve functional autonomy or quality of life, but peer-reviewed evaluations of these outcomes are lacking.

Section A: Comprehensive models of health care reported in peer-reviewed journals to produce statistically significant improvements in the quality of life or the functional autonomy of persons with chronic conditions.

MEDLINE reviews of the scientific literature from January 1987 through June 2011 identified 15 successful models of comprehensive care for persons with chronic conditions (Models A-O in Table B-1).

Nine of these models are based on either interdisciplinary primary care teams (Model A) or community-based supplemental health-related services that enhance traditional primary care (Models B-I).

Three successful models address the challenges that accompany care transitions, including one that facilitates transitions from hospital to home (Model J) and two that provide acute care in patients' homes, either in lieu of hospital care (Model K) or following brief hospital care (Model L).

Three institution-based models have improved care for residents of nursing homes (Model M) and for patients in acute care hospitals (Models N and O).

Note: Aside from meta-analyses and reviews, this paper summarizes only peer-reviewed studies that found that new models improved outcomes; it excludes "negative" studies. Thus, the evidence reported here should be construed primarily as preliminary findings, not as complete summaries of positive and negative studies of the models of care.

Below we summarize the models' goals, target populations, operations, and evidence of effectiveness in improving quality of life and functional autonomy—as well as in reducing the use and cost of health services. When appropriate, we note how these models incorporate community-based services.

Interdisciplinary Primary Care Models (Model A)

Each of these models (e.g., IMPACT, Guided Care, GRACE, PACE and others) strives to enhance chronically ill patients' functional autonomy and quality of life. In each, comprehensive care is provided by interdisciplinary teams composed of a primary care physician and one or more other co-located health care professionals, such as nurses, social workers, nurse practitioners, or rehabilitation therapists, who communicate regularly with each other. Many of these models coordinate medical care with supportive services provided by community-based agencies.

A related, recently popularized model is the patient-centered medical home (PCMH), which targets all patients in a primary care practice, including those with and those without chronic conditions (Berenson et al., 2011). Using interdisciplinary teams and electronic information technology, medical homes provide:

- Empanelment—each patient is assigned to a primary care provider who is responsible for that patient's care over time.
- Access—patients have access to health care 24/7/365 through same-day office visits and communication by telephone, email, and Internet.
- Diagnostic, therapeutic, and preventive services for addressing most of its patients' needs for acute and chronic health care.
- Coordination of all providers of care, especially through transitions between sites of care.
- Support for patient self-management of their health-related conditions.
- Clinical decision making that incorporates patients' goals, values, preferences, and culture.
- Periodic review of patient records to identify patients at high risk and those with gaps in their care.
- For high-risk patients, team-based comprehensive health assessment, evidence-based comprehensive care planning, proactive monitoring, transitional care, coordination of health care and community services, and support for family caregivers.

Although processes are available through which practices can be recognized as medical homes (e.g., the National Committee for Quality Assurance's PPC-PCMH recognition, levels 1-3), there is considerable heterogeneity among medical homes. For example, some medical homes are self-contained, that is, all staff members are co-located at the primary care practice, whereas others involve collaboration between practice and staff members who are located in community-based agencies. Two empirical studies of medical homes have undergone peer review and have been published in credible scientific journals; both were conducted in medical homes in which the health care teams were co-located in primary care practices. Obviously, studies of the effects of one type of medical homes may not apply to other types.

As shown in the table, most interdisciplinary primary care models have improved patients' quality of life and functional autonomy. Some types of teams have significantly reduced patients' use of selected health services. For most of these models, however, the available evidence of success is limited to a single randomized trial. Only teams focused on heart failure have improved patients' survival and have been evaluated in enough studies to allow a meta-analysis, which reported significant reductions in hospital admissions and total health care cost (Arean et al., 2005; Battersby et al., 2007; Beck et al., 1997; Bernabei et al., 1998; Boult et al., 2008, 2011; Boyd et al., 2008, 2010; Callahan et al., 2006; Chavannes et al., 2009; Counsell et al., 2007, 2009; Fann et al., 2009; Gilfillan et al., 2010; Hughes et al., 2000; Kane et al., 2006; Khunti et al., 2007; McAlister et al., 2004; Rabow et al., 2004; Reid et al., 2010; Rosemann et al., 2007; Sylvia et al., 2008; Unützer et al., 2002, 2008; van Orden et al., 2009; Windham et al., 2003; Yu et al., 2006).

Care/Case Management (Model B)

The overarching goal of care management (CM) programs is to improve the efficiency of health care by optimizing chronically ill patients' use of medical services. In most CM programs, a nurse or a social worker works as a care manager to help chronically ill patients and their families assess problems, communicate with health care providers, and navigate the health care system. The degree to which care managers coordinate patients' medical care with community-based supportive services varies from program to program. Care managers are usually employees of health insurers or capitated health care provider organizations. CM has been shown fairly consistently to improve patients' quality of life, less so their functional autonomy. Its effects on the use and cost of health services are mixed (Alkema et al., 2007; Anttila et al., 2000; de la Porte et al., 2007; Ducharme et al., 2005; Gagnon et al., 1999; Inglis et al., 2006; Kane et al., 2004b; Markle-Reid et al., 2006; Martin et al., 2004; Ojeda et al., 2005; Peters-Klimm et al., 2010; Rea et al., 2004; Vickrey et al., 2006).

Disease Management (Model C)

Disease management (DM) programs attempt to improve the quality and outcomes of health care for people who have a particular chronic condition (e.g., diabetes, heart failure). DM programs (now often called population management programs) supplement primary care by providing patients with support and information about their chronic conditions, either in writing or by telephone. Health insurers or capitated provider organizations contract with DM companies that employ nurses or other trained technicians to provide patients with health education and instructions for self-monitoring, following treatment guidelines, and participating in medical encounters. Few DM programs engage community-based services. One review that examined DM for heart failure, coronary disease, and diabetes reported no significant effect on any of the relevant outcomes. A meta-analysis of heart failure programs, however, reported that DM was associated with significantly fewer hospital admissions. A subsequent randomized controlled trial (RCT) found that DM for chronic obstructive pulmonary disease (COPD) patients was associated with better quality of care, better quality of life, improved COPD-related survival, and a shift from unscheduled to scheduled visits to physicians. Another RCT showed significant improvements in the quality of life and functional autonomy, as well as reduced use of hospitals by patients with angina (Holtz-Eakin, 2004; Sridhar et al., 2008; Whellan et al., 2005; Woodend et al., 2008).

Preventive Home Visits (Model D)

Preventive home visits are multidimensional, in-home assessments of older people performed by nurses, physicians, or other visitors that generate recommendations to primary care providers. Their goals are to improve the treatment of existing health problems, to prevent new ones, and thereby to enhance patients' quality of life and functional autonomy. Some of these programs integrate community-based supportive services with medical services, whereas others focus entirely on medical care. Meta-analyses have found that these programs can reduce disability, mortality, and nursing home admissions, especially when they target relatively healthy "young-old" persons, include a clinical examination with the initial assessment, or offer extended follow-up. The heterogeneity of the programs and populations studied creates considerable uncertainty about the generalizability of these results (Elkan et al., 2001; Huss et al., 2008; Stuck et al., 2002).

Outpatient Comprehensive Geriatric Assessment (CGA) and Geriatric Evaluation and Management (GEM) (Model E)

Outpatient CGA and GEM are supplemental services designed to improve the quality of life and functional autonomy of high-risk older persons. CGA and GEM programs are usually staffed by interdisciplinary teams of physicians, nurses, social workers, and, in some programs, also by rehabilitation therapists, pharmacists, dieticians, psychologists, or clergy. Most programs are sponsored by hospitals, academic health centers, or capitated health care provider organizations, such as the Veterans Administration. The programs identify the patient's health conditions, develop treatment plans for those conditions, and (in GEM) implement the treatment plans over weeks to months. They obtain information from and communicate their findings and recommendations to their patients' established primary care providers, and they include community-based supportive services in their plans and recommendations. In about half the RCTs that measured patients' quality of life and functional autonomy, outpatient GEM improved these outcomes. However, outpatient GEM does not consistently reduce the use or the cost of health care services (Boult et al., 2001; Burns et al., 2000; Caplan et al., 2004; Cohen et al., 2002; Epstein et al., 1990; Keeler et al., 1999; Nikolaus et al., 1999; Phibbs et al., 2006; Reuben et al., 1999a; Rubenstein et al., 2007; Rubin et al., 1993; Silverman et al., 1995; Toseland et al., 1996).

Pharmaceutical Care (Model F)

Pharmaceutical care is advice about medications provided by pharmacists to patients or interdisciplinary care teams. Pharmaceutical care programs aim to improve the use of medications and thereby to improve patients' health. Depending on the program, pharmacists' recommendations may be focused on a site of care (e.g., nursing home, patient's home), on a specific disease (e.g., heart failure, hypertension), or on specific patient profiles (e.g., patients receiving GEM, patients taking several medications). Such programs have been shown to improve appropriate prescribing, medication adherence, disease-specific outcomes, and, in some cases, survival. Quality of life has not been improved consistently, but some programs have reduced the use of hospitals (Crotty et al., 2004; Gattis et al., 1999; Lee et al., 2006; López et al., 2006; Spinewine et al., 2007; Wu et al., 2006)

Chronic Disease Self-Management (Model G)

Chronic disease self-management (CDSM) programs are structured, time-limited interventions designed to provide health information and empower patients to assume an active role in managing their chronic conditions, often through the use of community-based services. Their ultimate goal is to improve patients' quality of life and functional independence. Some programs, led by health professionals, focus on managing a specific condition, such as stroke, whereas others, led by trained lay persons, are aimed at addressing chronic conditions more generically. Most are sponsored by health insurers or community agencies; they communicate with primary care providers primarily through their clients. Numerous randomized controlled trials and a meta-analysis report that CDSM leads to better quality of life and greater functional autonomy. Several studies also report that CDSM reduces the use and cost of health services (Chodosh et al., 2005; Clark et al., 1992, 2000; Fu et al., 2003; Hughes et al., 2004; Janz et al., 1999; Leveille et al., 1998; Lorig et al., 1999; Maly et al., 1999; Swerissen et al., 2006; Wheeler et al., 2003).

Proactive Rehabilitation (Model H)

Proactive rehabilitation is a relatively new supplement to primary care in which rehabilitation therapists provide outpatient assessments and interventions designed to help physically disabled older persons to maximize their functional autonomy, quality of life, and safety at home. The few studies that have evaluated this intervention have consistently shown beneficial effects on physical function. In a quasi-experimental study, subjects receiving home restorative care had a significantly greater likelihood of remaining at home. Reductions in hospital, emergency department, or home care use have occurred less consistently (Gill et al., 2002; Gitlin et al., 2006a, 2006b; Griffiths et al., 2000; Mann et al., 1999; Tinetti et al., 2002).

Caregiver Education and Support (Model I)

Caregiver education and support programs are designed to help informal/family caregivers to enhance the well-being of their loved ones with chronic conditions. Led by psychologists, social workers, or rehabilitation therapists, these programs provide varying combinations of health information, training, access to professional and community resources, emotional support, counseling, and information about coping strategies. There is strong evidence, both in randomized studies and in two meta-analyses, that programs that support the caregivers of patients with dementia delay nursing home placement significantly, particularly programs that are structured and intensive. Similarly, all three studies, including one meta-analysis, that examined the effect of caregiver programs on patients' quality of life showed significant benefit (Brodaty et al., 2003; Kalra et al., 2004; Mittelman et al., 2006; Patel et al., 2004; Pinquart and Sörensen, 2006; Teri et al., 2003).

Transitional Care (Model J)

Most transitional care programs are designed to facilitate smoother and safer patient transitions from a hospital to another site of care (e.g., another health care setting, home), ultimately resulting in fewer readmissions to hospitals. Transitional care is typically provided by a nurse or an advance practice nurse (APN), who begins by preparing the hospitalized patient and informal caregiver for the coming transition. Depending on the program, the nurse, sometimes known as a "transition coach," may participate in the discharge planning, teach the patient about self-care (particularly about the use of medication), coach the patient and informal caregiver about communicating with health professionals effectively, visit the patient soon after discharge, and monitor the patient for days to weeks after the transition. A patient's transitional plan may include community-based resources, such as home health care, meals on wheels, or subsidized handicapped transportation. Most transitional care programs have been sponsored by health insurers or capitated health care provider organizations. Transitional care is consistently successful in improving patients' quality of life and reducing their readmissions to hospitals (Coleman et al., 2006; Naylor et al., 2004; Phillips et al., 2004).

Hospital-at-Home (Model K and Model L)

Hospital-at-Home (HaH) programs provide care for a limited number of acute medical conditions that have been traditionally treated in acute care hospitals. The goal is to resolve the acute condition more safely, comfortably, and inexpensively than inpatient hospital care can achieve. In the "substitutive" type of HaH (Model K), care is provided in the home in lieu of hospital care. After initial assessment confirms that a patient requires hospital-level treatment but can be treated safely at home, the patient returns home and is treated by an HaH team that includes a physician, nurses, technicians, and rehabilitative therapists. Tests and treatments that would otherwise be provided in a hospital are delivered in the home until the patient has recovered. Substitutive models differ in the intensity of the care they provide, particularly by physicians. Most models have improved patients' quality of life and reduced inpatient utilization and health care costs.

"Early discharge" models of HaH (Model L) provide acute care in the home following a brief hospitalization. In early discharge HaH models, after a patient's medical condition has stabilized in the hospital, the patient returns home and is treated there by an HaH team consisting chiefly of nurses, technicians, and rehabilitative therapists. Early discharge models have been evaluated following surgery, such as joint replacement, and for such medical conditions as rehabilitation after stroke. Most of these programs have reduced inpatient utilization but have had few measurable effects on quality of life or functional autonomy (Board et al., 2000; Caplan et al., 1999, 2005; Jones et al., 1999; Leff et al., 2005, 2006; Martin et al., 1994; Melin and Bygren, 1992; Ricauda et al., 2004, 2005, 2008; Rodgers et al., 1997; Rudd et al., 1997; Tibaldi et al., 2004; Wilson et al., 1999, 2002).

Care in Nursing Homes (Model M)

Several new models of care have been developed to improve the lives of nursing home residents. Most rely on primary care provided by an APN or physician assistant (PA) employed by an insurance company, the nursing home, or a provider organization. The APN or PA evaluates the resident every few weeks, trains the nursing home staff to recognize and respond to early signs of deterioration, assesses changes in the resident's status, communicates with the resident's family, and treats straightforward medical conditions at the nursing home (rather than admitting the resident to a hospital). The APN or PA usually works in partnership with a physician skilled in long-term care and who provides supplemental care as needed. Most such programs do not include community-based agencies. One model has been shown to improve residents' quality of life, and one improved residents' functional autonomy. Several models have reduced the frequency of residents' visits to hospitals and emergency departments (Kane and Homyak, 2003; Kane et al., 1989, 2003, 2004a, 2005, 2007; Morrison et al., 2005; Reuben et al., 1999b).

Prevention and Management of Delirium (Model N)

Special programs for hospitalized older patients have been designed to preserve quality of life and functional independence by reducing the effects of delirium. These programs usually involve training hospital staff, implementing preventive measures and routine screening for delirium, using evidence-based guidelines to address risk factors for delirium, assessing its causes, and treating it promptly when it appears. Studies of such programs have reported reductions in the incidence and complications of delirium, faster resolution of it, and shorter hospital stays, all of which are associated with better quality of life and greater recovery of functional abilities. Trials of delirium management programs have demonstrated fewer benefits, suggesting that programs designed to prevent delirium are more beneficial than those designed to treat it (Cole et al.,1994; Inouye et al., 1999; Leslie et al., 2005; Lundström et al., 2005, 2007; Pitkala et al., 2008; Rizzo et al., 2001).

Comprehensive Inpatient Care (Model O)

Comprehensive hospital care models include interdisciplinary geriatric consultation teams, acute care for elders (ACE) units, comprehensive pharmacy programs, inpatient comprehensive geriatric assessment (CGA), and inpatient geriatric evaluation and management (GEM) units. These interventions seek to improve the quality and outcomes of hospital care for chronically ill patients by preventing adverse events, facilitating transitions back to the community, and reducing readmissions to the hospital. An ACE unit is a medical ward with an elder-friendly environment, care by an interdisciplinary geriatric team, a philosophy of patient activation, and early discharge planning. A 1993 meta-analysis of eight studies concluded that inpatient consultation teams preserve older inpatients' cognition and ability to return to their own homes, but they have no effect on functional autonomy, survival, or hospital readmissions. Three RCTs and one quasi-experimental study suggest that ACE units may improve inpatients' health and functional autonomy without consistently affecting their survival or their use or cost of health services. A meta-analysis reported that inpatient CGA and GEM significantly improved patients' functional autonomy (after 12 months) and survival (after 6 months). Researchers in Sweden found that a comprehensive inpatient pharmacy program reduced adverse drug events and readmissions in older patients (Asplund et al., 2000; Counsell et al., 2000; Gillespie et al., 2009; Landefeld et al., 1995; Marcantonio et al., 2001; Mudge et al., 2006; Saltvedt et al., 2002, 2004; Stuck et al., 1993).

In Table B-1, an up-arrow indicates that a model has significantly improved an outcome. The fractions in parentheses indicate the number of studies that assessed an outcome (denominator) and the number that reported significantly positive effects (numerator). Asterisks indicate that at least one meta-analysis reported a significantly positive effect. Red letters highlight increases in the use or costs of certain health care services, some [of] which may be desirable, such as increases in outpatient visits that lead to fewer hospital admissions.

Section B: Comprehensive models of health care claimed in non-peer-reviewed reports to improve the quality of life or the functional autonomy of persons with chronic conditions.

Collaborative Medical Homes

Collaborative medical homes are primary care practices that collaborate with community-based agencies—rather than expanding their intramural staff and operations—to provide comprehensive medical home services to their patients. Examples described on the following pages include Community Care of North Carolina and the Vermont Blueprint for Health. Several reports of the effects of collaborative medical homes have been publicized recently. However, these reports have provided few scientific details, and their analyses have not been subjected to scientific peer review.

These reports have value, but they are limited by various combinations of (1) incomplete descriptions of the population served and the medical home services provided, (2) dissimilar (or no) comparison groups, (3) small sample sizes, (4) weak analytic approaches, (5) inappropriate statistical testing, and/or (6) selective reporting of only favorable results.

Community Care of North Carolina (CCNC) consists of 14 regional community health networks supported by a statewide administrative infrastructure. In each network, physician practices (medical homes) collaborate with hospitals, local health departments, and social service agencies to provide comprehensive care—including care management—for the majority of North Carolina's Medicaid enrollees. Most CCNC case managers are based in community settings. The CCNC program's effects on quality of life and functional independence have not been reported, but a management consulting firm estimates that the CCNC saved the state of North Carolina up to $300 million through reductions in hospitalizations and emergency room use (Community Care of North Carolina, 2010, 2011; Steiner et al., 2008).

The Vermont Blueprint for Health is one of eight state-based programs participating in the Centers for Medicare and Medicaid Services' Multi-Payer Advanced Primary Care Practice Demonstration. In this model, each advanced primary care practice (medical home) is supported by a community health team and a health information technology (HIT) infrastructure. Community health teams, composed of registered nurses, social workers, and behavioral health counselors, coordinate care; coach patients in self-care; ensure that they are up to date with appointments, tests, and prescriptions; and make referrals for mental health and substance abuse care. Public health specialists guide the community health teams toward meeting the goals of public health campaigns. Practices receive their usual fee-for-service health insurance payments, plus additional per person per month fees, which vary depending on the practice's degree of attainment of patient-centered medical home standards. The effects of the Vermont Blueprint for Health on patients' quality of life and functional autonomy have not been assessed, but preliminary intramural analysis of pre-post data suggest that the program has reduced hospitalizations and emergency room visits and generated an 11.6 percent cost savings in one community (Bielaszka-Du Vernay, 2011).

Complex Clinics

Complex clinics are multidisciplinary primary care practices that provide comprehensive care for people with complicated medical and psychosocial conditions. Some complex clinics treat only complex patients, and others treat the full range of patients, some of whom have complex needs. Such clinics have been launched and evaluated in several U.S. loca-

TABLE B-1 Summary of Evidence on Outcomes of 15 Models of Comprehensive Chronic Care

Model	Coordination with community-based services	Studies	Quality of life	Functional autonomy	Survival	Use/cost of health services
A. Interdisciplinary primary care	X	1 meta-analysis, 2 reviews, 10 RCTs, 6 QE studies, 1 XS time series	↑ (10/11)	↑ (6/9)	↑ (2*/14)	Lower use (12*/15), Lower costs (3*/11), Higher costs (1/7)
B. Care/case management	X	13 RCTs, 1 QE study	↑ (7/9)	↑ (1/4)	(4/8)	Lower use (6/10), More use (4/10), Lower costs (1/3)
C. Disease management		1 review, 1 meta-analysis, 2 RCTs	↑ (2/3)	↑ (1/1)	(1/3)	Lower use (2/3)
D. Preventive home visits		3 meta-analyses	NA	↑ (2*/3)	↑ (3*/3)	Lower use (2/3)
E. Comprehensive geriatric assessment, Geriatric evaluation and management	X	10 RCTs, 1 QE	↑ (7/10)	↑ (6/11)	↑ (1/9)	Lower use (4/9), More use (3/9), Higher costs (1/5)
F. Pharmaceutical care		6 RCTs	↑ (1/3)	NA	↑ (2/5)	Lower use (2/3)
G. Chronic disease self-management	X	1 meta-analysis, 10 RCTs	↑ (8*/9)	↑ (7*/7)	NA	Lower use (4/5), Lower costs (1/1)
H. Proactive rehabilitation		4 RCTs, 1 QE study	↑ (2/3)	↑ (4/5)	↑ (1/3)	Lower use (2/4), More use (1/4)

Category		Studies				Outcomes
I. Caregiver education and support	X	2 meta-analyses 3 RCTs	↑ (3*/3)	↑ (1/2)	ND (1/1)	Lower use (3*/4) Lower costs (1/1)
J. Transitional care	X	1 meta-analysis 2 RCTs	↑ (2*/2)	ND (1/1)	↑ (1/2)	Lower use (2/3) Lower costs (3*/3)
K. Substitutive hospital-at-home		5 RCTs 1 QE study	↑ (5/6)	↑ (1/6)	ND (5/5)	Shorter LOS (3/3) Lower costs (5/5)
L. Early discharge hospital-at-home		4 RCTs	↑ (1/4)	↑ (1/4)	ND (3/3)	Lower use (4/4)
M. Care in nursing homes		5 QE studies 1 RCT	↑ (1/1)	↑ (1/3)	↑ (1/2)	Lower use (4/4) More use (2/4) Lower costs (1/1)
N. Prevention and management of delirium		4 RCTs 2 QE studies	↑ (5/5)	↑ (1/1)	↑ (1/3)	Shorter LOS (2/3) Lower costs (1/3)
O. Comprehensive inpatient care		2 meta-analyses 6 RCTs 1 QE study	(3*/4)	(5*/6)	(3*/7)	Lower use (3/9) More use (1/8)

NOTE: * includes meta-analysis; ↑ = better outcome; LOS = length of stay in hospital; NA = not assessed; ND = no difference; QE = quasi-experimental, RCT = randomized controlled trial, XS = cross-sectional.

Fractions: numerator = number of studies showing significant difference, denominator = number of studies in which this outcome was assessed.

tions in recent years, and reports in the lay press assert that they have reduced chronically ill patients' use of emergency departments and hospitals, thereby reducing the overall cost of their health care (Gawande, 2011). Information that underlies such reports has been published in several trade publications, which are summarized here. As detailed below, these non-peer-reviewed reports tend to claim 20–30 percent savings for Medicare, but they do not report the level of detail that would be necessary to make independent determinations of the validity of these claims.

Examples of complex clinics that treat *only* complex patients:

- **Boeing's Intensive Outpatient Care Program (IOCP) in Puget Sound, WA**
  The IOCP aims to improve the quality of health care while reducing the costs of care for patients predicted to incur high health care costs. For each patient, a registered nurse/case manager conducts a comprehensive evaluation, develops a care plan, promotes patient self-management of chronic diseases, and confers with the patient's primary care physician through regular "huddles." IOCP patients' scores on functional independence and depression improved from baseline, but these scores were not compared with a control group. Preliminary results also suggest that the IOCP achieved a 20 percent reduction in spending compared with a propensity-matched control group, largely as a result of reduced use of emergency departments and hospitals. This difference was not statistically significant (Milstein and Kothari, 2009).

- **Four Medical Home Runs**
  Four practices were identified as medical home runs if health insurers reported that they had achieved similar quality of care compared with their local peers and at least 15 percent average annual per capita reductions in health care costs. All four models provided chronically ill patients with intensive, individualized care management and coordination with selected specialists (Milstein and Gilbertson, 2009).

- **The Citywide Care Management System in Camden, NJ**
  The Camden Coalition of Healthcare Providers (CCHP) developed the Citywide Care Management System (CCMS) to target "super-utilizers" of emergency departments and hospitals. A primary care team composed of a family physician, a nurse practitioner, a community health worker, and a social worker seeks to integrate solutions to patients' unmet medical and social needs and thereby

to reduce their use of acute care services. CCMS social workers, for example, help patients apply for public benefits, find housing, enroll in substance abuse counseling, manage legal issues, and arrange transportation to medical appointments. An internal pre-post analysis reports that CCMS patients had fewer emergency visits and hospitalizations, resulting in a 56 percent reduction in overall spending (Brenner, 2009; Green et al., 2010).

- **The Special Care Center in Atlantic City, NJ**
  AtlantiCare, the largest local health care provider in southern New Jersey, developed the Special Care Center (SCC) as a comprehensive clinic for patients with chronic conditions. The SCC is staffed by medical assistants and licensed practical nurses acting as health coaches who meet with patients individually and coordinate their care with physicians. Mental health and pharmacy staff also collaborate with the care team. Internal data suggest that compared with a similar AtlantiCare population that received usual care, SCC patients had better rates of cholesterol control, drug compliance, smoking cessation, and patient satisfaction, as well as fewer hospitalizations and emergency visits and shorter lengths of stay (Blash et al., 2010).

- **The CareMore Model**
  The CareMore model, implemented by a Medicare Advantage plan in Southern California, involves intensive case management for frail and chronically ill members and close monitoring of nonfrail members to prevent decline. CareMore patients undergo a comprehensive physical exam with a detailed medical history and are then triaged to appropriate chronic disease management teams. A nurse practitioner is the focal point of the care team, which relies on health information technology and remote monitoring to track patients' status. An "extensivist" physician supervises CareMore patients in the hospital and ensures smooth transitions to posthospital care. CareMore also refers its members to several community-based services to supplement their medical care, including transportation and fitness programs, home and respite care, and caregiver assistance. CareMore reports a 15 percent reduction in health care costs compared with regional averages, as well as superior diabetes control and lower rehospitalization rates compared with national averages (Reuben, 2011).

Examples of complex clinics that treat complex and noncomplex patients:

- **The Commonwealth Care Alliance's Senior Care Options program**
  Senior Care Options, a product of the Community Care Alliance in Boston, is a dual-eligible special needs plan that serves primarily older adults receiving Medicare and Medicaid—the dual eligible population. With capitated payments from Medicare and Medicaid, Senior Care Options provides clinical care in a variety of settings. A multidisciplinary team of nurse practitioners, geriatric social workers, and other clinic- and community-based staff conducts comprehensive assessments and arranges a wide array of services, including transportation and escorts to appointments, to promote independent functioning by patients with chronic conditions. Unpublished data suggest that Senior Care Options improves the quality of care for chronically ill patients and reduces their use of hospitals and nursing homes, as well as their overall health care costs (AHRQ; Meyer, 2011).

- **Clinica Family Health Services**
  Clinica Family Health Services is a community health center that serves a primarily low-income, Hispanic population near Denver, Colorado. It adopted the patient-centered medical home model to improve access to care for its patients, half of whom are uninsured. "Pods" of providers, including physicians, nurses, medical assistants, case managers, and behavioral health specialists, coordinate care and share responsibility for patients. Their work environment is open and accessible to facilitate communication. Clinica reports improved access to care and continuity of care, as well as better rates of immunizations and control of diabetes and hypertension compared with the average for Medicaid programs (Bodenheimer, 2011).

CONCLUSION

Fifteen new models of comprehensive chronic health care have been shown by at least one high-quality research study to be capable of making significant improvements in chronically ill patients' quality of life and functional autonomy. Six of these new models integrate community-based supportive services with medical care, making them attractive partners for collaboration with community-based public health initiatives:

- Transitional care
- Caregiver education and support
- Chronic disease self-management
- Interdisciplinary primary care
- Care/case management
- Geriatric evaluation and management

High-quality scientific evidence indicates that the first three—transitional care, caregiver education and support, and chronic disease self-management—may also reduce the use and cost of health care, which may facilitate their widespread dissemination in the future. The economic effects of the other three new models—interdisciplinary primary care, care/case management, and geriatric evaluation and management—are less clear and consistent. Additional new models of comprehensive chronic care (e.g., collaborative medical homes, complex clinics) may be shown in the future to improve chronically ill persons' functional autonomy and quality of life, but high-quality scientific evidence of such effects is currently lacking.

PROPOSALS

Public health initiatives that seek to improve the functional autonomy and quality of life of persons with chronic conditions should:

1. **Explore opportunities to collaborate** with organizations that pay for (i.e., insurers) or participate in (i.e., providers) these six successful new models of comprehensive chronic care. For example, a local public health department might broker collaborative agreements between local insurers that fund transitional care programs and local community-based service agencies, such as meals on wheels and handicapped transportation providers, who assist people who are making transitions from hospital to home. Similarly, state health departments might facilitate ongoing cooperative agreements between primary care practices that wish to upgrade their services to become medical homes and state-supported, community-based chronic disease self-management courses, caregiver support programs, and Area Agencies on Aging, all of which provide important medical home services. Facilitating such integration of medical and community-based supportive services is one of the foremost challenges identified by the Chronic Care Model and the Expanded Chronic Care Model for improving the outcomes of chronic care. Public health agencies, which fund or provide many community-based services, are ideally positioned to help bridge the gaps between these silos.

2. **Use mass media** to communicate public messages to chronically ill persons, their families, their health care providers, and their local community agencies about the importance of integrating medical and community-based care. Many people (and their families) who live with chronic conditions are unaware of the medical care models and/or the community-based services that could help improve their functional independence and the quality of their lives. As a result, they settle for "routine" health care, which is often fragmented and inattentive to mental health, self-management, family caregivers, community-based services, and patients' priorities for independence and quality of life. Similarly, chronically ill people may not take advantage of available resources, such as community-based transportation, meals, and volunteer chore programs. Public health organizations could partner with disability and disease-specific public advocacy groups—such as the American Diabetes Association, the Alzheimer's Association—to fund and provide informational communications through social and traditional media, such as Facebook, Twitter, print, television, radio and billboards. Messages could alert chronically ill persons and their families to the availability of local medical providers that coordinate their efforts with community-based services, as well as to the direct accessibility of community-based services that could meet their needs.

3. **Evaluate longitudinally** the effects of collaborations between medical and community-based care providers on the functional autonomy and quality of life of Americans living with chronic conditions. The concept of integrating medical and community-based services for the benefit of people with chronic illnesses has considerable appeal. There are formidable obstacles, however, to the practical implementation of this concept, not the least of which is the absence of credible scientific data supporting the value of such integration. We do not know, for example, whether the additional costs incurred by integrating community-based services into a primary care practice, most of which are driven by additional staff time, can be justified by better quality of life or greater functional independence for the practice's chronically ill patients. We also do not know whether such integration would increase, decrease, or have no effect on the overall costs of comprehensive care for such patients. Rhetorical arguments about the logic and wisdom of service integration can raise awareness, but they are unlikely to evoke difficult change without compelling supportive evidence. National public health entities, such as the Centers for Disease Control and Prevention, could facilitate the research necessary to provide such evidence. The CDC could sponsor, for example, a suite of demon-

stration projects designed to measure multiple effects of different approaches to service integration on the lives of Americans living with chronic conditions.

ACKNOWLEDGMENTS

The authors gratefully acknowledge the invaluable contributions to this report made by the IOM committee and staff, the myriad innovators and researchers who developed the models and compiled the evidence summarized here, and Ms. Taneka Lee, who word-processed the manuscript. The paper is the result of collegial, iterative collaboration by the committee, the IOM/NAS staff, and the authors. We hope that it succeeds in helping to improve the lives of millions of Americans who live with chronic conditions.

REFERENCES

AHRQ (Agency for Healthcare Research and Quality). AHRQ Health Care Innovations Exchange. http://www.innovations.ahrq.gov/ (accessed August 9, 2011).

Alkema, G.E., K.H. Wilber, G.R. Shannon, and D. Allen. 2007. Reduced mortality: The unexpected impact of a telephone-based care management intervention for older adults in managed care. *Health Services Research* 42(4):1632–1650.

Anttila, S.K., H.S. Huhtala, M.J. Pekurinen, and T.K. Pitkäjärvi. 2000. Cost-effectiveness of an innovative four-year post-discharge programme for elderly patients—prospective follow-up of hospital and nursing home use in project elderly and randomized controls. *Scandinavian Journal of Public Health* 28(1):41–46.

Arean, P.A., L. Ayalon, E. Hunkeler, E.H. Lin, L. Tang, L. Harpole, H. Hendrie, J.W. Jr. Williams, and J. Unützer; IMPACT Investigators. 2005. Improving depression care for older, minority patients in primary care. *Medical Care* 43(4):381–390.

Asplund, K., Y. Gustafson, C. Jacobsson, G. Bucht, A. Wahlin, J. Peterson, J.O. Blom, and K.A. Angquist. 2000. Geriatric-based versus general wards for older acute medical patients: A randomized comparison of outcomes and use of resources. *Journal of the American Geriatrics Society* 48(11):1381–1388.

Barr, V.J., S. Robinson, B. Marin-Link, L. Underhill, A. Dotts, D. Ravensdale, and S. Salivaras. 2003. The expanded Chronic Care Model: An integration of concepts and strategies from population health promotion and the Chronic Care Model. *Hospital Quarterly* 7(1):73–82.

Battersby, M., P. Harvey, P.D. Mills, E. Kalucy, R.G. Pols, P.A. Frith, P. McDonald, A. Esterman, G. Tsourtos, R. Donato, R. Pearce, and C. McGowan. 2007. SA HealthPlus: A controlled trial of a statewide application of a generic model of chronic illness care. *Milbank Quarterly* 85(1):37–67.

Beck, A., J. Scott, P. Williams, D. Jackson, G. Gade, and P. Cowan. 1997. A randomized trial of group outpatient visits for chronically ill older HMO members: The Cooperative Health Care Clinic. *Journal of the American Geriatrics Society* 45(5):543–549.

Berenson, R., K. Devers, and R. Burton. 2011. *Will the Patient-Centered Medical Home Transform the Delivery of Health Care? Timely Analysis of Immediate Health Policy Issues.* Washington, DC: Urban Institute.

Bernabei, R., F. Landi, G. Gambassi, A. Sgadari, G. Zuccala, V. Mor, L.Z. Rubenstein, and P. Carbonin. 1998. Randomised trial of impact of model of integrated care and case management for older people living in the community. *British Medical Journal* 316(7141):1348–1351.

Bielaszka-DuVernay, C. 2011. Vermont's blueprint for medical homes, community health teams, and better health at lower cost. *Health Affairs* 30(3):383–386.

Blash, L., S.A. Chapman, and C. Dower. 2010. *The Special Care Center: A Joint Venture to Address Chronic Disease.* San Francisco, CA: Center for the Health Professions. http://www.futurehealth.ucsf.edu/Content/29/2010-11_The_Special_Care_Center_A_Joint_Venture_to_Address_Chronic _Disease.pdf (accessed August 8, 2011).

Board, N., N. Brennan, and G.A. Caplan. 2000. A randomised controlled trial of the costs of hospital as compared with hospital in the home for acute medical patients. *Australian and New Zealand Journal of Public Health* 24(3):305–311.

Bodenheimer, T. 2011. Lessons from the trenches—a high-functioning primary care clinic. *New England Journal of Medicine* 365(1):5–8.

Bodenheimer, T., E.H. Wagner, and K. Grumbach. 2002. Improving primary care for patients with chronic illness: The chronic care model, Part 2. *Journal of the American Medical Association* 288(15):1909–1914.

Boult, C., L.B. Boult, L. Morishita, B. Dowd, R.L. Kane, and C.F. Urdangarin. 2001. A randomized clinical trial of outpatient geriatric evaluation and management. *Journal of the American Geriatrics Society* 49(4):351–359.

Boult, C., L. Reider, K. Frey, B. Leff, C.M. Boyd, J.L. Wolff, S. Wegener, J. Marsteller, L. Karm, and D. Scharfstein D. 2008. The early effects of "Guided Care" on the quality of health care for multi-morbid older persons: A cluster-randomized controlled trial. *Journals of Gerontology, Series A, Biological Sciences and Medical Sciences* 63(3):321–327.

Boult, C., A. Frank, L. Boult, J.T. Pacala, C. Snyder, and B. Leff. 2009.Successful models of comprehensive care for older adults with chronic conditions: evidence for the Institute of Medicine's "Retooling for an Aging America" report. *Journal of the American Geriatrics Society* 57:2328–2337.

Boult, C., L. Reider, B. Leff, K.D. Frick, C.M. Boyd, J.L. Wolff, K. Frey, L. Karm, S.T. Wegener, T. Mroz, and D.O. Scharfstein. 2011. The effect of guided care teams on the use of health services: Results from a cluster-randomized controlled trial. *Archives of Internal Medicine* 171(5):460–466.

Boyd, C.M., E. Shadmi, L.J. Conwell, M. Griswold, B. Leff, R. Brager, M. Sylvia, and C. Boult. 2008. A pilot test of the effect of Guided Care on the quality of primary care experiences for multi-morbid older adults. *Journal of General Internal Medicine* 23(5):536–542.

Boyd, C.M., L. Reider, K. Frey, D. Scharfstein, B. Leff, J. Wolff, C. Groves, L. Karm, S. Wegener, J. Marsteller, and C. Boult. 2010. The effects of Guided Care on the perceived quality of health care for multi-morbid older persons: 18-month outcomes from a cluster-randomized controlled trial. *Journal of General Internal Medicine* 25(3):235–242.

Brenner, J. 2009. *Reforming Camden's Health Care System—One Patient at a Time. Prescriptions for Excellence in Health Care.* http://jdc.jefferson.edu/cgi/viewcontent.cgi?article=1047&context=pehc (accessed August 11, 2011).

Brodaty, H., A. Green, and A. Koschera. 2003. Meta-analysis of psychosocial interventions for caregivers of people with dementia. *Journal of the American Geriatrics Society* 51(5):657–664.

Burns, R., L.O. Nichols, J. Martindale-Adams, and M.J. Graney. 2000. Interdisciplinary geriatric primary care evaluation and management: Two-year outcomes. *Journal of the American Geriatrics Society* 48(1):8–13.

Callahan, C.M., M.A. Boustani, F.W. Unverzagt, M.G. Austrom, T.M. Damush, A.J. Perkins, B.A. Fultz, S.L. Hui, S.R. Counsell, and H.C. Hendrie. 2006. Effectiveness of collaborative care for older adults with Alzheimer's disease in primary care: A randomized controlled trial. *Journal of the American Medical Association* 295(18):2148–2157.

Caplan, G.A., J.A. Ward, N.J. Brennan, J. Coconis, N. Board, and A. Brown. 1999. Hospital in the home: A randomised controlled trial. *Medical Journal of Australia* 170(4):156–160.

Caplan, G.A., A.J. Williams, B. Daly and K. Abraham. 2004. A randomized, controlled trial of comprehensive geriatric assessment and multidisciplinary intervention after discharge of elderly from the emergency department—the DEED II study. *Journal of the American Geriatrics Society* 52(9):1417–1423.

Caplan, G.A., J. Coconis, and J. Woods. 2005. Effect of hospital in the home treatment on physical and cognitive function: A randomized controlled trial. *Journals of Gerontology. Series A, Biological Sciences and Medical Sciences* 60(8):1035–1038.

Chavannes, N.H., M. Grijsen, M. van den Akker, H. Schepers, M. Nijdam, B. Tiep, and J. Muris. 2009. Integrated disease management improves one-year quality of life in primary care COPD patients: A controlled clinical trial. *Primary Care Respiratory Journal* 18(3):171–176.

Chodosh, J., S.C. Morton, W. Mojica, M. Maglione, M.J. Suttorp, L. Hilton, S. Rhodes, and P. Shekelle. 2005. Meta-analysis: Chronic disease self-management programs for older adults. *Annals of Internal Medicine* 143(6):427–438.

Clark, N.M., N.K. Janz, M.H. Becker, M.A. Schork, J. Wheeler, J. Liang, J.A. Dodge, S. Keteyian, K.L. Rhoads, and J.T. Santinga. 1992. Impact of self-management education on the functional health status of older adults with heart disease. *Gerontologist* 32(4):438–443.

Clark, N.M., N.K. Janz, J.A. Dodge, M.A. Schork, T.E. Fingerlin, J.R. Wheeler, J. Liang, S.J. Keteyian, and J.T. Santinga. 2000. Changes in functional health status of older women with heart disease: Evaluation of a program based on self-regulation. *Journals of Gerontology, Series B, Psychological Sciences and Social Sciences* 55(2):S117–S126.

Cohen, H.J., J.R. Feussner, M. Weinberger, M. Carnes, R.C. Hamdy, F. Hsieh, C. Phibbs, D. Courtney, K.W. Lyles, C. May, C. McMurtry, L. Pennypacker, D.M. Smith, N. Ainslie, T. Hornick, K. Brodkin, and P. Lavori. 2002. A controlled trial of inpatient and outpatient geriatric evaluation and management. *New England Journal of Medicine* 346(12):905–912.

Cole, M.G., F.J. Primeau, R.F. Bailey, M.J. Bonnycastle, F. Masciarelli, F. Engelsmann, M.J. Pepin, and D. Ducic. 1994. Systematic intervention for elderly inpatients with delirium: A randomized trial. *CMAJ* 151(7):965–970.

Coleman, E.A., C. Parry, S. Chalmers, and S.J. Min. 2006. The care transitions intervention: Results of a randomized controlled trial. *Archives of Internal Medicine* 166(17):1822–1828.

Community Care of North Carolina. 2010. *Treo Solutions Report*. Raleigh, NC: North Carolina Community Care Networks, Inc. http://www.communitycarenc.org/elements/media/related-downloads/treo-analysis-of-ccnc-performance.pdf (accessed August 11, 2011).

Community Care of North Carolina. 2011. *Enhanced Primary Care Case Management System: Legislative Report*. Raleigh, NC: North Carolina Community Care Networks, Inc. http://www.communitycarenc.org/elements/media/publications/report-to-the-nc-general-assembly-january-2011.pdf (accessed August 11, 2011).

Counsell, S.R., C.M. Holder, L.L. Liebenauer, R.M. Palmer, R.H. Fortinsky, D.M. Kresevic, L.M. Quinn, K.R. Allen, K.E. Covinsky, and C.S. Landefeld. 2000. Effects of a multicomponent intervention on functional outcomes and process of care in hospitalized older patients: A randomized controlled trial of Acute Care for Elders (ACE) in a community hospital. *Journal of the American Geriatrics Society* 48(12):1572–1581.

Counsell, S.R., C.M. Callahan, D.O. Clark, W. Tu, A.B. Buttar, T.E. Stump, and G.D. Ricketts. 2007. Geriatric care management for low-income seniors: A randomized controlled trial. *Journal of the American Medical Association* 298(22):2623–2633.

Counsell, S.R., C.M. Callahan, W. Tu, T.E. Stump, and G.W. Arling. 2009. Cost analysis of the Geriatric Resources for Assessment and Care of Elders care management intervention. *Journal of the American Geriatrics Society* 57(8):1420–1426.

CMS (Center for Medicare and Medicaid Services). 2009. *Annual Report of the Board of Trustees of the Federal Hospital Insurance and Federal Supplementary Medicare Insurance Trust Funds.* Baltimore, MD: Centers for Medicare and Medicaid Services. http://www.cms.hhs.gov/ReportsTrustFunds/ downloads/tr2009.pdf (accessed August 11, 2011).

Crotty, M., J. Halbert, D. Rowett, L. Giles L, R. Birks, H. Williams, and C. Whitehead. 2004. An outreach geriatric medication advisory service in residential aged care: A randomised controlled trial of case conferencing. *Age and Ageing* 33(6):612–617.

Davis, K., C. Schoen, and K. Stremikis. 2010. *Mirror, Mirror on the Wall: How the Performance on the U.S. Health Care System Compares Internationally.* New York: The Commonwealth Fund. http://www.commonwealthfund.org/~/media/Files/Publications/Fund%20Report/2010/Jun/1400_Davis_Mirror_Mirror_on_the_wall_2010.pdf (accessed August 8, 2011).

de la Porte, P.W., D.J. Lok, D.J. van Veldhuisen, J. van Wijngaarden, J.H. Cornel, N.P. Zuithoff, E. Badings, and A.W. Hoes. 2007. Added value of a physician-and-nurse-directed heart failure clinic: Results from the Deventer-Alkmaar heart failure study. *Heart* 93(7):819–825.

Ducharme, A., O. Doyon, M. White, J.L. Rouleau, and J.M. Brophy. 2005. Impact of care at a multidisciplinary congestive heart failure clinic: A randomized trial. *Canadian Medical Association Journal* 173(1):40–45.

Elkan, R., D. Kendrick, M. Dewey, M. Hewitt, J. Robinson, M. Blair, D. Williams, and K. Brummell. 2001. Effectiveness of home based support for older people: Systematic review and meta-analysis. *British Medical Journal* 323(7315):719–725.

Epstein, A.M., J.A. Hall, M. Fretwell, M. Feldstein, M.L. DeCiantis, J. Tognetti, C. Cutler, M. Constantine, R. Besdine, and J. Rowe. 1990. Consultative geriatric assessment for ambulatory patients. A randomized trial in a health maintenance organization. *Journal of the American Medical Association* 263(4):538–544.

Fann, J.R., M.Y. Fan, and J. Unützer. 2009. Improving primary care for older adults with cancer and depression. *Journal of General Internal Medicine* 24(Suppl 2):S417–S424.

Fu, D., H. Fu, P. McGowan, Y.E. Shen, L. Zhu, H. Yang, J. Mao, S. Zhu, Y. Ding, and Z. Wei. 2003. Implementation and quantitative evaluation of chronic disease self-management programme in Shanghai, China: Randomized controlled trial. *Bulletin of the World Health Organization* 81(3):174–182.

Gagnon, A.J., C. Schein, L. McVey, and H. Bergman. 1999. Randomized controlled trial of nurse case management of frail older people. *Journal of the American Geriatrics Society* 47(9):1118–1124.

Gattis, W.A., V. Hasselblad, D.J. Whellan, and C.M. O'Connor. 1999. Reduction in heart failure events by the addition of a clinical pharmacist to the heart failure management team: Results of the Pharmacist in Heart Failure Assessment Recommendation and Monitoring (PHARM) Study. *Archives of Internal Medicine* 159(16):1939–1945.

Gawande, A. 2011. The hot spotters: Can we lower medical costs by giving the neediest patients better care? *The New Yorker* January 24.

Gilfillan, R.J., J. Tomcavage, M.B. Rosenthal, D.E. Davis, J. Graham, J.A. Roy, S.B. Pierdon, F.J. Jr., Bloom, T.R. Graf, R. Goldman, K.M. Weikel, B.H. Hamory, R.A. Paulus, and G.D. Jr., Steele 2010. Value and the medical home: Effects of transformed primary care. *American Journal of Managed Care* 16(8):607–614.

Gill, T.M., D.I. Baker, M. Gottschalk, P.N. Peduzzi, H. Allore, and A. Byers. 2002. A program to prevent functional decline in physically frail, elderly persons who live at home. *New England Journal of Medicine* 347(14):1068–1074.

Gillespie, U., A. Alassaad, D. Henrohn, H. Garmo, M. Hammarlund-Udenaes, H. Toss, A. Kettis-Lindblad, H. Melhus, and C. Mörlin. 2009. A comprehensive pharmacist intervention to reduce morbidity in patients 80 years or older: A randomized controlled trial. *Archives of Internal Medicine* 169(9):894–900.

Gitlin, L.N., L. Winter, M.P. Dennis, M. Corcoran, S. Schinfeld, and W.W. Hauck. 2006a. A randomized trial of a multicomponent home intervention to reduce functional difficulties in older adults. *Journal of the American Geriatrics Society* 54(5):809–816.

Gitlin, L.N., W.W. Hauck, L. Winter, M.P. Dennis, and R. Schulz. 2006b. Effect of an in-home occupational and physical therapy intervention on reducing mortality in functionally vulnerable older people: Preliminary findings. *Journal of the American Geriatrics Society* 54(6):950–955.

Green, S.R., V. Singh, and W. O'Byrne. 2010. Hope for New Jersey's city hospitals: The Camden Initiative. *Perspectives in Health Information Management* (Spring 2010):1–14.

Griffiths, T.L., M.L. Burr, I.A. Campbell, V. Lewis-Jenkins, J. Mullins, K. Shiels, P.J. Turner-Lawlor, N. Payne, R.G. Newcombe, A.A. Ionescu, J. Thomas, and J. Tunbridge. 2000. Results at 1 year of outpatient multidisciplinary pulmonary rehabilitation: A randomised controlled trial. *Lancet* 355(9201):362–368.

Holtz-Eakin, D. 2004. *An Analysis of the Literature on Disease Management Programs.* Washington, DC: Congressional Budget Office.

Hughes, S.L., F.M. Weaver, A. Giobbie-Hurder, L. Manheim, W. Henderson, J.D. Kubal, A. Ulasevich, and J. Cummings; Department of Veterans Affairs Cooperative Study Group on Home-Based Primary Care. 2000. Effectiveness of team-managed home-based primary care: A randomized multicenter trial. *Journal of the American Medical Association* 284(22):2877–2885.

Hughes, S.L., R.B. Seymour, R. Campbell, N. Pollak, G. Huber, and L. Sharma. 2004. Impact of the fit and strong intervention on older adults with osteoarthritis. *Gerontologist* 44(2):217–228.

Huss, A., A.E. Stuck, L.Z. Rubenstein, M. Egger, and K.M. Clough-Gorr. 2008. Multidimensional preventive home visit programs for community-dwelling older adults: A systematic review and meta-analysis of randomized controlled trials. *Journals of Gerontology. Series A, Biological Sciences and Medical Sciences* 63(3):298–307.

Inglis, S.C., S. Pearson, S. Treen, T. Gallasch, J.D. Horowitz, and S. Stewart. 2006. Extending the horizon in chronic heart failure: Effects of multidisciplinary, home-based intervention relative to usual care. *Circulation* 114(23):2466–2473.

Inouye, S.K., S.T. Bogardus, Jr., P.A. Charpentier, L. Leo-Summers, D. Acampora, T.R. Holford, and L.M. Cooney, Jr. 1999. A multicomponent intervention to prevent delirium in hospitalized older patients. *New England Journal of Medicine* 340(9):669–676.

IOM (Institute of Medicine). 1978. *Aging and Medical Education.* Washington, DC: National Academy of Sciences.

IOM. 1987. Report of the Institute of Medicine: Academic geriatrics for the year 2000. *Journal of the American Geriatrics Society* 35(8):773–791.

IOM. 2001. *Crossing the Quality Chasm: A New Health System for the 21st Century.* Washington, DC: National Academy Press.

IOM. 2008. *Retooling for an Aging America: Building the Health Care Workforce.* Washington, DC: The National Academies Press.

Janz, N.K., N.M. Clark, J.A. Dodge, M.A. Schork, L. Mosca, and T.E. Fingerlin. 1999. The impact of a disease-management program on the symptom experience of older women with heart disease. *Women & Health* 30(2):1–24.

Jones, J., A. Wilson, H. Parker, A. Wynn, C. Jagger, N. Spiers, and G. Parker. 1999. Economic evaluation of hospital at home versus hospital care: Cost minimisation analysis of data from randomised controlled trial. *BMJ* 319(7224):1547–1550.

Kalra, L., A. Evans, I. Perez, A. Melbourn, A. Patel, M. Knapp, and N. Donaldson. 2004. Training carers of stroke patients: Randomised controlled trial. *BMJ* 328(7448):1099. http://www.bmj.com/content/328/7448/1099.abstract (accessed January 6, 2012).

Kane, R.L., and P. Homyak. 2003. *Multi State Evaluation of Dual Eligibles Demonstration: Minnesota Senior Health Options Evaluation Focusing on Utilization, Cost, and Quality of Care.* Minneapolis, MN: University of Minnesota School of Public Health. http://www. cms.gov/reports/downloads/kane2003_1.pdf (accessed January 6, 2012).

Kane, R.L., J. Garrard, C.L. Skay, D.M. Radosevich, J.L. Buchanan, S.M. McDermott, S.B. Arnold, and L. Kepferle. 1989. Effects of a geriatric nurse practitioner on process and outcome of nursing home care. *American Journal of Public Health* 79(9):1271–1277.

Kane, R.L., G. Keckhafer, S. Flood, B. Bershadsky, and M.S. Siadaty. 2003. The effect of Evercare on hospital use. *Journal of the American Geriatrics Society* 51(10):1427–1434.

Kane, R.L., S. Flood, B. Bershadsky, and G. Keckhafer. 2004a. Effect of an innovative Medicare managed care program on the quality of care for nursing home residents. *Gerontologist* 44(1):95–103.

Kane, R.L., P. Homyak, B. Bershadsky, S. Flood, and H. Zhang. 2004b. Patterns of utilization for the Minnesota Senior Health Options Program. *Journal of the American Geriatrics Society* 52(12):2039–2044.

Kane, R.L., P. Homyak, B. Bershadsky, T. Lum, S. Flood, and H. Zhang. 2005. The quality of care under a managed-care program for dual eligibles. *Gerontologist* 45(4):496–504.

Kane, R.L., P. Homyak, B. Bershadsky, and S. Flood. 2006. Variations on a theme called PACE. *Journals of Gerontology. Series A, Biological Sciences and Medical Sciences* 61(7):689–693.

Kane, R.A., T.Y. Lum, L.J. Cutler, H.B. Degenholtz, and T.C. Yu. 2007. Resident outcomes in small-house nursing homes: A longitudinal evaluation of the initial green house program. *Journal of the American Geriatrics Society* 55(6):832–839.

Keeler, E.B., D.A. Robalino, J.C. Frank, S.H. Hirsch, R.C. Maly, and D.B. Reuben. 1999. Cost-effectiveness of outpatient geriatric assessment with an intervention to increase adherence. *Medical Care* 37(12):1199–1206.

Khunti, K., M. Stone, S. Paul, J. Baines, L. Gisborne, A. Farooqi, X. Luan, and I. Squire. 2007. Disease management programme for secondary prevention of coronary heart disease and heart failure in primary care: a cluster randomised controlled trial. *Heart* 93(11):1398–1405.

Landefeld, C.S., R.M. Palmer, D.M. Kresevic, R.H. Fortinsky, and J. Kowal. 1995. A randomized trial of care in a hospital medical unit especially designed to improve the functional outcomes of acutely ill older patients. *New England Journal of Medicine* 332(20):1338–1344.

Lee, J.K., K.A. Grace, and A.J. Taylor. 2006. Effect of a pharmacy care program on medication adherence and persistence, blood pressure, and low-density lipoprotein cholesterol: A randomized controlled trial. *Journal of the American Medical Association* 296(21):2563–2571.

Leff, B., L. Burton, S.L. Mader, B. Naughton, J. Burl, S.K. Inouye, W.B. Greenough, III, S. Guido, C. Langston, K.D. Frick, D. Steinwachs, and J.R. Burton. 2005. Hospital at home: Feasibility and outcomes of a program to provide hospital-level care at home for acutely ill older patients. *Annals of Internal Medicine* 143(11):798–808.

Leff, B., L. Burton, S. Mader, B. Naughton, J. Burl, R. Clark, W.B. Greenough, III, S. Guido, D. Steinwachs, and J.R. Burton. 2006. Satisfaction with hospital at home care. *Journal of American Geriatrics Society* 54(9):1355–1363.

Leslie, D.L., Y. Zhang, S.T. Bogardus, T.R. Holford, L.S. Leo-Summers, and S.K. Inouye. 2005. Consequences of preventing delirium in hospitalized older adults on nursing home costs. *Journal of the American Geriatrics Society* 53(3):405–409.

Leveille, S.G., E.H. Wagner, C. Davis, L. Grothaus, J. Wallace, M. LoGerfo, and D. Kent. 1998. Preventing disability and managing chronic illness in frail older adults: A randomized trial of a community-based partnership with primary care. *Journal of the American Geriatrics Society* 46(10):1191–1198.

López Cabezas, C., C. Falces Salvador, D. Cubí Quadrada, A. Arnau Bartés, M. Ylla Boré, N. Muro Perea, and E. Homs Peipoch. 2006. Randomized clinical trial of a postdischarge pharmaceutical care program vs regular follow-up in patients with heart failure. *Farmacia Hospitaliaria* 30(6):328–342.

Lorig, K.R., D.S. Sobel, A.L. Stewart, B.W. Brown, Jr., A. Bandura, P. Ritter, V.M. Gonzalez, D.D. Laurent, and H.R. Holman. 1999. Evidence suggesting that a chronic disease self-management program can improve health status while reducing hospitalization: A randomized trial. *Medical Care* 37(1):5–14.

Lundström, M., A. Edlund, S. Karlsson, B. Brännström, G. Bucht, and Y. Gustafson. 2005. A multifactorial intervention program reduces the duration of delirium, length of hospitalization, and mortality in delirious patients. *Journal of the American Geriatrics Society* 53(4):622–628.

Lundström, M., B. Olofsson, M. Stenvall, S. Karlsson, L. Nyberg, U. Englund, B. Borssén, O. Svensson, and Y. Gustafson. 2007. Postoperative delirium in old patients with femoral neck fracture: a randomized intervention study. *Aging Clinical and Experimental Research* 19(3):178–186.

Maly, R.C., L.B. Bourque, and R.F. Engelhardt. 1999. A randomized controlled trial of facilitating information giving to patients with chronic medical conditions: Effects on outcomes of care. *Journal of Family Practice* 48(5):356–363.

Mann, W.C., K.J. Ottenbacher, L. Fraas, M. Tomita, and C.V. Granger. 1999. Effectiveness of assistive technology and environmental interventions in maintaining independence and reducing home care costs for the frail elderly. A randomized controlled trial. *Archives of Family Medicine* 8(3):210–217.

Marcantonio, E.R., J.M. Flacker, R.J. Wright, and N.M. Resnick. 2001. Reducing delirium after hip fracture: A randomized trial. *Journal of the American Geriatrics Society* 49(5):516–522.

Markle-Reid, M., R. Weir, G. Browne, J. Roberts, A. Gafni, and S. Henderson. 2006. Health promotion for frail older home care clients. *Journal of Advanced Nursing* 54(3):381–395.

Martin, D.C., M.L. Berger, D.T. Anstatt, J. Wofford, D. Warfel, R.S. Turpin, C.C. Cannuscio, S.M. Teutsch, and B.J. Mansheim. 2004. A randomized controlled open trial of population-based disease and case management in a Medicare Plus Choice health maintenance organization. *Preventing Chronic Disease* 1(4):A05.

Martin, F., A. Oyewole, and A. Moloney. 1994. A randomized controlled trial of a high support hospital discharge team for elderly people. *Age and Ageing* 23(3):228–234.

McAlister, F.A., S. Stewart, S. Ferrua, and J.J. McMurray. 2004. Multidisciplinary strategies for the management of heart failure patients at high risk for admission: A systematic review of randomized trials. *Journal of the American College of Cardiology* 44(4):810–819.

Melin, A.L., and L.O. Bygren. 1992. Efficacy of the rehabilitation of elderly primary health care patients after short-stay hospital treatment. *Medical Care* 30(11):1004–1015.

Meyer, H. 2011. A new care paradigm slashes hospital use and nursing home stays for the elderly and the physically and mentally disabled. *Health Affairs* 30(3):408–411.

Milstein, A., and E. Gilbertson. 2009. American medical homes runs: Four real-life examples of primary care practices that show a better way to substantial savings. *Health Affairs* 28(5):1317–1326.

Milstein, A., and P. Kothari. 2009. Are higher-value care models replicable? *Health Affairs Blog.* http://healthaffairs.org/blog/2009/10/20/are-higher-value-care-models-replicable/ (accessed August 8, 2011).

Mittelman, M.S., W.E. Haley, O.J. Clay, and D.L. Roth. 2006. Improving caregiver well-being delays nursing home placement of patients with Alzheimer disease. *Neurology* 67(9):1592–1599.

Morrison, R.S., E. Chichin, J. Carter, O. Burack, M. Lantz, and D.E. Meier. 2005. The effect of a social work intervention to enhance advance care planning documentation in the nursing home. *Journal of the American Geriatrics Society* 53(2):290–294.

Mudge, A., S. Laracy, K. Richter, and C. Denaro. 2006. Controlled trial of multidisciplinary care teams for acutely ill medical inpatients: Enhanced multidisciplinary care. *Internal Medicine Journal* 36(9):558–563.

Naylor, M.D., D.A. Brooten, R.L. Campbell, G. Maislin, K.M. McCauley, and J.S. Schwartz. 2004. Transitional care of older adults hospitalized with heart failure: A randomized, controlled trial. *Journal of the American Geriatrics Society* 52(5):675–684.

Nikolaus, T., N. Specht-Leible, M. Bach, P. Oster, and G. Schlierf. 1999. A randomized trial of comprehensive geriatric assessment and home intervention in the care of hospitalized patients. *Age and Ageing* 28(6):543–550.

Ojeda, S., M. Anguita, M. Delgado, F. Atienza, C. Rus, A.L. Granados, F. Ridocci, F. Vallés, and J.A. Velasco. 2005. Short- and long-term results of a programme for the prevention of readmissions and mortality in patients with heart failure: Are effects maintained after stopping the programme? *European Journal of Heart Failure* 7(5):921–926.

Patel, A., M. Knapp, A. Evans, I. Perez, and L. Kalra. 2004. Training care givers of stroke patients: Economic evaluation. *BMJ* 328(7448):1102. http://www.bmj.com/content/328/7448/1102.full (accessed January 6, 2012).

Peters-Klimm, F., S. Campbell, K. Hermann, C.U. Kunz, T. Müller-Tasch, J. Szecsenyi, and Competence Network Heart Failure. 2010. Case management for patients with chronic systolic heart failure in primary care: The HICMan exploratory randomised controlled trial. *Trials* 11:56.

Phibbs, C.S., J.E. Holty, M.K. Goldstein, A.M. Garber, Y. Wang, J.R. Feussner, and H.J. Cohen. 2006. The effect of geriatrics evaluation and management on nursing home use and health care costs: Results from a randomized trial. *Medical Care* 44(1):91–95.

Phillips, C.O., S.M. Wright, D.E. Kern, R.M. Singa, S. Shepperd, and H.R. Rubin. 2004. Comprehensive discharge planning with postdischarge support for older patients with congestive heart failure: A meta-analysis. *Journal of the American Medical Association* 291(11):1358–1367.

Pinquart, M., and S. Sörensen. 2006. Helping caregivers of persons with dementia: Which interventions work and how large are their effects? *International Psychogeriatrics* 18(4):577–595.

Pitkala, K.H., J.V. Laurila, T.E. Strandberg, H. Kautiainen, H. Sintonen, and R.S. Tilvis. 2008. Multicomponent geriatric intervention for elderly inpatients with delirium: Effects on costs and health-related quality of life. *Journals of Gerontology. Series A, Biological Sciences and Medical Sciences* 63(1):56–61.

Rabow, M.W., S.L. Dibble, S.Z. Pantilat, and S.J. McPhee. 2004. The comprehensive care team: A controlled trial of outpatient palliative medicine consultation. *Archives of Internal Medicine* 164(1):83–91.

Rea, H., S. McAuley, A. Stewart, C. Lamont, P. Roseman, and P. Didsbury. 2004. A chronic disease management programme can reduce days in hospital for patients with chronic obstructive pulmonary disease. *Internal Medicine Journal* 34(11):608–614.

Reid, R.J., K. Coleman, E.A. Johnson, P.A. Fishman, C. Hsu, M.P. Soman, C.E. Trescott, M. Erikson, and E.B. Larson. 2010. The group health medical home at year two: Cost savings, higher patient satisfaction, and less burnout for providers. *Health Affairs (Millwood)* 29(5):835–843.

Reuben, D.B. 2011. Physicians in supporting roles in chronic disease care: The CareMore model. *Journal of the American Geriatrics Society* 59(1):158–160.

Reuben, D.B., J.C. Frank, S.H. Hirsch, K.A. McGuigan, and R.C. Maly. 1999a. A randomized clinical trial of outpatient comprehensive geriatric assessment coupled with an intervention to increase adherence to recommendations. *Journal of the American Geriatrics Society* 47(3):269–276.

Reuben, D.B., J.F. Schnelle, J.L. Buchanan, R.S. Kington, G.L. Zellman, D.O. Farley, S.H. Hirsch, and J.G. Ouslander. 1999b. Primary care of long-stay nursing home residents: Approaches of three health maintenance organizations. *Journal of the American Geriatrics Society* 17(2):131–138.

Ricauda, N.A., M. Bo, M. Molaschi, M. Massaia, D. Salerno, D. Amati, V. Tibaldi, and F. Fabris. 2004. Home hospitalization service for acute uncomplicated first ischemic stroke in elderly patients: A randomized trial. *Journal of the American Geriatrics Society* 52(2):278–283.

Ricauda, N.A., V. Tibaldi, R. Marinello, M. Bo, G. Isaia, C. Scarafiotti, and M. Molaschi. 2005. Acute ischemic stroke in elderly patients treated in Hospital at Home: A cost minimization analysis. *Journal of the American Geriatrics Society* 53(8):1442–1443.

Ricauda, N.A., V. Tibaldi, B. Leff, C. Scarafiotti, R. Marinello, M. Zanocchi, and M. Molaschi. 2008. Substitutive "hospital at home" versus inpatient care for elderly patients with exacerbations of chronic obstructive pulmonary disease: A prospective randomized, controlled trial. *Journal of the American Geriatrics Society* 56(3):493–500.

Rizzo, J.A., S.T. Bogardus, Jr., L. Leo-Summers, C.S. Williams, D. Acampora, and S.K. Inouye. 2001. Multicomponent targeted intervention to prevent delirium in hospitalized older patients: What is the economic value? *Medical Care* 39(7):740–752.

Rodgers, H., J. Soutter, W. Kaiser, P. Pearson, R. Dobson, C. Skilbeck, and J. Bond. 1997. Early supported hospital discharge following acute stroke: Pilot study results. *Clinical Rehabilitation* 11(4):280–287.

Rosemann, T., S. Joos, G. Laux, J. Gensichen, and J. Szecsenyi. 2007. Case management of arthritis patients in primary care: A cluster-randomized controlled trial. *Arthritis and Rheumatism* 57(8):1390–1397.

Rubenstein, L.Z., C.A. Alessi, K.R. Josephson, M. Trinidad Hoyl, J.O. Harker, and F.M. Pietruszka. 2007. A randomized trial of a screening, case finding, and referral system for older veterans in primary care. *Journal of the American Geriatrics Society* 55(2):166–174.

Rubin, H.R., B. Gandek, W.H. Rogers, M. Kosinski, C.A. McHorney, and J.E. Ware, Jr. 1993. Patients' ratings of outpatient visits in different practice settings. Results from the Medical Outcomes Study. *Journal of the American Medical Association* 270(7):835–840.

Rudd, A.G., C.D. Wolfe, K. Tilling, and R. Beech. 1997. Randomised controlled trial to evaluate early discharge scheme for patients with stroke. *BMJ* 315(7115):1039–1044.

Salsberg, E., and A. Grover. 2006. Physician workforce shortages: Implications and issues for academic health centers and policymakers. *Academic Medicine* 81(9):782–787.

Saltvedt, I., E.S. Mo, P. Fayers, S. Kaasa, and O. Sletvold. 2002. Reduced mortality in treating acutely sick, frail older patients in a geriatric evaluation and management unit. A prospective randomized trial. *Journal of the American Geriatrics Society* 50(5):792–798.

Saltvedt, I., T. Saltnes, E.S. Mo, P. Fayers, S. Kaasa, and O. Sletvold. 2004. Acute geriatric intervention increases the number of patients able to live at home. A prospective randomized study. *Aging Clinical and Experimental Research* 16(4):300–306.

Shea, K., A. Shih, and K. Davis. 2008. *Health Care Opinion Leaders' Views on Health Care Delivery System Reform. Commonwealth Fund Commission on a High Performance Health System Data Brief.* New York: The Commonwealth Fund.

Silverman, M., D. Musa, D.C. Martin, J.R. Lave, J. Adams, and E.M. Ricci. 1995. Evaluation of outpatient geriatric assessment: A randomized multi-site trial. *Journal of the American Geriatrics Society* 43(7):733–740.

Spinewine, A., C. Swine, S. Dhillon, P. Lambert, J.B. Nachega, L. Wilmotte, and P.M. Tulkens. 2007. Effect of a collaborative approach on the quality of prescribing for geriatric inpatients: A randomized, controlled trial. *Journal of the American Geriatrics Society* 55(5):658–665.

Sridhar, M., R. Taylor, S. Dawson, N.J. Roberts, and M.R. Partridge. 2008. A nurse led intermediate care package in patients who have been hospitalised with an acute exacerbation of chronic obstructive pulmonary disease. *Thorax* 63(3):194–200.

Steiner, B.D., A.C. Denham, E. Ashkin, W.P. Newton, T. Wroth, and L.A. Dobson, Jr. 2008. Community care of North Carolina: Improving care through community health networks. *Annals of Family Medicine* 6(4):361–367.

Stuck, A.E., M. Egger, A. Hammer, C.E. Minder, and J.C. Beck. 2002. Home visits to prevent nursing home admission and functional decline in elderly people: Systematic review and meta-regression analysis. *Journal of the American Medical Association* 287(8): 1022–1028.

Stuck, A.E., A.L. Siu, G.D. Wieland, J. Adams, and L.Z. Rubenstein. 1993. Comprehensive geriatric assessment: A meta-analysis of controlled trials. *Lancet* 342(8878):1032–1036.

Swerissen, H., J. Belfrage, A. Weeks, L. Jordan, C. Walker, J. Furler, B. McAvoy, M. Carter, and C. Peterson. 2006. A randomised control trial of a self-management program for people with a chronic illness from Vietnamese, Chinese, Italian and Greek backgrounds. *Patient Education and Counseling* 64(1-3):360–368.

Sylvia, M.L., M. Griswold, L. Dunbar, C.M. Boyd, M. Park, and C. Boult. 2008. Guided Care: Cost and utilization outcomes in a pilot study. *Disease Management* 11(1):29–36.

Teri, L., L.E. Gibbons, S.M. McCurry, R.G. Logsdon, D.M. Buchner, W.E. Barlow, W.A. Kukull, A.Z. LaCroix, W. McCormick, and E.B. Larson. 2003. Exercise plus behavioral management in patients with Alzheimer disease: A randomized controlled trial. *Journal of the American Medical Association* 290(15):2015–2022.

Tibaldi, V., N. Aimonino, M. Ponzetto, M.F. Stasi, D. Amati, S. Raspo, D. Roglia, M. Molaschi, and F. Fabris. 2004. A randomized controlled trial of a home hospital intervention for frail elderly demented patients: Behavioral disturbances and caregiver's stress. *Archives of Gerontology and Geriatrics Supplement* (9)(9):431–436.

Tinetti, M.E., D. Baker, W.T. Gallo, A. Nanda, P. Charpentier, and J. O'Leary. 2002. Evaluation of restorative care vs usual care for older adults receiving an acute episode of home care. *Journal of the American Medical Association* 287(16):2098–2105.

Toseland, R.W., J.C. O'Donnell, J.B. Engelhardt, S.A. Hendler, J.T. Richie, and D. Jue. 1996. Outpatient geriatric evaluation and management. Results of a randomized trial. *Medical Care* 34(6):624–640.

Unützer, J., W. Katon, C.M. Callahan, J.W. Williams, Jr., E. Hunkeler, L. Harpole, M. Hoffing, R.D. Della Penna, P.H. Noël, E.H. Lin, P.A. Areán, M.T. Hegel, L. Tang, T.R. Belin, S. Oishi, C. Langston, and IMPACT Investigators. Improving Mood-Promoting Access to Collaborative Treatment. 2002. Collaborative care management of late-life depression in the primary care setting: A randomized controlled trial. *Journal of the American Medical Association* 288(22):2836–2845.

Unützer, J., W.J. Katon, M.Y. Fan, M.C. Schoenbaum, E.H. Lin, R.D. Della Penna, and D. Powers. 2008. Long-term cost effects of collaborative care for late-life depression. *American Journal of Managed Care* 14(2):95–100.

U.S. Census Bureau. 2004. *Population Projections.* www.census.gov/population/www/projections/usinterimproj/natprojtab02a.pdf (accessed August 8, 2011).

van Orden, M., T. Hoffman, J. Haffmans, P. Spinhoven, and E. Hoencamp. 2009. Collaborative mental health care versus care as usual in a primary care setting: A randomized controlled trial. *Psychiatric Services* 60(1):74–79.

Vickrey, B.G., B.S. Mittman, K.I. Connor, M.L. Pearson, R.D. Della Penna, T.G. Ganiats, R.W. Demonte, Jr., J. Chodosh, X. Cui, S. Vassar, N. Duan, and M. Lee. 2006. The effect of a disease management intervention on quality and outcomes of dementia care: A randomized, controlled trial. *Annals of Internal Medicine* 145(10):713–726.

Wagner, E.H., C. Davis, J. Schaefer, M. Von Korff, and A. Brian. 1999. A survey of leading chronic disease management programs: Are they consistent with the literature? *Managed Care Quarterly* 7(3):58.

Wenger, N.S., D.H. Solomon, C.P. Roth, C.H. MacLean, D. Saliba, C.J. Kamberg, L.Z. Rubenstein, R.T. Young, E.M. Sloss, R. Louie, J. Adams, J.T. Chang, P.J. Venus, J.F. Schnelle, and P.G. Shekelle. 2003. The quality of medical care provided to vulnerable community-dwelling older patients. *Annals of Internal Medicine* 139(9):740–747.

Wheeler, J.R., N.K. Janz, and J.A. Dodge. 2003. Can a disease self-management program reduce health care costs? The case of older women with heart disease. *Medical Care* 41(6):706–715.

Whellan, D.J., V. Hasselblad, E. Peterson, C.M. O'Connor, and K.A. Schulman. 2005. Meta-analysis and review of heart failure disease management randomized controlled clinical trials. *American Heart Journal* 149(4):722–729.

Wilson, A., H. Parker, A. Wynn, C. Jagger, N. Spiers, J. Jones, and G. Parker. 1999. Randomised controlled trial of effectiveness of Leicester hospital at home scheme compared with hospital care. *British Medical Journal* 319(7224):1542–1546.

Wilson, A., A. Wynn, and H. Parker. 2002. Patient and carer satisfaction with "hospital at home": Quantitative and qualitative results from a randomised controlled trial. *British Journal of General Practice* 52(474):9–13.

Windham, B.G., R.G. Bennett, and S. Gottlieb. 2003. Care management interventions for older patients with congestive heart failure. *American Journal of Managed Care* 9(6):447–459.

Wolff, J.L., B. Starfield, and G. Anderson. 2002. Prevalence, expenditures, and complications of multiple chronic conditions in the elderly. *Archives of Internal Medicine* 162:2269–2276.

Woodend, A.K., H. Sherrard, M. Fraser, L. Stuewe, T. Cheung, and C. Struthers. 2008. Telehome monitoring in patients with cardiac disease who are at high risk of readmission. *Heart and Lung* 37(1):36–45.

Wu, J.Y., W.Y. Leung, S. Chang, B. Lee, B. Zee, P.C. Tong, and J.C. Chan. 2006. Effectiveness of telephone counselling by a pharmacist in reducing mortality in patients receiving polypharmacy: Randomised controlled trial. *BMJ* 333(7567):522.

Yu, D.S., D.R. Thompson, and D.T. Lee. 2006. Disease management programmes for older people with heart failure: Crucial characteristics which improve post-discharge outcomes. *European Heart Journal* 27(5):596–612.

Appendix C

Agendas of Public Meetings
Held by the Committee

First Meeting
January 20, 2011
The Keck Building
Washington, DC

Presentation of the Charge

Wayne H. Giles, M.D., M.S.
Director, Division of Adult and Community Health
National Center for Chronic Disease Prevention and Health
Promotion
Centers for Disease Control and Prevention

Patience White, M.D., M.A.
Chief Public Health Officer
The Arthritis Foundation

Committee Discussion

Public Comment

Presentations

Anand Parekh, M.D., M.P.H.
U.S. Department of Health and Human Services

Donald Lyman, M.D., D.T.P.H.
National Association of Chronic Disease Directors

Committee Discussion

Public Comment

Second Meeting
March 22, 2011
The Keck Building
Washington, DC

Presentations

James Marks, M.D., M.P.H.
Senior Vice President
Robert Wood Johnson Foundation

A. Seiji Hayashi, M.D., M.P.H.
Chief Medical Officer, Bureau of Primary Health Care
Health Resources and Services Administration
U.S. Department of Health and Human Services

Charles Boult, M.D., M.P.H., M.B.A.
Professor of Health Policy and Management
The Johns Hopkins Bloomberg School of Public Health

Committee Discussion

Presentations

Jack Clark, Ph.D.
Associate Professor and Senior Medical Sociologist
Boston University School of Public Health;
Center for Health Quality, Outcomes, and Economic Research

Nancy Whitelaw, Ph.D.
Senior Vice President and Director
National Council on Aging

Janet S. Wyatt, Ph.D., R.N.
Board of Directors
The Arthritis Foundation

Committee Discussion

Public Comment

Presentations

> Jeffrey Levi, Ph.D.
> *Executive Director*
> *Trust for America's Health*

> Terry Dwelle, M.D., M.P.H.T.M.
> *North Dakota State Health Officer*

> Mark Horton, M.D.
> *Former, California State Health Officer (2007–2011)*

> Denise Levis Hewson, R.N., B.S.N., M.S.P.H.
> *Director of Clinical Programs and Quality Improvement for*
> *Community Care of North Carolina*

Committee Discussion

Presentations

> Helen Darling, M.A.
> *President and CEO of the National Business Group on Health*

> Wayne Burton, M.D.
> *Global Corporate Medical Director for American Express*
> *Corporation*

> Katie Lorig, Ph.D., R.N.
> *Director of the Stanford Patient Education Research Center and*
> *Professor of Medicine at Stanford University*

> Suzanne G. Mintz, M.S.
> *President/CEO*
> *National Family Caregivers Association*

Committee Discussion

Public Comment

Appendix D

Committee Biographies

Robert B. Wallace, M.Sc., M.D., is the Irene Ensminger Stecher Professor of epidemiology and internal medicine at the University of Iowa Colleges of Public Health and Medicine, and director of the University's Center on Aging. He has been a member of the U.S. Preventive Services Task Force (USPSTF) and the National Advisory Council on Aging of the National Institutes of Health. He is a member of the Institute of Medicine (IOM), past chair of IOM's Board on Health Promotion and Disease Prevention, and current chair of IOM's Board on the Health of Select Populations. He is the author or coauthor of over 300 publications and 22 book chapters and has been the editor of 4 books, including the current edition of Maxcy-Rosenau-Last's *Public Health and Preventive Medicine.* Dr. Wallace's research interests are in clinical and population epidemiology and focus on the causes and prevention of disabling conditions of older persons. He has had substantial experience in the conduct of both observational cohort studies of older persons and clinical trials, including preventive interventions related to fracture, cancer, coronary disease, and women's health. He is an investigator in the Health Initiative, a national intervention trial exploring the prevention of breast and colon cancer and coronary disease. He is also a co-principal investigator of the Health and Retirement Study, a national cohort study of the health and economic status of older Americans, and a co-investigator of the National Health and Aging Trends Study, a national cohort study of the causes and prevention of disability among older Americans. Dr. Wallace received an M.Sc. from SUNY Buffalo and his M.D. degree from Northwestern University Medical School.

Ronald T. Ackermann, M.D., M.P.H., F.A.C.P., is a general internist, population health researcher, and associate professor of medicine at the Northwestern University Feinberg School of Medicine. He is director of the Community Engaged Research Center at the Northwestern University Clinical and Translational Sciences Institute and is considered a national expert in health care–community partnerships to address unhealthy lifestyle behaviors and improve the prevention and control of common chronic illnesses such as asthma, congestive heart failure, and diabetes. He is the principal architect and director of a large ongoing research program to evaluate the feasibility, costs, and effectiveness of partnered approaches for preventing and managing type 2 diabetes. He has also served as a lead evaluation consultant for AHRQ, the Lewin Group, and the Center for Health Care Strategies in a series of learning initiatives designed to improve the implementation and evaluation of disease and care management interventions by both Medicaid and commercial managed care programs in 20 U.S. states.

Karen Basen-Engquist, Ph.D., M.P.H., is a professor in the Department of Behavioral Science at the University of Texas MD Anderson Cancer Center, Houston. She received her doctoral degree in psychology from the University of Texas at Austin, and an M.P.H. in health promotion and health education from the University of Texas School of Public Health. Her research focuses on cancer survivors and the role of health behavior interventions in decreasing the severity of late effects of cancer, improving physical functioning, optimizing their quality of life, and reducing their risk of developing other chronic diseases. In particular she has led several studies of the effect of exercise interventions on physical functioning, symptoms, and cardiovascular health in breast, endometrial, and colorectal cancer survivors. Dr. Basen-Engquist chairs MD Anderson's working group for cancer survivorship research and in that role is in charge of organizing the development of a survivorship research center, which will provide seed money funding to researchers and provide research symposia on cancer survivorship. In addition, she directs the Patient-Reported Outcomes, Survey, and Population Shared Resource, which provides technical assistance and support for investigators who conduct clinical, behavioral, and survivorship research that uses participant-reported outcomes. Dr. Basen-Engquist also chairs MD Anderson's Comprehensive Cancer Control committee on energy balance and obesity, which involves collaboration with researchers and community members to develop and implement evidence-based population interventions to increase physical activity and diet quality and decrease obesity in the greater Houston area. Dr. Basen-Engquist also has expertise in both assessment and intervention related to chronic diseases and other problems experienced by cancer survivors.

Bobbie A. Berkowitz, Ph.D., R.N., FAAN, is currently the Dean and Mary O'Neil Mundinger Professor of Nursing at Columbia University School of Nursing and senior vice president of the Columbia University Medical Center. She was previously the Alumni Endowed Professor of Nursing and Chair of the Department of Psychosocial and Community Health at the University of Washington School of Nursing and adjunct professor in the School of Public Health and Community Medicine. In addition, she served as a consulting professor with Duke University and the University of California at Davis. Dr. Berkowitz directed the NIH/NINR funded Center for the Advancement of Health Disparities Research and the National Program Office for the RWJF funded Turning Point Initiative. She joined the faculty at the University of Washington after having served as deputy secretary for the Washington State Department of Health and chief of nursing services for the Seattle-King County Department of Public Health. Dr. Berkowitz has been a member of the Washington State Board of Health, the Washington Health Care Commission, the board of the American Academy of Nursing, and chaired the Board of Trustees of Group Health Cooperative. She serves on a number of editorial boards, including the *Journal of Public Health Management and Practice,* and *American Journal of Public Health, Policy, Politics, and Nursing Practice,* and as associate editor of *Nursing Outlook.* Dr. Berkowitz is an elected fellow in the American Academy of Nursing and elected member of the Institute of Medicine. She holds a Ph.D. in nursing science from Case Western Reserve University and an M.A. in nursing and a B.S. in nursing from the University of Washington. Her areas of expertise and research include public health systems and health equity.

Leigh F. Callahan, Ph.D., has research interests including self-management of disease outcomes, musculoskeletal outcomes, evaluation of exercise and arthritis, and social predictors of chronic disease outcomes. Dr. Callahan has 20-plus years of experience in arthritis and health outcomes research, and experience in public health as a former arthritis epidemiologist with the Centers for Disease Control and Prevention. She has authored more than 170 publications and articles, is a frequent presenter at conferences and meetings worldwide, and continues to spearhead a number of projects examining the factors surrounding arthritis and physical activity, health outcomes, and health disparities. Dr. Callahan received her B.S. in radiologic science from the University of North Carolina and her Ph.D. in public policy from Vanderbilt University. She is an associate professor in the Departments of Medicine and Social Medicine and an adjunct associate professor in the Department of Epidemiology at the University of North Carolina at Chapel Hill. She is the director of the Multidisciplinary Clinical Research Center's Methodology Core at the Thurston Arthritis Research Center, codirector of the North Carolina Family Medicine Research

Network, and has taught Clinical Epidemiology and Aging and Health courses at UNC Chapel Hill.

Ronni Chernoff, Ph.D., R.D., FADA, CSG, is the associate director of the Geriatric Research, Education & Clinical Center for Education and Evaluation for the Central Arkansas Veterans Healthcare System, director of the Arkansas Geriatric Education Center, and professor of geriatrics at the University of Arkansas for Medical Sciences. She is past president of the American Dietetic Association, where she also served as chair, Council on Research, and chair of the Commission on Dietetic Registration. Dr. Chernoff has published numerous abstracts, journal articles, and book chapters and is editor of the text *Geriatric Nutrition: The Health Professional's Handbook*, third edition (2006). She has served as editor-in-chief of *Perspectives in Applied Nutrition;* section coeditor of *Current Opinions in Clinical Nutrition and Metabolic Care;* on the editorial board of the *Journal of Parenteral and Enteral Nutrition* and the *Journal of the American Dietetic Association;* and associate editor of *Nutrition in Clinical Practice.* She also served on the editorial boards of *Topics in Geriatric Rehabilitation, Nutrition Support Services, Clinical Management Newsletter, Directions in Clinical Nutrition, Senior Patient (Postgraduate Medicine),* and the *Journal of Nutrition for the Elderly.* Her primary research interests are nutrition and aging and health promotion and nutrition and wound healing. Dr. Chernoff received her B.S. from Cornell University and her Ph.D. from the University of Pennsylvania. She is also professor of health behavior and health education in the College of Public Health at the University of Arkansas for Medical Sciences.

David B. Coultas, M.D., is currently Vice President for Clinical Affairs and Professor and Chairman of the Department of Medicine at the University of Texas Health Science Center at Tyler. He completed training in internal medicine and pulmonary disease at the University of New Mexico and was a member of the University of New Mexico faculty for 16 years and Chief of the Division of Epidemiology and Preventive Medicine for 6 years. Subsequently, he was Associate Chairman of Internal Medicine at the University of Florida HSC/Jacksonville. His personal research interests include the epidemiology of pulmonary diseases and health outcomes research, and his projects have focused on patients with interstitial lung diseases, environmental and occupational lung diseases, and chronic obstructive pulmonary disease.

Sherita Hill Golden, M.D., M.H.S., is an associate professor of medicine in the division of endocrinology and metabolism at the Johns Hopkins University School of Medicine. She also holds joint appointments in the Welch Center for Prevention, Epidemiology, and Clinical Research, and in the department of epidemiology at the Johns Hopkins University Bloomberg School of Public Health. She is the director of the Johns Hopkins Inpatient Diabetes Management Service, serves as a chairperson of the Glucose Steering Committee for the Johns Hopkins Hospital, is chairperson of the Epidemiology and Biostatistics Interest Group of the American Diabetes Association, and is vice chair of the Diabetes Committee for the American Heart Association's Council on Nutrition, Physical Activity, and Metabolism. Dr. Golden's primary research interest centers around identifying endocrine risk factors associated with the development of diabetes and cardiovascular disease. Her current research focuses on studying the neuroendocrine response to chronic psychological stress as a risk factor for diabetes and cardiovascular disease. She is a former Robert Wood Johnson Minority Medical Faculty Career Development Award recipient, and her current research is funded through the National Institute of Diabetes, Digestive, and Kidney Diseases, the National Heart, Lung, and Blood Institute, and the Agency for Healthcare Research and Quality. Dr. Golden graduated Phi Beta Kappa and summa cum laude from the University of Maryland, College Park, and alpha omega alpha from the University of Virginia School of Medicine before training in internal medicine and endocrinology and metabolism at the Johns Hopkins Hospital. During her fellowship in endocrinology, she received an M.H.S. in clinical epidemiology from the Johns Hopkins University Bloomberg School of Public Health.

Jeffrey R. Harris, M.D., M.P.H., M.B.A., is a professor of health services in the School of Public Health at the University of Washington (UW). He moved to the UW in 2001 after a 20-year career at the Centers for Disease Control and Prevention (CDC), where he began as an epidemic intelligence service officer. His research focuses on healthy aging, community-based prevention of chronic diseases, and dissemination and adoption of best practices. His research methods include dissemination and implementation research, epidemiology, and evaluation. Dr. Harris serves as director and PI for the Health Promotion Research Center (HPRC), a CDC Prevention Research Center. The mission of the HPRC is to improve health by conducting high-quality prevention research that has an emphasis on healthy aging and can be incorporated into community practice. Teaching interests include the history, organization, and effectiveness of the U.S. health care system. Board-certified in both internal medicine and preventive medicine, Dr. Harris received his M.D. from the University of Texas Southwestern Medical School, his M.P.H. from Johns Hopkins University Bloomberg School of Public Health, and his M.B.A. from UW.

Russell Harris, M.D., M.P.H., is professor of medicine and adjunct professor of epidemiology at the University of North Carolina at Chapel Hill.

He is director of the M.D.-M.P.H. Program at UNC. He has worked with the U.S. Preventive Services Task Force (USPSTF) since 1997, including conducting systematic reviews, consulting on methods, and serving a 5-year term as a member of the USPSTF. He has led five large studies of improving preventive care in community primary-care practice. He is board certified in both internal medicine and preventive medicine. He is interested in preventive medicine, heart disease, cancer, stroke, diabetes, and high blood pressure. His research interests include preventive care, screening, health disparities, and cost of care. He is principal investigator and director of the UNC Research Center for Excellence in Clinical Preventive Services within the Cecil G. Sheps Center for Health Services Research at UNC. He received his M.D. degree from Johns Hopkins University School of Medicine and his M.P.H. from UNC School of Public Health. He is a former Robert Wood Johnson Clinical Scholar at Case-Western Reserve University and UNC.

Katie B. Horton, R.N., M.P.H., J.D., is a research professor at George Washington University's School of Public Health and Health Services, Department of Health Policy. Professor Horton's research focuses primarily on the implementation of health reform, specifically issues that relate to public health, health insurance coverage, quality of and access to care—especially for those with chronic disease. Prior to joining GW, Ms. Horton was president of Health Policy R&D, a health policy firm in Washington, DC, and spent more than a decade on Capitol Hill working for the Senate Finance Committee and Congressman Pete Stark (D-CA) where she was responsible for the member's legislative agenda. Ms. Horton has broad experience working with congressional advisory organizations such as the Medicare Payment Advisory Commission, the Government Accountability Office, and the Congressional Budget Office and has also worked extensively with the Centers for Medicare and Medicaid Services. Ms. Horton also served as director of clinical services for Operation Smile, a humanitarian organization providing health services to indigent children in developing countries.

M. Jeanne Miranda, Ph.D., is professor, Department of Psychiatry and Biobehavioral Sciences and assistant director of the Center for Health Services at the University of California, Los Angeles. Dr. Miranda is a mental health services researcher who has focused her work on providing mental health care to low-income and minority communities. Dr. Miranda's major research contributions have been in evaluating the impact of mental health care for ethnic minority communities. Her research has demonstrated the effectiveness of care for depression in impoverished women, but that outreach is necessary to engage these women in care. Dr. Miranda is an investigator in three UCLA centers focusing on improving disparities in health care for ethnic minorities. She directs community cores and an innovative research core focusing on translating lifestyle interventions (diet and exercise) for low-income and minority communities. She was the senior scientific editor of *Mental Health: Culture, Race and Ethnicity, A Supplement to Mental Health: A Report of the Surgeon General,* published August 2001. She is currently developing and testing interventions to improve outcomes for older children adopted from foster care. Dr. Miranda received her Ph.D. in clinical psychology from University of Kansas and completed post-doctoral training at University of California, San Francisco. She served on the IOM Committee on Crossing the Quality Chasm: Adaptation to Mental Health and Addictive Disorders and the IOM Committee, Review and Assessment of the NIH's Strategic Research Plan and Budget to Reduce and Ultimately Eliminate Health Disparities. She has been a member of the Institute of Medicine since 2005.

Marcia Nielsen, Ph.D., M.P.H., is the executive director of the Patient Centered Primary Care Collaborative, a large coalition of provider, purchaser, and consumer stakeholders who have joined together to develop and advance the patient centered medical home model of health care delivery. She previously served as associate dean for Health Policy, vice chair, and associate professor within the Department of Health Policy and Management at the University of Kansas School of Medicine where her research and teaching focused on health system reform at the federal and state level, the relationship between socioeconomic disparities and health, access to primary health care and the patient centered medical home, and public health. Prior to rejoining the KU faculty, she was the first executive director (2006–2009) and board chair (2005) of Kansas's health care agency, the Kansas Health Policy Authority (KHPA). While at KHPA, Dr. Nielsen oversaw Kansas Medicaid, the State Children's Health Insurance Program, the State Employee Health Program, and developed a coordinated health policy agenda for the state. Prior to moving to Kansas in 2002, Dr. Nielsen spent 10 years in Washington, DC. During the debate over comprehensive health care reform in the 1990s, she worked as a legislative assistant to then U.S. Senator Bob Kerrey (D-NE). She later served as the health lobbyist and assistant director of legislation for the AFL-CIO. Dr. Nielsen has a B.S. in biology and psychology from Briar Cliff College, an M.P.H. from the George Washington University, and a Ph.D. in health policy and management from the Johns Hopkins University Bloomberg School of Public Health. She served as a Peace Corps volunteer working for Ministry of Public Health in Thailand, and also served for 6 years in the U.S. Army Reserves.

Olugbenga G. Ogedegbe, M.D., M.P.H., M.S., is an assistant professor of medicine in the Department of Medicine and the director of the Center for

Healthful Behavior Change at NYU Lagone Medical Center. His research interest is focused primarily on minority health with special emphasis on the mechanisms and reduction of health disparities in hypertension-related outcomes. Specifically, he is conducting multi- and interdisciplinary behavioral interventions targeted at improving medication adherence and blood pressure control among hypertensive African American patients who receive care in community-based primary care settings. This line of research will ultimately lead to the development and implementation of community-based behavioral interventions targeted at cardiovascular risk reduction in minority patients. Dr. Ogedegbe is the principal investigator on two NHLBI-funded R01 behavioral intervention trials. Using a multidisciplinary focus, one of such studies will investigate the effectiveness of interventions targeted at both patients and physicians in improving BP control among 1,058 hypertensive African Americans in 30 community-health centers in New York City. Co-investigators in this endeavor include clinical psychologists, clinical hypertension specialists, social epidemiologist, registered dieticians/nutritionist and health educators. Other behavioral intervention studies are focused on blood pressure reduction among minority elders in senior centers and faith-based organizations. To this end, Dr. Ogedegbe has formed community-based partnerships with several organizations, including the New York City Department of Health's Office of Minority Health, several senior centers, and faith-based organizations in New York City. His long-term goal is to develop a cadre of effective practice-based behavioral approaches that are easily sustainable and can be translated into practice among low-income minority patients with uncontrolled hypertension.

Patrick Remington, M.D., M.P.H., is associate dean for public health and professor of population health sciences at the School of Medicine and Public Health, University of Wisconsin–Madison. His research interests are on methods used to measure the health of communities and communicate this information to the public and policy makers. He is currently codirecting an RWJ-funded project entitled Mobilizing Action Toward Community Health (MATCH). This 3-year, $5-million project ranks the health of the counties in all 50 states and examines strategies to improve population health. Dr. Remington worked for 15 years practicing public health, first at the CDC (1982–1988) and then at the Wisconsin Division of Public Health (1988–1997). Since joining the Department of Population Health Sciences in 1997, he has directed the UW Population Health Institute and was the founding director of the Master of Public Health Program. Dr. Remington earned a B.S. in molecular biology (1976) and an M.D. (1981) from the University of Wisconsin–Madison; completed an internal medicine internship at the Virginia Mason Medical Center in Seattle (1982); the Epidemic Intelligence Service (EIS) (1984) and Preventive Medicine Residency (1985) at the CDC;

and an M.P.H. degree (1986) from the University of Minnesota. He has authored or coauthored over 300 publications and teaches courses on public health practice to undergraduate, medical, and public health students.

David B. Reuben, M.D., is director, Multicampus Program in Geriatrics Medicine and Gerontology, and chief, Division of Geriatrics at the University of California, Los Angeles (UCLA) Center for Health Sciences. He is the Archstone Foundation Chair and Professor at the David Geffen School of Medicine at UCLA and director of the UCLA Claude D. Pepper Older Americans Independence Center. Dr. Reuben sustains professional interests in clinical care, education, research, and administrative aspects of geriatrics. He has won seven awards for excellence in teaching and maintains a clinical primary care practice of frail older persons and attends on inpatient, and geriatric psychiatry units at UCLA. Dr. Reuben is a geriatrician-researcher with expertise in studies linking common geriatric syndromes (e.g., functional impairment, sensory impairment, malnutrition) to health outcomes such as mortality, costs, and functional decline. He also has extensive experience with interventional research (e.g., comprehensive geriatric assessment) that has focused on health care delivery to older persons. His most recent work focuses on developing and testing interventions to improve the quality of care that primary care physicians provide for geriatric conditions.

In 2000, Dr. Reuben was given the Dennis H. Jahnigen Memorial Award for outstanding contributions to education in the field of geriatrics, and in 2008, he received the Joseph T. Freeman Award by the Gerontological Society of America. Dr. Reuben was part of the team that received the 2008 John M. Eisenberg Patient Safety and Quality Award for Research—Joint Commission and National Quality Forum (NQF), for Assessing Care of the Vulnerable Elderly (ACOVE). He is a past-president of the American Geriatrics Society and the Association of Directors of Geriatric Academic Programs (ADGAP). Dr. Reuben is past-chair of the board of directors of the American Board of Internal Medicine. He is lead author of the widely distributed book *Geriatrics at Your Fingertips*. Dr. Reuben has served on four previous IOM committees and a NAS committee.

Michael Schoenbaum, Ph.D., is senior advisor for mental health services, epidemiology, and economics in the Office of the Director at the National Institute of Mental Health. In that capacity, he directs a unit charged with conducting analyses of mental health burden, service use and costs, intervention opportunities, and other policy-related issues, in support of institute decision making. Dr. Schoenbaum's research has focused particularly on the costs and benefits of interventions to improve health and health care, evaluated from the perspectives of patients, providers, payers, and society. Prior to joining NIMH, Dr. Schoenbaum spent 9 years at the

RAND Corporation, where his work included studies of the feasibility and consequences of improving care for common mental disorders, particularly depression; studies of the social epidemiology and economic consequences of chronic illness and disability; design and evaluation of decision-support tools to help consumers make health benefits choices; and international health sector development projects. Dr. Schoenbaum was a Robert Wood Johnson Scholar in health policy at the University of California, Berkeley, from 1995–1997. Dr. Schoenbaum received his Ph.D. in Economics from the University of Michigan.